The Biopolitics of Dementia

This book explores how dementia studies relates to dementia's growing public profile and corresponding research economy.

The book argues that a neuropsychiatric biopolitics of dementia positions dementia as a syndrome of cognitive decline, caused by discrete brain diseases, distinct from ageing, widely misunderstood by the public, that will one day be overcome through technoscience. This biopolitics generates dementia's public profile and is implicated in several problems, including the failure of drug discovery, the spread of stigma, the perpetuation of social inequalities and the lack of support that is available to people affected by dementia. Through a failure to critically engage with neuropsychiatric biopolitics, much dementia studies is complicit in these problems.

Drawing on insights from critical psychiatry and critical gerontology, this book explores these problems and the relations between them, revealing how they are facilitated by neuro-agnostic dementia studies work that lacks robust biopolitical critiques and sociopolitical alternatives. In response, the book makes the case for a more biopolitically engaged "neurocritical" dementia studies and shows how such a tradition might be realised through the promotion of a promissory sociopolitics of dementia.

James Rupert Fletcher is Wellcome Fellow in the Department of Sociology at the University of Manchester, UK. His research covers several areas of the dementia economy, with an emphasis on using social theory and methods to understand dementia as a political entity. He has published on subjects including informal dementia care networks, mental capacity legislation and its influence on research governance, the anti-ageing technoscience market, anti-stigma and awareness-raising campaigns regarding psychiatric disorder, the operationalisation of ethnicity and age in research, the biomarker discovery economy, the curation of dementia-friendly cultural events, dementia prevention public health strategies and environmental effects on cognition in urban settings. His lecturing spans medical sociology, the sociology of ageing, social research methods and ethical governance.

Dementia in Critical Dialogue

This series will bring together diverse and multidisciplinary commentators around key areas for development in the field of dementia studies. It will include, but not be restricted to edited collections and monographs that will embrace a dialogic and relational approach where writers from within the field of dementia studies engage in a critical exchange with those from other fields.

The series will offer a critical perspective on key and emerging issues for the field of dementia with relevance to research, policy and practice. It contains a reasonable mix of theoretical, policy-related, methodological and applied research contributions. We would like to encourage texts that incorporate transnational and majority world/Global South perspectives in the understanding of dementia. The series editors will appoint a volume editor(s) and work closely with them to help bring together an appropriate mix of authors for each edition.

Series Editors:

Richard Ward (richard.ward1@stir.ac.uk)
Linn J. Sandberg (linn.sandberg@sh.se)
James Fletcher (james.fletcher@manchester.ac.uk)
Andrea Capstick (A.J.Capstick@bradford.ac.uk)

If you wish to submit a book proposal for the series, please contact the Series Editors or Emily Briggs emily.briggs@tandf.co.uk

Critical Dementia Studies
An Introduction
Edited by Richard Ward and Linn J. Sandberg

A Critical History of Dementia Studies
Edited By James Rupert Fletcher, Andrea Capstick

The Biopolitics of Dementia
A Neurocritical Perspective
James Rupert Fletcher

For more information on the series please visit: https://www.routledge.com/Dementia-in-Critical -Dialogue/book-series/DCD

The Biopolitics of Dementia

A Neurocritical Perspective

James Rupert Fletcher

Routledge
Taylor & Francis Group
LONDON AND NEW YORK

First published 2024
by Routledge
4 Park Square, Milton Park, Abingdon, Oxon OX14 4RN

and by Routledge
605 Third Avenue, New York, NY 10158

Routledge is an imprint of the Taylor & Francis Group, an informa business

© 2024 James Rupert Fletcher

British Library Cataloguing-in-Publication Data
A catalogue record for this book is available from the British Library

Library of Congress Cataloging-in-Publication Data
Names: Fletcher, James Rupert, author.
Title: The biopolitics of dementia: a neurocritical perspective/James Rupert Fletcher.
Other titles: Dementia in critical dialogue.
Description: Abingdon, Oxon; New York, NY: Routledge, 2024. |
Series: Dementia in critical dialogue | Includes bibliographical references and index.
Identifiers: LCCN 2023027491 (print) | LCCN 2023027492 (ebook) |
ISBN 9781032504469 (hardback) | ISBN 9781032504483 (paperback) |
ISBN 9781003398523 (ebook)
Subjects: MESH: Dementia–psychology | Research | Socioeconomic Factors | Politics
Classification: LCC RC523 (print) | LCC RC523 (ebook) | NLM WM 220 |
DDC 616.8/31–dc23/eng/20230727
LC record available at https://lccn.loc.gov/2023027491
LC ebook record available at https://lccn.loc.gov/2023027492

ISBN: 978-1-032-50446-9 (hbk)
ISBN: 978-1-032-50448-3 (pbk)
ISBN: 978-1-003-39852-3 (ebk)

DOI: 10.4324/9781003398523

Typeset in Sabon
by Deanta Global Publishing Services, Chennai, India

For nans, big and little.

Contents

Preface

In 2010, I asked my undergraduate personal tutor how I could get his job. In answer, he introduced me to the academic career path and the idea of doing a PhD. My two potential topics were immediately obvious, both stemming from my personal life: (1) construction labour during the Great Recession and (2) unpaid dementia care. Intuitively, these topics seem rather dissimilar. However, they are curiously entangled. The existence of this book is a hint that I opted for dementia research. Seemingly by chance, that decision coincided with a period of remarkable growth in British dementia research that is bound up with the Great Recession and its political consequences, particularly for shaping key industries. That growth of dementia research partially explains why I am here, qualified, employed and writing this book. Without it, ironically, I would probably be working in construction. So, strangely enough, my original choice to study dementia has circuitously brought me back to studying the post-2008 political economic re-constitution of key industries and the people affected by them. I, like many of my peers (and this book), am a product of the resulting political economy of dementia.

This is a book about dementia research and its relationship with its core research problem: dementia. More specifically, it is a book about dementia studies, a diverse and loose collection of social scientific, humanities and arts scholarship with which I self-identify. My holding-together of dementia studies as an entity throughout this book is contestable, but for me, it has sufficient coherence as an institutionalised intellectual and political pursuit that it makes sense for me to speak to it as my audience. For a more nuanced overview of dementia studies, I recommend the earlier books in this series.[1,2] While often separated out as the poorer relation in a "cure vs care" binary of research types, I think that dementia studies can be better understood as an outgrowth of the wider dementia research economy. Dementia studies is both symbolically and materially indebted to that economy. So, while my attention is primarily focused on dementia studies, and it is those scholars in particular that I am speaking to, it would be a mistake to approach dementia studies as being somehow isolated from dementia research in general and from dementia as an entity. Indeed, much of this book is dedicated to interrogating those relationships: dementia studies ~ dementia research ~ dementia itself.

I argue that dementia studies is too often constrained by anti-(bio)medi-calisation sensibilities, critiquing the dehumanisation and institutional control of people affected by dementia. This focus has rendered our scholarship troublingly uncritical of, and somewhat complicit in, the neuropsychiatric biopolitics of dementia. Since the late-20th century, this biopolitics has reified a dementia that is familiar to us today: syndrome of cognitive decline, caused by discrete brain diseases, distinct from normal ageing, major global health challenge, widely misunderstood by the public, to be cured by future technoscientific advances, requiring significant investment. Such reification should not be conflated with constructionism. Rather, it is the biopolitical cultivation of a peculiar economy based on a very real phenomenon: dysfunctional cognitive decline in later life. This biopolitics facilitates a range of problems, from the erosion of social support, to the spread of dangerous and ineffective drugs and the moralised racialisation of inequalities. I am confident most of my dementia studies peers would not wish to contribute to these developments, yet we risk doing so when we uncritically accept the neuropsychiatric biopolitics of dementia.

In response, I argue that we might build a neurocritical dementia studies dedicated to deconstructing biopolitics and offering alternatives, particularly by cultivating affinities with the rich sub-traditions of critical gerontology and critical psychiatry. Those alternatives take the form of a promissory sociopolitics of dementia that is primarily dedicated to nurturing the welfare of people affected by dementia. This sociopolitics is promissory in as much as it foregrounds a hopeful future and works to make that future feel realistic, even inevitable, so that it might improve our symbolic and material conditions in the present. It is sociopolitical in as much as it foregrounds sociogenic and political-economic causes of and responses to dementia, offering alternatives to the (often rather anti-social) biogenic and scientistic aesthetics that typify the neuropsychiatric biopolitics of dementia.

There are a lot of ideas here that require substantial exposition. In this book, I will progress through each to build my argument for a neurocritical dementia studies as a means of pursuing a better dementia research economy and a better dementia, that is, better for those affected by it. Along the way, I hope to enlist, or at least provoke, some of you.

References

1. Ward, R., and Sandberg, L. (2023). *Critical Dementia Studies* (Routledge).
2. Fletcher, J.R., and Capstick, A. (2023). *A Critical History of Dementia Studies* (Routledge).

Acknowledgements

Research is often a collective effort with an individual's name stamped on it. In that vein, this book represents contributions from a large group of people and organisations. I am grateful for the financial support given to me by the Economic and Social Research Council and the Wellcome Trust. From the Critical Dementia Network, I have been expertly guided through the world of publishing by Andrea Capstick, Linn Sandberg and Richard Ward, and have developed my thinking on racialisation alongside Maria Zubair and Moïse Roche. Through the British Society of Gerontology, I have gained from the insights of Carol Maddock, Martin Hyde and Kellyn Lee on questions of stigma, awareness and ethics. Contrary to many, I find Twitter a remarkable resource for support, and my particular thanks go to Timothy Daly for his feedback. I have benefitted from the support and wisdom of various colleagues at the Department of Global Health and Social Medicine and the Institute of Gerontology at King's College London, including Nick Manning, Karen Glaser, Nik Rose, Laurie Corna and Anthea Tinker, as well as my examiners Paul Higgs and Heather Wilkinson. Special thanks go to Rasmus Birk and Giuli Cavaliere. At the Manchester Urban Ageing Research Group, Tine Buffel, Chris Phillipson and James Nazroo have welcomed me into Manchester's research networks, Mao Deng and David Dobson have supported my work on friendliness, and Miriam Tenquist's work-in-progress sessions have helped refine this text. From the Morgan Centre for Research into Everyday Lives, Vanessa May and Andy Balmer have been terrific advisors. Elsewhere at the University of Manchester, Josh Bunting, Sofia Doyle, Dharmi Kapadia, John Keady and Jennifer Mason have all offered constructive input into my work, and I am especially thankful to Debbie Price for her longstanding mentorship. Finally, I want to thank Rosanna Lush McCrum for supporting me through the years of work contained herein.

Abbreviations

AD	Alzheimer's disease
US	United States
NIA	National Institutes on Aging
NIH	National Institute of Health
UK	United Kingdom
ARUK	Alzheimer's Research UK
LATE	Limbic-predominant age-associated TDP-43 encephalopathy
Aβ	Amyloid-beta
FDA	US Food and Drug Administration
APP	Amyloid-beta precursor protein
PSEN1	Presenilin 1
PSEN2	Presenilin 2
APOE	Apolipoprotein E
APOEε4	Apolipoprotein E ε4 allele
GWAS	Genome-wide association studies
DSM	Diagnostic and Statistical Manual of Mental Disorders
MCI	Mild cognitive impairment
UNCRPD	United Nations Convention on the Rights of Persons with Disabilities
DNA	Deoxyribonucleic acid
EMA	European Medicines Agency
JPAD	The Journal of Prevention of Alzheimer's Disease
ARIA	Amyloid-related imaging abnormalities
CMS	Centers for Medicare & Medicaid Services
BBC	British Broadcasting Corporation
GP	General practitioner
NHS	National Health Service
BLM	Black Lives Matter
BAME	Black, Asian and minority ethnic
APPG	All Party Parliamentary Group
WHO	World Health Organisation
PPI	Patient and public involvement
SCIE	Social Care Institute for Excellence
BME	Black and minority ethnic

R&D	Research and design
CEO	Chief Executive Officer
AIDS	Acquired immune deficiency syndrome
DFI	Dementia-friendly initiative
DFC	Dementia-friendly community
UNICEF	United Nations Children's Fund
UNESCO	United Nations Educational, Scientific and Cultural Organization
NICE	National Institute for Health and Care Excellence
FA	Football Association

1 Introduction

The Successful Failure of Dementia Research

Historical introductions to dementia often begin with one of two jumping-off points, either early mentions of dementia-like conditions in ancient texts[1–3] or the work of Alois Alzheimer at the beginning of the 20th century.[4, 5] Each of these approaches does a particular type of work. The former shows that the relationship between mental decline and ageing has long been a human concern. The latter provides some perspective on how dementia came to be formally recognised as a neurological phenomenon, divided into senile (in older people) and presenile (in younger people) varieties.[1] These are themes that I will return to repeatedly throughout the book. Here, however, I want to take a third approach to this history-telling by attributing the sociopolitical beginnings of the thing that most of us consider "dementia" to the 1970s and 1980s.[6] This is central to my critical standpoint for three reasons. First, it indicates the transience of dementia as a continuously changing thing or rather a collection of historically, socially, economically and politically contingent things.[2] Dementia in the post–1970s period overlaps its equivalents in 2000 BC Egypt and 1910 AD Germany, yet it is also distinct, and it is those peculiarities that I focus on. Second, the demarcation of a late 20th-century evolution of dementia places it within a wider social and political history of neuropsychiatric research that helps to understand why and how our versions of dementia occurred (and are still occurring). Third, my interest in dementia's broad history is a route into a more particular history of social dementia research, which was comparatively a rather niche affair before the late 20th century.

This introductory chapter opens with a brief appraisal of the remarkable expansion of dementia research over recent decades. It focuses on the late 20th- and early 21st-century development of what Patrick Fox has called the "Alzheimer's movement".[7] This movement has generated significant increases in dementia research funding, related initiatives and research outputs. Having outlined the growth of dementia research over this time, I argue that this movement has, to date, largely failed to achieve its explicit primary aims. These aims are the development of effective treatments (especially cures), high standards of care and good quality of life for those affected by dementia. This introductory depiction

DOI: 10.4324/9781003398523-1

of the dementia research landscape provides the basis for the book's identification of problems that are generated by mainstream research itself. It highlights how the nature of dementia and dementia research, often naturalised under the rubrics of "disease" and "science", are intimately bound up with and dictated by political processes. Indeed, I will argue that they are political forms. That is essentially what this book is about – the ways in which dementia studies (which I will argue can be understood as an offshoot of the Alzheimer's movement) has sometimes appeared naïve, or even complicit, in the political making and remaking of dementia and associated research initiatives. By itself, this is not necessarily problematic, beyond the aforementioned failure of research to achieve its aims, at least so far. However, as will become apparent, the resulting circumstances of dementia and research may too often come at the expense of people affected by dementia. It is here, I will argue, that the relations between dementia studies and the wider political machinations surrounding dementia do become problematic.

Before I begin, I must acknowledge the shortcomings of grand historic narratives. They simplify multifaceted realities into linear character-driven plots. They offer pale reflections of the phenomena they pertain to represent and are perhaps better reflections of the storytellers themselves. With this in mind, a far more authentically multiple and developed historical perspective on dementia studies can be found in an earlier volume in this series entitled *A Critical History of Dementia Studies*.[8] Nonetheless, some brief reflection is needed to contextualise dementia today, particularly the relations between social science and dementia that are central to this text. I do this because some historical appreciation of the machinations of dementia and associated research are crucial to nurturing a sense of their deeply political nature. Ultimately, if there is one thing that I would like this book to do, it is to unsettle any predilections toward the depoliticisation and naturalisation of dementia and human responses to it.

1.1 The Rise of the Dementia Research

In the mid-20th century, dementia was publicly, and somewhat medically and scientifically, an age-differentiated problem. Alzheimer's disease[3] (AD) was a distinct illness in people aged under 60, and hence often referred to as presenile dementia, whereas senile dementia affected those over 60.[9] Senile dementia was widely deemed more inevitable and less problematic than its presenile analogue, in line with the *abiotrophic* view that certain forms of deterioration are normal in old age, originally characterised by Sir William Gower as "an essential failure of vitality".[10] This notion of abiotrophy pushed much of what we now consider AD to the edges of legitimate medical interest and intervention because as a feature of ageing, and particularly old age, it was widely considered unamenable to treatment.[11] Rosamond

Robbert has charted the conflation of dementia with ageing, and by extension, the assumption that it is untreatable, as far back as Hippocrates's psychiatric writing in the 5th century BC, which had a lasting legacy amidst a general lack of medical interest in later-life mental disorder.[12] Distinguishing AD by age has important epidemiological implications because dementia is heavily associated with ageing. The vast majority of cases occur in older populations, while younger people are rarely affected.[13] Therefore, if we only consider cases among younger people to be a legitimate illness, it follows that the illness is rare. Typically, rare illnesses warrant little mainstream attention, and AD was hence a relatively niche health concern. Scientifically, the age differentiation of senile and presenile dementia has long been suspect. Criticisms stem back to the earliest days of "Alzheimer's disease." Researchers in the 1910s noted that the clinical and physiological characteristics of AD were the same irrespective of whether a person was aged 50 or 70.[14, 15] Despite this criticism, the age distinction survived. Indeed, the notion of senile dementia remained in the *Diagnostic and Statistical Manual* in some form until 1994.[16]

The beginning of the end for this questionable age-based system was also the beginning of a dementia that is recognisable today. In the 1970s, scientific scepticism and neurological evidence generated by new technologies, such as electron-microscopy,[17, 18] united to fatally undermine the notion that dementias were age-differentiated. Neurologist Robert Katzman combined two strands of evidence: novel neurological findings questioning the status of senile dementia and epidemiological descriptions of dementia among the older population. The neuroscientific evidence seemed to show that, at a molecular level, AD was the same thing irrespective of whether the person was aged above or below 60. The epidemiological evidence showed that this ageless AD was common in older people. Combining these two observations enabled Katzman to extend the AD classification to encompass large numbers of older people. By including older people, AD was transformed from a rare disease into a highly prevalent condition. Indeed, Katzman claimed that AD was the fourth or fifth biggest killer in the United States (US). He delivered this revelation to the Houston Neurological Symposium in 1974 and published a corresponding paper in the Archives of Neurology.[19] This work is a conceptual foundation of contemporary AD, and by extension, much dementia, as a common disease (and syndrome) of later life.[12]

It is important to understand these events in a political context. Katzman's apparently revolutionary argument was essentially a reiteration of widespread scepticism toward age differentiation. Such scepticism had long been supported by a weight of logic and scientific evidence. This raises the question of why Katzman's argument would transform dementia in the 1970s when those same ideas had had little effect over the previous half century. The answer is likely that Katzman was in the right place at the right time. His work coincided with the establishment of the US National Institute on Aging (NIA), and the two became entwined in a singular fate. The founding of the NIA was opposed by many stakeholders due to concerns that too many institutes were being created, that a new institute would compete with existing institutes for funding, that ageing was being adequately addressed elsewhere and that successful biomedical interventions into ageing were improbable and potentially undesirable. As such, the fledging institution had to justify its existence. This was hampered by a lack of focus.

Ageing is a broad topic, and the NIA initially struggled to identify a central issue around which to organise. The early NIA was also beset by internal arguments over whether to pursue a purely biomedical research agenda or to develop a broader portfolio covering economic and psychosocial concerns.[7] The NIA found inspiration in the post-war success of the National Institutes of Health's (NIH) work on cancer, which was aided by positive public sentiment toward biomedical research following various war-time breakthroughs. As a result, the NIH budget increased from $46 million in 1950 to $400 million in 1960, much of that being directed to its new National Cancer Institute.[20] In 1974, the first director of the NIA, renowned gerontologist and psychiatrist Robert Butler, identified dementia as a research priority for the institute.[21] In his own words, he set about answering the question: "How do you sell Alzheimer's disease?"[22] Under his stewardship, emulating the NIH's strategy, the NIA was instrumental in promoting Katzman's version of AD as a major health and social problem that could be overcome through research. Corralling around AD gifted the NIA with a clear development strategy and a strong justification for resource allocation. Ultimately, Katzman's concept of AD provided solutions to the NIA's problems, to some extent, by enabling the NIA to remake ageing into AD.

The NIA's AD strategy was implemented in various ways throughout the late 1970s. Dedicated conferences were held, bringing scientists together to define the problem, propose a means of addressing it, plan for accessing the required resources, stimulate further interest and garner NIH support. A "Neurobiology of Aging" funding programme was established to encourage research into the physiology of age-related cognitive decline and to attract researchers into the as-yet underpopulated field. The US[4] "Alzheimer's Disease Society" was created to coordinate a grassroots advocacy movement for families affected by AD. Its two aims were to disseminate information to medical professionals and the general public and to raise public and governmental support for research. The "Alzheimer's Disease and Related Disorders Association" – later to become the "Alzheimer's Association" – was formed to promote research, advocacy, organisational development and fundraising. Its role was to publicise research findings and emotive accounts from people affected by AD, recruit notable figureheads and lobby congress members.[24] Overall, the NIA's efforts were extremely successful. Their federal funding increased 304%, from $19 million in 1976 to $77 million in 1986.[25] In turn, NIA funding for AD research increased by 2000%, from $4 million in 1976 to $80 million in 1989.[7] The US Congress convened 12 hearings dedicated to AD between 1980 and 1985,[12] and in 1986 mandated that the NIA should prioritise AD research.[26] Under NIA stewardship, Katzman's AD quickly transitioned from a rare disease affecting people aged under 60 into one of the world's most pressing health and social problems, affecting a large and rapidly increasing population of older people. In 1980, the third edition of the American Psychiatric Association's *Diagnostic and Statistical Manual of Mental Disorders* replaced "presenile" and "senile" dementia with "primary degenerative dementia," explicitly rejecting age-based categorisation:[5]

> The Dementias associated with Alzheimer's and Pick's diseases have been referred to as Senile and Presenile Dementias, the former arbitrarily signifying an age of onset over 65. Since nearly all cases of these Dementias are associated with Alzheimer's disease and the identification of Alzheimer's ... is largely or entirely dependent on histopathological data, it seems more useful to have in a clinical classification of mental disorders a single category that encompasses the syndrome of Primary Degenerative Dementia.[28]

For more details, I recommend Rosamond Robbert's extensive analysis of various bibliographic, media, financial and political metrics related to the development of interest in AD through the late 1970s and early 1980s.[12] AD's transition during this time took dementia with it, similarly propelling it toward notoriety, the two entities already being widely conflated. In sum, these political machinations formed the basis for a flourishing research industry.[24]

Since the transformative period of the late 20th century, dementia research has broadly continued to grow, and in the early 21st century, it has become a significant international industry. In 2020, the NIA's federal budget grew to $3.5 billion, with the NIH dedicating $3.1 billion to AD research in 2021.[29], [30] In the United Kingdom (UK), a national "Dementia Research Institute" was established in 2017 with combined backing of £290 million from the Medical Research Council, the Alzheimer's Society and Alzheimer's Research UK (ARUK).[31] Outside of this investment, British government funding for dementia research increased from £28 million in 2009–2010 to £83 million in 2017–2018[32] and the number of dementia researchers in the UK doubled between 2008–2009 and 2014–2015.[33] The Conservative Party pledged to double dementia research funding during the 2019 election campaign.[34] These increases have been particularly pronounced in the US and UK,[35] but the growing dementia economy is evident in other countries. For instance, the Australian National Health and Medical Research Council increased its spending on dementia research from $22 million in 2000 to $55 million in 2019.[36] Of course, such government figures do not take into account the third sector, which has been integral to the development of dementia research. Donations to dementia charities represent a substantial source of research funding. In 2019–2020, ARUK spent £21 million on dementia research, up from £9 million in 2015–2016.[37] The Alzheimer's Association dedicated $47 million to research in 2019–2020, up from $25 million in 2015–2016.[38] The dementia research economy is sizeable, and this size has been attained relatively quickly.

While the scale of growth in dementia research is impressive in absolute terms, it should also be appraised relatively. To this end, many stakeholders argue that it is underdeveloped compared with other fields. The successes of cancer research, which initially inspired the NIA's AD strategy, remain integral to appeals for more dementia research funding. Indeed, the 2022 Alzheimer's Society conference included a session in which Professor Sir Mike Richards, who is credited with making cancer a British government priority, provided advice on how to similarly popularise dementia among policy makers. Cancer receives far more governmental and charitable research funding than dementia. Stakeholders in the dementia research economy repeatedly use this comparison to argue for more resources. For example, ARUK's 2017 report on dementia research capacity offered comparisons with the cancer research economy across several metrics. They note that, in the UK in 2014–2015, there were 3,169 publications on dementia and 15,697 on cancer, and that there were 6,141 dementia researchers compared with 26,266 cancer researchers. Statistics regarding this uneven distribution are used to support the conclusion that "dementia research can be described as being 30 years behind cancer" and that "dementia research investment remains significantly behind other disease fields, particularly when the scale of the economic burden of the condition is considered. Further investments in dementia research must be made".[33] Similarly, the opening sentence of a 2021 report by the All-Party Parliamentary Group on Dementia (APPG) reads: "dementia research in the UK has been historically under-funded; with just 31p spent on dementia research for every £1 spent on cancer research".[39]

While the cited differences are evidently large, comparative appeals to absolute figures downplay the remarkable growth of dementia research relative to cancer research. The APPG report notes that between 2008–2009 and 2014–2015 the number of dementia researchers and publications increased 91% and 96%, respectively, compared with 42% and 46% for cancer. This growth rate is tempered with the observation that "while dementia has made the greatest relative progress in terms of increasing numbers of publications and researchers, it has started from the lowest baseline". Similar cancer comparisons are commonplace. The Alzheimer's Society notes:

> Progress is being made in securing further investment in dementia research. Since 2009/10, annual government and charity spend on dementia research has increased from £43.6 million to almost £74 million in 2013. However, in 2012/13 cancer research still received seven times that spent on dementia.[40]

Cancer research is a particularly useful comparator because it enables the large and rapidly developing field of dementia research to simultaneously acknowledge its recent progress while also positioning itself as a poor rela-tion. These appeals typically speak to dementia research as a single grand enterprise (echoing appeals to "cancer research"). In practice, dementia research spans many distinct subfields, which I will consider shortly, but it is important to recognise this characteristic presentation of a unified field in funding appeals. Hence, despite impressive expansion, advocacy for further growth in dementia research continues.

Another component of sustained advocacy for the dementia research economy is, somewhat paradoxically, the observation that its efforts have so far failed. These efforts span the development of cures, high standards of care and good quality of life for those affected by dementia. Despite decades of investment, we have not yet met these targets, and frankly, the outlook is poor. Only five symptom-modifying treatments of short-term benefit are cur-rently available in the US and most of Europe, where a new treatment has not been approved since 2003.[41–43] These offer short-term benefits, come with various negative side effects and are ineffective for many people.[44, 45] AD is considered to be among the most high-risk areas of pharmaceutical research, with a 99.6% phase-three failure rate.[46] This is reflected in pharmaceutical giant Pfizer's decision to abandon its AD research programme in 2018, echo-ing a general turn away from neuropsychiatric drug discovery investment in response to longstanding costly failures.[47] The US approvals of aduca-numab and lecanemab in 2021 and 2023, respectively (discussed at length in Chapter 4), as the first disease-modifying treatments for AD have been marred by controversy, largely because they have little effect on cognition combined with severe side effects.

In lieu of effective treatments, people with dementia are frequently pre-scribed more general antipsychotics, often as a means of dealing with symp-toms that have not been addressed through non-pharmacological treatments, e.g. music therapy or exercise, which are recommended by various profes-sional bodies.[48, 49] Antipsychotic prescribing in dementia has limited effi-cacy and is associated with a range of adverse effects, including infections, falls and increased mortality.[50, 51] Sadly, in resource-constrained healthcare settings, antipsychotics are often used as first-line treatments in response to behaviours that staff find challenging.[52] This association with institutional pressures likely explains recent evidence showing that rates of antipsychotic prescribing to people with dementia increased during the COVID pandemic and have not subsequently decreased.[53–55] Exacerbating the problem, people with dementia are especially susceptible to adverse effects owing to polyp-harmacy,[56] and research reveals high rates of psychotropic polypharmacy among people with dementia, combined with poor review and deprescribing practices.[57, 58] Hence, people with dementia face the counterintuitive phar-maceutical problem of a lack of treatment and over-treatment.

Beyond the grim pharmaceutical landscape, dementia care quality is also often found wanting. It is important to recognise that there is a lot of good-quality care and many people trying their best to support those in need.

However, most people with dementia are likely to experience poor care, or rather, a distinct lack of care.[59] Indeed, as I will unpack at length in Chapter 8, around the world, both historically and today, dementia is a largely informal affair, experienced and responded to in isolation from services by the majority of those affected. A recent national assessment by the Alzheimer's Society concluded that people affected by dementia in the UK struggle to access services and face "catastrophic costs" for poor-quality care. In another common type of cancer comparison, the report suggests that "people with dementia inevitably experience worse care and support than people with other long-term conditions, like cancer."[60] It will likely take several years to fully research the impact of the COVID pandemic on the provision of care for dementia. That said, early indications are that the quarantining of care institutions, coupled with the relaxation of statutory responsibilities, retraction of domiciliary services and corresponding long-term isolation, have all dramatically worsened what was already a challenging social care environment for people affected by dementia.[61]

Given decades of investment, one might ask why so little progress has been made in meeting the core targets of dementia research, even before a pandemic. Such disappointment could feasibly be framed as a damning indictment of the dementia research economy. Yet the failure to attain its targets is often used as a justification for why dementia research is so vital and why its efforts should be increased. At a foundational level, this manifests a basic tension, wherein the existence of research seeking to solve the dementia problem is predicated on the existence of a dementia problem. More immediately, it shows that the failures of research can be turned to the service of that research, furnishing further justifications for resource accrual. The struggle for resource increases has been exacerbated by COVID. Fears that the pandemic's economic consequences will impact research budgets prompted organisations to issue statements and promote petitions calling for sustained government commitments to funding, as politicians' commitments have seemed to falter.[62] Yet, COVID has also painfully catalysed the importance of attending to dementia and those affected by it, with dementia being by far the leading pre-existing condition associated with COVID-related deaths.[63] In Northern Ireland, more than a third of people who are reported to have died with COVID up to November 2020 had dementia.[64] The actual total may be even higher. Two-thirds of non-COVID excess mortality from March to May 2020 were attributed to dementia, leading ARUK to call for research into whether the increases concealed undiagnosed COVID.[65] Writing in the *Lancet* in the autumn of 2021, Lalli and colleagues turned to COVID itself to argue for funding: "Now, more than ever, is the time to invest in dementia research. COVID has shown the world how science can tackle major health challenges, which should set an example to learn from".[63] Hence, there remain many rationales for supporting the continued growth of dementia research.

This rapid history of the dementia research economy and its contemporary status provides an origin story for my main focus in this text: *dementia studies*.

While the expansion of dementia research has largely played out across the natural sciences and associated institutional infrastructures, a notable body of humanities and social scientific work has developed in relation to it, or at least around its fringes. This field of "dementia studies" partly emerged in the 1980s in response to the AD movement outlined above. That responsive disposition was manifest as a collection of sociological and psychological critiques of (bio)medicalisation[6] in relation to dementia and old age, particularly regarding the fear that people diagnosed with dementia were being dehumanised. I will outline this background extensively in the next chapter because its intellectual development has profound implications for contemporary dementia studies and the wider dementia research economy.

As I will repeatedly clarify, this story is one of several that can be told about the development of dementia studies and attends to the particular attributes that most concern my arguments. Hence, it should in no way be read as a definitive history of dementia studies nor an authoritative account of its contemporary form. For instance, in the UK, another major influence on the development of dementia studies was the political drive toward university-based nurse training,[66] bringing what had traditionally been the vocational territory of healthcare professionals into the world of higher education – infiltrating faculties, syllabi, research programmes, grant bids, journal articles, conferences, etc.[67] This political remaking of nursing as a university subject has subsequently been strengthened through the Bologna Process, which has sought to enhance and standardise nursing higher education across the European Union, further cementing dementia as a scholarly matter.[68] I am also keen to emphasise that forms of somewhat psychological and sociological dementia scholarship also preceded the AD movement.[69–71] Indeed, I will delve into these histories in the concluding chapter as a source of inspiration for reimaging dementia studies.

Nonetheless, over the past several decades, dementia studies has matured into a meaningful area of social science and humanities scholarship, and increasingly activism, attending to a range of dementia-related topics, typically with a marked commitment to improving the general well-being of people affected by dementia. It is now institutionalised in journals,[72] books,[73], [74] book series,[75] networks,[76, 77] conferences,[78, 79] university courses,[80–83] centres[84, 85] and institutes[86] and has evolved into a diverse amalgamation of scholarship and activism. This book is primarily concerned with dementia studies, broadly conceived as social scientific and humanities work that attends to dementia, engages with key forums and often self-identifies as such. It is a field that I will consider in far greater detail in the next chapter, in the context of dementia research generally, as a means of providing background for my argument throughout this text. Ultimately, that argument contends that too much dementia studies scholarship has, by virtue of a strong attentiveness to dehumanising (bio)medicalisation, been naïve to the political machinations of dementia research. At worst, it has become complicit in furthering initiatives that are unconducive to the welfare of people affected by dementia – e.g. racialising education campaigns and austere friendliness agendas – as will become apparent throughout this book.

1.2 Book Layout

The book proceeds as follows. By way of background, Chapter 2 offers a more detailed overview of the post-1980s development of dementia studies in relation to the ongoing machinations of dementia research more broadly, providing much-needed context. This begins with a broad overview of notable developments in mainstream dementia research through cholinesterase inhibitors and proteinopathic hypotheses, leading to contemporary interest in biomarkers and pre-symptomatic dementias. I develop a tandem account of dementia studies, contending that the field has repeatedly defined itself in response to (bio)medicalisation across the wider dementia research economy. I conclude by arguing that, while dementia studies has often explicitly positioned itself as resisting, and hence in relation to (bio)medicalisation, this has primarily developed in line with concerns regarding dehumanisation and associated implications. This position has generated some worthwhile intellectual and practical developments, but when read in relation to what has actually been happening in the wider dementia research economy, it is a limited and often underwhelming stance.

Chapter 3 picks up where Chapter 2 concludes, suggesting that the attentiveness of dementia studies to a dehumanising (bio)medical model, while helpful in many respects, has obscured a deeper focus on the underlying biopolitics that a (bio)medical model might manifest in some respects. I suggest several reasons why traditional anti-(bio)medicalisation critiques are of limited use to understanding and addressing the contemporary status of dementia. I argue that it could prove more fruitful to conceive of dementia and associated research as being beholden to a neuropsychiatric biopolitics, with diverse stakeholders cultivating the self-governance of public thought and conduct, as opposed to a (bio)medical model. To nurture more biopolitical critiques, I turn to critical theory. Specifically, I employ the sub-disciplines of critical psychiatry and critical gerontology, which have much to offer to dementia studies but are bizarrely under-utilised given the characteristic breadth and richness of our field. Together, I argue, they offer the intellectual tools for deconstructing and reimaging dementia and the study thereof.

Chapter 4 puts this deconstruction into practice. I consider three core biopolitical claims regarding dementia: "dementia is caused by diseases of the brain", "dementia is not a normal part of ageing" and "research will discover a cure". Together, I argue, these familiar claims are indicative of the imposition of normative commitments intended to alter public thought and action, but they are typically naturalised through the cultivation of a scientistic aesthetic as though they are somehow above or beyond the realm of politics. In each instance, I draw on critical psychiatry and critical gerontology to deconstruct the normativities at stake, with the aim of providing a reinvigorated critical dementia studies with the intellectual tools for more robust engagements with the neuropsychiatric biopolitics of dementia. I return to these three core claims throughout the book due to their far-reaching influence.

Having set out the historical, institutional and conceptual foundations of my argument, in Chapter 5, I turn my attention to perhaps the most profound repercussion of the neuropsychiatric biopolitics of dementia. I argue that dementia has been reconfigured into forms that are irreconcilable with most people's experiences of dementia but which are conducive to biopolitical enterprises that have proliferated around dementia. Using the example of Biogen's controversial anti-Alzheimer drug aducanumab, I argue that dementia has been reworked into a new entity that is more amenable to biopolitical interventions. This is the case to such an extent that we have now effectively *cured* dementia in several instances, but of course, such success depends on how one defines "cured". I argue that this phenomenon can be understood in terms of circularity, a form of back-to-front problem solving whereby the problem is made to fit the solution. A circularity-based assessment of aducanumab reveals a lot about the neuropsychiatric biopolitics of dementia, its disaggregation from the interests of people affected by dementia and the extent to which it can be successful irrespective of seemingly contradictory clinical and scientific contexts.

Chapters 6 and 7 focus more tightly on the role that an uncritical dementia studies plays in facilitating and even furthering the neuropsychiatric biopolitics of dementia. To do so, I consider the subgenres of dementia studies scholarship attending to stigma and ethnicity. In recent years, both these topics have gained considerable attention in dementia studies, partly in response to social contexts of wider public concern with mental health awareness, and ethnicity and racism. Stigma research has imposed poor conceptualisations of stigma onto a wide range of phenomena as a means of justifying public-facing interventions, e.g. edutainment ad-campaigns, to increase compliance with neuropsychiatric biopolitics. Ironically, those interventions may themselves exacerbate forms of stigma. Similarly, crude conceptualisations of ethnicity have been used to problematise specific cultures in relation to a range of outcome measures that draw uncritically on biopolitical commitments. The flourishing of both stigma and ethnicity scholarship in dementia studies offers two instructive examples of how we are, as a research community, inevitably tied to the wider tides of neuropsychiatric biopolitics and corresponding public consciousness. We are a vital component of that ecosystem and can inadvertently reproduce its norms in an uncritical manner.

Chapter 8 turns to the bigger picture, outlining how the neuropsychiatric biopolitics of dementia, and the complicity of an uncritical dementia studies in that biopolitics, becomes most problematic when it reproduces our contemporary political economy of dementia. This political economy is too often opposed to the interests of people affected by dementia. It is principally a post–financial-crisis intensification of late 20th-century trends toward lesser social support, heightened personal responsibility and greater capital accumulation. Here, social support is delegated to family members while formal provision becomes increasingly limited to information provision. Just as idealised notions of "community" have driven historic service retrenchments, so are similar ideas of "friendliness" bound up with contemporary withdrawals of support. At the same time, dementia research has flourished as an investment opportunity, with high-profile appeals to the certitude of future cures facilitating substantial capital accumulation. Regrettably, again, we too often find an uncritical dementia studies being complicit in sustaining this political economy.

In the final chapter, I conclude by attempting to reconcile my general pessimism regarding our contemporary circumstances with the observation that we have done good things in the past and can do so again, and by outlining various entirely feasible means of developing what I call a "neuro-critical dementia studies", better able to resist some of the more damaging characteristics of the neuropsychiatric biopolitics of dementia. I argue that contemporary epidemiological evidence regarding declining dementia incidence in high-income countries, coupled with mid-20th-century scholarship in social psychiatry and social gerontology, provides hard evidence that a neuro-critical dementia studies has the conceptual and technical tools at its disposal for pursuing a genuinely substantive sociopolitics of dementia. This sociopolitics could enrich dementia research and make real inroads into dementia itself in ways that centre on nurturing the welfare of people affected by dementia. To this end, I outline several things we can do, collectively and individually, practically, right now.

* * *

As noted in the preface, the main purpose of this book is to propose that much dementia studies is too often problematically uncritical of neuropsychiatric biopolitics. It is neuro-agnostic. By this, I mean that social scientific and humanities scholarship often reflects too little on the biopolitical nature of the entity around which it revolves: dementia. I aim to show how that is manifest, why it matters and to advocate for new approaches. I am critical of the dementia research economy throughout, perhaps overly, but this is not to be read as an argument against dementia research. Even if one takes a bluntly sceptical view of our field in its entirety, there are many far worse things that vast sums of money could be spent on and human energies dedicated to than most dementia research (excluding some contemporary drug trials with worrying side effects, as I will discuss in Chapter 5). My aim, then, is limited and pragmatic. I hope that some dementia studies scholars find the work stimulating and that it inspires some improvements in their own practice. On a personal note, this text may read as something of an indictment of dementia studies in particular, but this is not my intention at all. In dementia studies, I have found a wonderful community of like-minded peers, united around supporting one another, furthering knowledge, improving the circumstances of disadvantaged people and generally pursuing a better world. I hope and fully expect to see the field flourish.

Notes

1 Of course, this formalisation and division are not the product of Alzheimer alone. Other well-known figures such as Binswanger and Kraepelin were instrumental, but the eponymous Alzheimer offers a centrepiece for traditional one-man historical narratives. We might also question the relative invisibility of Auguste Deter, Alzheimer's first documented case, in many such histories.
2 I will reiterate throughout this text that I am not making a constructionist argument. Later-life cognitive decline manifestly exists and can be deeply traumatising for those affected. My concerns are with shifting symbolic and institutional uses of cognitive impairment to suit various ideological and material interests.
3 A word on terminology. Clinically, AD is a common subtype of dementia characterised by particular protein aggregations. Colloquially, AD is often used to refer to dementia generally, especially in the US. Sociologically, AD is a diagnostic catch-all where we put all later-life dementias that are not attributed to other subtypes. In this text, when I am not echoing a particular author's language, I use AD in the sociological sense.
4 In the UK, the distinct but identically named "Alzheimer's Disease Society" was established in 1979 by professor of geratology Gordon Wilcock and ex-carer Cora Phillips. This Society performed similar functions to emerging US organisations – raising public and political awareness, funding research, etc. – and would later become the "Alzheimer's Society" in 1999.[23]
5 There was, however, some disagreement over this explicit rejection of age, and authors cautioned that, clinically, AD should typically still be referred to as a "presenile dementia".[16] The previous "presenile" and "senile" dementia nomenclature was also partially maintained in the phrasing: "Dementias arising in the senium and presenium".[12] Hence, in the DSM-III, one gets a sense of the hesitant and equivocal institutionalisation of a new ageless dementia. Indeed, during consultation for the DSM-III, Katzman and Terry suggested that the authors should include "Senile dementia of the Alzheimer type", with Terry suggesting that, "In this way we don't necessarily lock ourselves into believing absolutely that the senile Alzheimer is exactly the same as the presenile Alzheimer".[27]
6 I bracket "bio" throughout because "biomedicalisation" and "medicalisation", while conceptually distinct, are often used interchangeably in dementia studies (discussed further in Chapter 2).

References

1. Boller, F., and Forbes, M.M. (1998). History of dementia and dementia in history: An overview. *Journal of the Neurological Sciences 158*, 125–133. doi: 10.1016/S0022-510X(98)00128-2.
2. Berchtold, N.C., and Cotman, C.W. (1998). Evolution in the conceptualization of Dementia and Alzheimer's disease: Greco-Roman period to the 1960s. *Neurobiology of Aging 19*, 173–189. doi: 10.1016/S0197-4580(98)00052-9.
3. Papavramidou, N. (2018). The ancient history of dementia. *Neurological Sciences 39*, 2011–2016. doi: 10.1007/s10072-018-3501-4.

4. Cipriani, G., Dolciotti, C., Picchi, L., and Bonuccelli, U. (2011). Alzheimer and his disease: A brief history. *Neurological Sciences 32*, 275–279. doi: 10.1007/s10072-010-0454-7.

5. Román, G. (2003). Vascular Dementia: A historical background. *International Psychogeriatrics 15* Supplement 1, 11–13. doi: 10.1017/S1041610203008901.

6. Zeilig, H. (2014). Dementia as a cultural metaphor. *The Gerontologist 54*, 258–267. doi: 10.1093/geront/gns203.

7. Fox, P. (1989). From senility to Alzheimer's disease: The rise of the Alzheimer's disease movement. *The Milbank Quarterly 67*, 58–102. doi: 10.2307/3350070.

8. Fletcher, J.R., and Capstick, A. (2023). *A Critical History of Dementia Studies*. Routledge.

9. Yang, H.D., Kim, D.H., Lee, S.B., and Young, L.D. (2016). History of Alzheimer's disease. *Dementia and Neurocognitive Disorders 15*, 115–121. doi: 10.12779/dnd.2016.15.4.115.

10. Levy, G., Levin, B., and Engelhardt, E. (2022). Echoes of William Gowers's concept of abiotrophy. *Journal of the History of the Neurosciences 31*, 425–449. doi: 10.1080/0964704X.2021.1989649.

11. Beard, R.L. (2016). *Living with Alzheimer's: Managing Memory Loss, Identity, and Illness*. New York University Press.

12. Robbert, R. (1989). *The Medicalization of Senile Dementia: From "Normality" to "Pathology"*. Western Michigan University.

13. Hebert, L.E., Weuve, J., Scherr, P.A., and Evans, D.A. (2013). Alzheimer disease in the United States (2010–2050) estimated using the 2010 census. *Neurology 80*, 1778–1783. doi: 10.1212/WNL.0b013e31828726f5.

14. Barrett, A. (1913). A case of Alzheimer's disease with unusual neurological disturbances. *The Journal of Nervous and Mental Disease 40*, 361–374. doi: 10.1097/00005053-191306000-00001.

15. Fuller, S.C., and Klopp, H.I. (1912). Further observations on Alzheimer's disease. *American Journal of Insanity 69*, 17–29.

16. George, D.R., Whitehouse, P.J., and Ballenger, J. (2011). The evolving classification of Dementia: Placing the DSM-V in a meaningful historical and cultural context and pondering the future of "Alzheimer's." *Culture, Medicine, and Psychiatry 35*, 417–435. doi: 10.1007/s11013-011-9219-x.

17. Kidd, M. (1963). Paired helical filaments in electron microscopy of Alzheimer's disease. *Nature 197*, 192–193. doi: 10.1038/197192b0.

18. Terry, R.D. (1963). The Fine Structure of Neurofibrilliary Tangles in Alzheimer's Disease. *Journal of Neuropathology and Experimental Neurology 22*, 629–642. doi: 10.1097/00005072-196310000-00005.

19. Katzman, R. (1976). The prevalence and malignancy of Alzheimer disease: A major killer. *Archives of Neurology 33*, 217–218. doi: 10.1001/archneur.1976.00500040001001.

20. Rettig, R.A. (2005). *Cancer Crusade: The Story of the National Cancer Act of 1971* iUniverse.

21. Butler, R.N. (1984). Critical examination of contemporary progress in dementia research. In: J. Wertheimer and M. Marois (eds.), *Senile Dementia: Outlook for the Future*. Alan R. Liss.

22. Butler, R.N. (1984). How Alzheimer's became a public issue. *Generations: Journal of the American Society on Aging 9*, 33–35.

23. Alzheimer's Society (2019). *Our History: 40 Years of Alzheimer's Society*. Alzheimer's Society.
24. Chaufan, C., Hollister, B., Nazareno, J., and Fox, P. (2012). Medical ideology as a double-edged sword: The politics of cure and care in the making of Alzheimer's disease. *Social Science & Medicine 74*, 788–795. doi: 10.1016/j.socscimed.2011.10.033.
25. Kerin, P.B., Estes, C.L., and Douglass, E.B. (1989). Federal funding for aging education and research: A decade Analysis1. *The Gerontologist 29*, 606–614. doi: 10.1093/geront/29.5.606.
26. Estes, C.L., and Binney, E.A. (1989). The biomedicalization of aging: Dangers and dilemmas. *The Gerontologist 29*, 587–596. doi: 10.1093/geront/29.5.587.
27. Katzman, R., Terry, R.D., and Bick, K.L. (1978). *Alzheimer's Disease: Senile Dementia and Related Disorders*. Raven Press.
28. American Psychiatric Association (1980). *Diagnostic and Statistical Manual*. APA Press.
29. NIA (2020). September 2020 Director's Status Report. National Institute on Aging. http://www.nia.nih.gov/about/naca/september-2020-directors-status-report.
30. AIM (2021). Check out the latest from @alzimpact. *The Alzheimer's Impact Movement*. https://www.alzimpact.org.
31. UK DRI (2021). About us. UK Dementia Research Institute. https://ukdri.ac.uk/about-us.
32. UK Parliament (2018). Dementia and Parkinson's Disease: Question for Department of Health and Social Care. UK Parliament. https://questions-statements.parliament.uk/written-questions/detail/2018-11-19/HL11541.
33. ARUK (2017). Keeping pace: Progress in dementia research capacity. Alzheimer's Research UK. https://www.alzheimersresearchuk.org/about-us/our-influence/policy-work/reports/keeping-pace-progress-dementia-research-capacity/.
34. ARUK (2021). Alzheimer's Research UK disappointed as pledge to double dementia research funding omitted from Spring Budget. Alzheimer's Research UK. https://www.alzheimersresearchuk.org/alzheimers-research-uk-disappointed-as-pledge-to-double-dementia-research-funding-omitted-from-spring-budget/.
35. Walton, C. (2019). Dementia research investment needs to reflect the enormous cost of dementia care. Alzheimer's Society. https://www.alzheimers.org.uk/for-researchers/election-manifesto-dementia-research-investment.
36. NHMRC (2022). Dementia research. National Health and Medical Research Council. https://www.nhmrc.gov.au/research-policy/research-priorities/dementia-research.
37. ARUK (2022). Annual reports. Alzheimer's Research UK. https://www.alzheimersresearchuk.org/about-us/who-we-are/our-history/annual-reports/.
38. Alzheimer's Association (2021). Annual Report. Alzheimer's Association. https://alz.org/about/annual-report.
39. UK DRI (2021). "Fuelling the Moonshot": MPs call for ten years of UK DRI funding. UK DRI: UK Dementia Research Institute. https://ukdri.ac.uk/news-and-events/fuelling-the-moonshot-mps-call-for-ten-years-of-uk-dri-funding.
40. Alzheimer's Society (n.d.). Alzheimer's Society's view on dementia research. Alzheimer's Society. https://www.alzheimers.org.uk/about-us/policy-and-influencing/what-we-think/dementia-research.

41. Herrmann, N., Chau, S.A., Kircanski, I., and Lanctôt, K.L. (2011). Current and emerging drug treatment options for Alzheimer's disease. *Drugs 71*, 2031–2065. doi: 10.2165/11595870-000000000-00000.
42. Salomone, S., Caraci, F., Leggio, G.M., Fedotova, J., and Drago, F. (2012). New pharmacological strategies for treatment of Alzheimer's disease: Focus on disease modifying drugs. *British Journal of Clinical Pharmacology 73*, 504–517. doi: 10.1111/j.1365-2125.2011.04134.x.
43. Schneider, L.S., Mangialasche, F., Andreasen, N., Feldman, H., Giacobini, E., Jones, R., Mantua, V., Mecocci, P., Pani, L., Winblad, B., et al. (2014). Clinical trials and late-stage drug development for Alzheimer's disease: An appraisal from 1984 to 2014. *Journal of Internal Medicine 275*, 251–283. doi: 10.1111/joim.12191.
44. Vaci, N., Koychev, I., Kim, C.-H., Kormilitzin, A., Liu, Q., Lucas, C., Dehghan, A., Nenadic, G., and Nevado-Holgado, A. (2021). Real-world effectiveness, its predictors and onset of action of cholinesterase inhibitors and memantine in dementia: Retrospective health record study. *The British Journal of Psychiatry 218*, 261–267. doi: 10.1192/bjp.2020.136.
45. Valenzuela, M., Sachdev, P., and Brodaty, H. (2021). Concerns about cholinesterase inhibitor recommendations. *Neurology.* https://n.neurology.org/content/concerns-about-cholinesterase-inhibitor-recommendations.
46. Cummings, J.L., Morstorf, T., and Zhong, K. (2014). Alzheimer's disease drug-development pipeline: Few candidates, frequent failures. *Alzheimer's Research & Therapy 6*, 37. doi: 10.1186/alzrt269.
47. BBC (2018). Pharma giant Pfizer pulls out of research into Alzheimer's. *BBC News.* https://www.bbc.com/news/health-42633871.
48. NICE (2023). Spotlight on antipsychotic medicines. National Institute for Health and Care Excellence. https://www.nice.org.uk/about/what-we-do/into-practice/measuring-the-use-of-nice-guidance/impact-of-our-guidance/niceimpact-dementia/ch6-spotlight-on-antipsychotic-medicines.
49. Pink, J., O'Brien, J., Robinson, L., and Longson, D. (2018). Dementia: Assessment, management and support: Summary of updated NICE guidance. *BMJ 361*, k2438. doi: 10.1136/bmj.k2438.
50. Maust, D.T., Kim, H.M., Seyfried, L.S., Chiang, C., Kavanagh, J., Schneider, L.S., and Kales, H.C. (2015). Antipsychotics, other psychotropics, and the risk of death in patients with Dementia: Number needed to harm. *JAMA Psychiatry 72*, 438–445. doi: 10.1001/jamapsychiatry.2014.3018.
51. Tampi, R.R., Tampi, D.J., Balachandran, S., and Srinivasan, S. (2016). Antipsychotic use in dementia: A systematic review of benefits and risks from meta-analyses. *Therapeutic Advances in Chronic Disease 7*, 229–245. doi: 10.1177/2040622316658463.
52. NHS (2022). *London: Appropriate Prescribing of Antipsychotic Medication in Dementia.* NHS.
53. Luo, H., Lau, W.C.Y., Chai, Y., Torre, C.O., Howard, R., Liu, K.Y., Lin, X., Yin, C., Fortin, S., Kern, D.M., et al. (2023). Rates of antipsychotic drug prescribing among people living with Dementia during the COVID-19 pandemic. *JAMA Psychiatry 80*, 211–219. doi: 10.1001/jamapsychiatry.2022.4448.
54. Howard, R., Burns, A., and Schneider, L. (2020). Antipsychotic prescribing to people with dementia during COVID-19. *The Lancet Neurology 19*, 892. doi: 10.1016/S1474-4422(20)30370-7.

55. Harrison, S.L., Buckley, B.J.R., Lane, D.A., Underhill, P., and Lip, G.Y.H. (2021). Associations between COVID-19 and 30-day thromboembolic events and mortality in people with dementia receiving antipsychotic medications. *Pharmacological Research 167*, 105534. doi: 10.1016/j.phrs.2021.105534.

56. Mullan, J., Burns, P., Mohanan, L., Lago, L., Jordan, M., and Potter, J. (2019). Hospitalisation for medication misadventures among older adults with and without dementia: A 5-year retrospective study. *Australasian Journal on Ageing 38*, e135–e141. doi: 10.1111/ajag.12712.

57. Riedl, L., Kiesel, E., Hartmann, J., Fischer, J., Roßmeier, C., Haller, B., Kehl, V., Priller, J., Trojan, M., and Diehl-Schmid, J. (2022). A bitter pill to swallow - Polypharmacy and psychotropic treatment in people with advanced dementia. *BMC Geriatrics 22*, 214. doi: 10.1186/s12877-022-02914-x.

58. Jester, D.J., Molinari, V., Zgibor, J.C., and Volicer, L. (2021). Prevalence of psychotropic polypharmacy in nursing home residents with dementia: A meta-analysis. *International Psychogeriatrics 33*, 1083–1098. doi: 10.1017/S1041610220004032.

59. CQC (2022). Cracks in the pathway. Care Quality Commission. https://www.cqc.org.uk/publications/themed-inspection/cracks-pathway.

60. Alzheimer's Society (2018). Dementia – The true cost: Fixing the care crisis. Alzheimer's Society. https://www.alzheimers.org.uk/about-us/policy-and-influencing/dementia-true-cost-fixing-care-crisis.

61. Liu, K.Y., Howard, R., Banerjee, S., Comas-Herrera, A., Goddard, J., Knapp, M., Livingston, G., Manthorpe, J., O'Brien, J.T., Paterson, R.W., et al. (2021). Dementia wellbeing and COVID-19: Review and expert consensus on current research and knowledge gaps. *International Journal of Geriatric Psychiatry 36*, 1597–1639. doi: 10.1002/gps.5567.

62. ARUK (2021). Alzheimer's Research UK disappointed as pledge to double dementia research funding omitted from Spring Budget. Alzheimer's Research UK. https://www.alzheimersresearchuk.org/alzheimers-research-uk-disappointed-as-pledge-to-double-dementia-research-funding-omitted-from-spring-budget/.

63. Lalli, G., Rossor, M., Rowe, J.B., and Strooper, B.D. (2021). The Dementia UK ecosystem: A call to action. *The Lancet Neurology 20*, 699–700. doi: 10.1016/S1474-4422(21)00246-5.

64. NISRA (2020). Covid-19 related deaths and pre-existing conditions March to November 2020. Northern Ireland Statistics and Research Agency. https://www.nisra.gov.uk/publications/covid-19-related-deaths-and-pre-existing-conditions-march-november-2020.

65. ARUK (2020). Two thirds of non-COVID-19 deaths are caused by dementia, but more testing is needed. Alzheimer's Research UK. https://www.alzheimersresearchuk.org/two-thirds-of-non-covid-19-deaths-dementia/.

66. Sturgeon, D. (2010). Transforming higher education and the professional preparation of nurses. *British Journal of Nursing 19*, 180–184. doi: 10.12968/bjon.2010.19.3.46539.

67. Prescott, S.F. (2017). *The Nursing Profession and Graduate Status in England: Perspectives from Student Nurses and Health Professional Educators*. University of Huddersfield.

68. Capstick, A., and Fletcher, J.R. (2023). Introduction. In *A Critical History of Dementia Studies*. Routledge.

69. Ballenger, J.F. (2017). Framing confusion: Dementia, society, and history. *AMA Journal of Ethics 19*, 713–719. doi: 10.1001/journalofethics.2017.19.7.mhst1-1707.

70. Ballenger, J. (2000). Beyond the characteristic plaques and tangles: Mid-twentieth century US psychiatry and the fight against senility. In: P. J. Whitehouse, K. Maurer, and J. F. Ballenger (eds.), *Concepts of Alzheimer Disease: Biological, Clinical, and Cultural Perspectives*. Johns Hopkins University Press.

71. Ballenger, J. (2006). Progress in the history of Alzheimer's disease: The importance of context. In: G. Perry, J. Avila, J. Kinoshita, and M. A. Smith (eds.), *Alzheimer's Disease: A Century of Scientific and Clinical Research*. IOS Press.

72. Dementia SAGE Journals. https://journals.sagepub.com/home/dem.

73. Innes, A. (2009). *Dementia Studies: A Social Science Perspective*. SAGE. doi: 10.4135/9781446213599.

74. Keady, J., Hydén, L.-C., Johnson, A., and Swarbrick, C. (2017). *Social Research Methods in Dementia Studies: Inclusion and Innovation*. Routledge.

75. Ward, R., and Sandberg, L. (2023). *Critical Dementia Studies*. Routledge.

76. Critical Dementia Network https://memoryfriendly.org.uk/programmes/critical-dementia-network/.

77. *Alzheimer's Disease International* (2015). 10/66 Dementia Research Group. https://1066.alzint.org/.

78. Alzheimer's Society Conferences and events. Alzheimer's Society. https://www.alzheimers.org.uk/dementia-professionals/conferences-and-events.

79. The Dementia Centre (2022). International Dementia Conference. https://www.dementiaconference.com/speakers.

80. MSc Dementia Studies University of Stirling. https://www.stir.ac.uk/courses/pg-taught/dementia-studies/.

81. Texas State University (2023). Interdisciplinary MS in Dementia and Aging Studies. //www.soci.txst.edu/Graduate-Degree/msda.html.

82. St. Lawrence College (2022). Dementia Studies. https://www.stlawrencecollege.ca/programs/dementia-studies/part-time/tri-campus.

83. University of Tasmania (2021). M3V Bachelor of Ageing and Dementia Studies. https://www.utas.edu.au/courses/chm/courses/m3v-bachelor-of-ageing-and-dementia-studies.

84. Centre for Applied Dementia Studies https://www.bradford.ac.uk/dementia/.

85. Linköping University (2023). Center for dementia research (CEDER). https://liu.se/en/research/ceder.

86. Salford Institute for Dementia and Ageing. https://www.salford.ac.uk/salford-institute-for-dementia.

2 Studying Dementia

Post-1970s Divergences in Dementia Studies and the Alzheimer's Movement

In this chapter, I outline and contextualise dementia studies as a social scientific, humanities and arts sub-tradition in relation to the broader development of dementia research over the past several decades. Throughout the chapter, I show that major traditions of dementia studies have repeatedly positioned themselves in opposition to (bio)medicalisation and adopted humanist stances that have largely overlooked matters of ageing, disease and cognition, often by taking them for granted. I begin by outlining the historic development of neurocognitive approaches to dementia. I argue that while many introductory histories of dementia begin with Alzheimer, the contemporary version of dementia that is most familiar to us, and the associated AD movement, can be best understood as a post-1970s development, albeit with conceptual roots that extend back to the early 19th century. I chart the progression of this dementia from powerful molecular and epidemiological critiques of "senile dementia" in the 1970s to contemporary efforts to delineate typologies of dementias, such as the recent announcement of the LATE subtype. Throughout, issues of ageing and time, biogenic cognitive disease, population typification and interprofessional contests have defined what we too often simplify as "the science".

In the second half of the chapter, I position dementia studies in response to these developments. In particular, I highlight the centrality of anti-(bio)medicalisation arguments to the foundational work of scholars such as Kitwood, Bond and Lyman in the late 1980s. I argue that the turn to anti-(bio)medicalisation critiques fostered an emphasis on addressing the purported dehumanising qualities of a (bio)medical model. As new areas of dementia studies have emerged, the tendency has persisted for anti-(bio)medicalisation perspectives to focus our attention on dehumanisation. To a considerable extent, an alertness to dehumanisation has provided a useful intellectual footing for cultivating dementia studies. However, there are intertwined dangers here. First, by leaning into humanism (or contestations thereof) as the legitimate terrain of social science and the humanities, dementia studies has potentially drifted away from a robust relationship with neurocognitive research. Second, anti-(bio)medicalisation scholarships were originally

DOI: 10.4324/9781003398523-2

appropriated from modernist social theory and have been developed by dementia studies as a means of interrogating social phenomena that may be more post-structural in nature.

In sum, this chapter demonstrates how early iterations of anti-(bio) medicalisation critique in dementia studies embedded humanist pre-dilections across influential sub-traditions. The issue of humanism remains poignant today, manifest in relational notions of citizenship, flourishing human rights activism and emerging posthumanist critiques. As dementia studies scholarships have developed in relation to the (bio) medical model and its supposedly dehumanising effects, many of the aforementioned occurrences in neurocognitive research have received comparably little attention. This is a shame because issues such as normative lifecourse timings and interprofessional conflicts are fundamentally social scientific issues. Dementia studies, though having diverged from neurocognitive research, could be ideally placed to speak to such developments if only it pursued closer engagement. The story of how different intellectual traditions study dementia provides an informative background for the rest of this book. It reveals how, despite having emerged from the same late-20th-century occurrences described in the previous chapter, different areas of dementia research have travelled markedly different routes. In response, much of this book will be dedicated to reuniting those travellers.

2.1 Ageing and Nosology

In the previous chapter, I offered a limited overview of the recent history of the dementia research economy in the broadest possible sense. My aim there was to emphasise the fundamentally political nature of that economy and to provide an accessible overview of how we got to where we are today, with our institutional successes and therapeutic failures. In this chapter, I want to introduce some important differentiations into that rather sweeping account, beginning with the neurocognitive tradition of dementia research. I do so because the dementia studies tradition that I will focus on throughout the majority of this text can only be understood in reference to the developments of the far more substantial[1] neurocognitive tradition. In developing this account, I wish to counter any sense in which that latter tradition is outside of the remit of dementia studies and to emphasise how, (bio)medical model aside, a range of sociopolitical considerations have shaped the recent trajectories of neurocognitive research. With this in mind, I will outline some notable developments in dementia research that have contributed to shaping our current situation.

The first recognisable and serious attempts to classify dementia as a distinct condition came in the 19th century.[1] Early French psychiatrists Phillipe Pinel and Jean-Étienne Esquirol applied the term dementia to a group of people characterised by "insanity", "incompetence" and "incapacity", partly caused by old age.[2, 3] Both Pinel and Esquirol thought that people with dementia suffered from a problem of the emotions as much as any disease, heavily associated with ageing and later life.[1] However, their creation of a distinct category of dementia was transformed into a more specific disease during the mid-19th century, as the idea became popular that distinct nosologies[2] represented localised disease entities.[4] To this end, Samuel Wilks produced the first account of brain atrophy in dementia in 1864, establishing dementia as a phenomenon stemming from physiological problems in the brain.[5] The nosological turn was similarly influential in transforming conceptualisations of ageing. Mid-19th-century research into age-associated cell degeneration positioned ageing as a process of broad physiological deterioration which led to various diseases.[4] In this context, Otto Binswanger introduced the term "presenile dementia" in 1894, differentiating those aged below 60 from those aged above 60, who had "senile dementia" attributed to ageing.[6] This dementia age distinction was grounded in abiotrophy, the notion that a certain range of physiological deterioration is normal as people age, but when this senescence occurs prematurely it is pathological.[4] It is also likely that what Binswanger was describing was akin to contemporary concepts of vascular dementia, now attributed to blood vessel deterioration in the brain.[6] These developments – neurocentric nosology, ageing and normal ranges – have been central to dementia ever since.

Alois Alzheimer was inspired by Binswanger's abiotrophic approach during his own observations of Auguste Deter in 1901. Frau Deter was a 51-year-old woman who experienced memory loss, personality changes and delusions. As a result, her husband confined her to the asylum in Frankfurt,[3] where the psychiatrist Alois Alzheimer took an interest in her. Following Deter's death in 1906, Alzheimer performed anatomical and histological studies on her brain. He discovered the neuropathological features that still characterise AD today – neurofibrillary tangles and amyloid plaques. Alzheimer published his findings in a short report in 1907 but received little attention. This changed in 1910 when renowned psychiatrist Emil Kraepelin included "Alzheimer's disease" in his textbook on psychiatry[7–9]. Here, AD was portrayed as a distinct disease, separate from ageing and senile dementia. However, there remains debate regarding whether Alzheimer and Kraepelin genuinely subscribed to this distinction. Both scholars noted their uncertainties.[4, 10] It is possible that competition between rival institutes, all working on similar phenomena of neuropsychiatric deterioration, incentivised the presenile/senile distinction. By tightening the defining criteria of AD, Kraepelin and Alzheimer ensured that their institute could claim full responsibility for the discovery of a novel and specific illness.[11] Irrespective of how intentional the distinction was and what the driving forces behind it were, AD became categorised as a discrete disease in people aged below 60.

The distinction between AD and senility was immediately subject to debate.[12, 13] It was already known that plaques and tangles characterised both presenile and senile dementia. Kraepelin's rather tenuous distinction was that plaques and tangles were less present in senile dementia, though this was a difficult claim to appraise.[14] By 1912, the American pathologist Solomon Carter Fuller had developed in-depth evaluations, concluding that there was insufficient evidence for AD as a specific disease entity.[15] During the early 20th century, studies revealed that neurofibrillary tangles and amyloid plaques were present in many conditions that caused dementia symptoms and were sometimes not present in those deemed to have AD. One study in 1933 showed that 80% of people aged over 65 had evidence of plaques and tangles post-mortem[14] However, the notion of AD as a specific condition affecting people aged below 60 continued as a clinical entity throughout the mid-20th century. At the same time, senile dementia provided a clinical and public explanation for similar symptoms in older people. AD was hence a kind of accelerated ageing in the brains of younger people. As noted in the previous chapter, this age distinction meant that AD remained a rare condition, with few people below the age of 60 ever developing the symptoms that would warrant diagnosis.[4]

Throughout this time, technological advances facilitated new insights into the molecular makeup of AD neuropathology, establishing a more detailed physiological basis for classifying the disease. However, such developments were of little consequence, given AD's relative obscurity. One development that would come to have particular importance in the development of contemporary AD was the application of electron microscopy to AD. In the early 1960s, an American associate professor, Robert Terry, was tasked with applying new electron microscope technology to the examination of neurological disorders. This required biopsy-collected tissue, which meant that the disease had to be fatal and present throughout the brain. Only two diseases were appropriate, storage diseases (which are rare inherited metabolic diseases) and dementias, such as the rare presenile disorder AD. Storage diseases were chosen because Terry's partner, Saul Korey, had relevant expertise in neurochemistry. However, Korey died unexpectedly. This left Terry with no option but to redirect his studies toward dementia, and specifically AD. Doing so, Terry refined descriptions of AD pathophysiology in patients aged 52–63. His resulting papers, published in the early 1960s, shed new light on the plaques and tangles of AD.[16, 17]

The accumulation of increasingly detailed accounts of AD neuropathology steadily substantiated longstanding scepticism toward the age-based distinction of presenile and senile dementias. Indeed, from a contemporary perspective, it can seem remarkable that this distinction remained for so long. The work of scientists such as Terry was pivotal to Robert Katzman's arguments against age discrimination. Indeed, in the early 1970s, Katzman and Terry worked together clinically. As discussed in the previous chapter, Katzman combined epidemiological descriptions of dementia incidence with biological depictions of presenile neuropathology to conceptualise the version of AD that remains influential today. By the end of the 1980s, AD was publicly and institutionally regarded as a hugely important disease.[18] Indeed, Robbert

Rosamond's sociological history of AD identifies the period 1980 to 1985 as the key point of consolidation, wherein AD became institutionalised at a remarkable pace and scale.[1] For instance, the US federal budget for AD research increased twenty-fold from $4 million in 1980 to $80 million in 1989.[4] It was a condition marked by plaques, tangles, atrophy and cognitive decline, which affected people the same, regardless of their age. Indeed, in response to the historic age-categorisation of AD, this new conceptualisation leaned heavily in the opposite direction, downplaying differences between early-onset and late-onset AD and potentially conflating the two misleadingly, opening up new problems that I will discuss in Chapter 4. The political process that developed around this new disease, as outlined in Chapter 1, fuelled a proliferation of resource investment and research interest in AD, further cementing its status. Critically, that politics centred on downplaying the influence of ageing and emphasising the role of discrete neuropathologies, creating an aetiological story that was more conducive to resource accumulation.

2.2 Contesting Aetiologies

One of the earliest breakthroughs in this new research landscape was the cholinergic hypothesis. This proposed that AD was caused by a lack of acetylcholine, a neurotransmitter that facilitates the transfer of information between neurons. By the 1970s, animal and drug studies suggested that acetylcholine had important relationships with memory and ageing.[19] In 1976, research showed that people diagnosed with AD had depleted acetylcholine at post-mortem.[20, 21] The cholinergic hypothesis inspired the development of cholinesterase inhibitors, the first of which (tacrine) was approved by the US Food and Drug Administration (FDA) in 1995. Today, the second-generation drugs donepezil, rivastigmine and galantamine are typically prescribed. This group of medications prevents enzymes from breaking down acetylcholine. They can modestly improve dementia symptoms and remain the most successful treatments available. Unfortunately, they only work for a brief period of time, and most experts now consider them to be symptom-modifying rather than disease-modifying. This means that they mask some of the effects of AD but do not attend to its underlying causes. While still regularly prescribed, early hope has steadily waned, and they are now widely considered to offer limited benefit.[19, 22] Cholinesterase inhibitors first exemplified the uncertainties of what constitutes disease-modification and clinically meaningful benefit when intervening in cognitive impairment. These thorny issues remain pertinent today, and we will return to them in Chapter 5.

By far, the most influential aetiological theory of AD concerns the protein amyloid-beta (Aβ). As noted, aggregations of protein (most notably plaques) in the brains of people with AD have long been suspected of playing some causative role.[23] In 1992, these suspicions were formalised in John Hardy and Gerald Higgins's paper on the amyloid cascade hypothesis.[24] They suggested that AD is caused by a build-up of Aβ, which aggregates into toxic clumps that lead to neuronal death. Aβ aggregation occurs when a protein called amyloid precursor is processed abnormally. It is usually broken up by α-secretase and cleared naturally. In AD, the protein is broken down by β-secretase instead. The resulting peptide (a fragment of the original protein) cannot be easily dealt with by the body and therefore accumulates.[22] This Aβ aggregation largely comprises the infamous plaques that have long been a cornerstone of AD research. Hardy and Higgins firmly pointed the finger at Aβ as the first stage of AD pathology. I was two months old at the time. More than three decades later, this same claim remains at the heart of various controversies in dementia research, and much of my professional life has been shaped by it.

The amyloid cascade hypothesis has inspired a flurry of drug discovery research (as well as criticism and heated debate). Anti-amyloid monoclonal antibodies have dominated the field. They work by either preventing the accumulation of Aβ or removing existing aggregations. To date, 23 candidates have successfully cleared Aβ, including six monoclonal antibodies, but this has not translated into substantive clinical improvements.[25, 26] The recent US FDA approval of the monoclonal antibody *aducanumab* for the treatment of AD has catalysed the issue because it was approved based on its removal of Aβ, despite showing little effect on cognition.[27] The implications of this decision, as well as the even more complicated case of the recent lecanemab FDA approval, will be discussed extensively in Chapter 5, which returns us to questions of *meaningful clinical effect*. Despite disappointing results so far, the amyloid cascade hypothesis continues to dominate AD research, a situation that the regulatory approvals of aducanumab and lecanemab will likely sustain. A 2021 review of the drug development pipeline found that amyloid-targeting candidates still made up the largest proportion of candidates at the preclinical trial stage.[28] Interestingly, a recent survey of 173 dementia researchers found that only 22% of respondents supported the amyloid hypothesis, but that members of this group were typically more senior, well-published and funded by pharmaceutical companies, possibly explaining the sustained potency of the hypothesis in lieu of, and even contradiction of, the existing evidence base.[29]

While secondary to amyloid, tau has been another major target in drug discovery research. Tau is a protein that is normally integral to a functioning brain, but in certain circumstances, it can be transformed into the hallmark neurofibrillary tangles of AD. As with Aβ, the accumulation of tangles in the brain is hypothesised to cause neuronal death and hence cognitive decline, though the mechanics of this process are less formalised than the amyloid cascade hypothesis. Tau has typically been thought of as a downstream effect by amyloid advocates because it emerges much closer to the onset of symptoms. However, this later development means that tau is actually more closely correlated with cognitive impairment than Aβ and is better correlated with specific brain regions associated with dysfunction.[30, 31] Throughout the 21st century, Aβ and tau enthusiasts have sometimes descended into ill-mannered arguments, characterised by commentators as a religious war between the Tauists and the βaptists.[31, 32] Aβ has generally triumphed, but tau has remained a primary target for many. In a manner disappointingly reminiscent of the anti-Aβ field, the first anti-tau antibody, *semorinemab*, failed to improve cognition in phase-II trials in 2020.[33] However, a number of anti-tau agents remain in development.[28]

Beyond the hotly contested proteinopathies of Aβ and tau, genetics has been another key concern in AD research. This has largely been fuelled by two discoveries. First, the flourishing field of molecular genetic research in the 1990s revealed that various mutations in three genes (APP, PSEN1 and PSEN2) were directly responsible for inherited young-onset AD.[4] Such instances of AD are rare, accounting for less than 1% of all AD, but they have been an important referent in general AD research because they occur predictably in select families. That predictability means that researchers can be relatively sure that those people will develop AD within a certain number of years. This is practically useful because dementia research is generally impeded by the typical lengthiness and unpredictability of prognoses. APP also encodes the Aβ peptide and is hence concordant with the amyloid cascade hypothesis.[34, 35] The second discovery, likewise in the context of early 1990s genetic optimism, was that one of three different variations of the APOE gene (specifically APOEε4) is a risk factor for AD. APOEε4 differs from the aforementioned genes in that it only influences susceptibility to AD in later life rather than being reliably associated with AD at relatively young ages. The proportions are debated, with studies offering wildly different estimates, but perhaps 50% of people with APOEε4 do not develop AD, and perhaps 50% of people with AD do not have APOEε4. This suggests that various other interactions are likely at play, but APOE stratification has nonetheless become an important component of contemporary drug trials.[32]

Since the 1990s, the genetic approach to AD has evolved in line with genetic science more broadly, from the pursuit of unilinear gene-outcome causation to more multifaceted and probabilistic causation. Early candidate gene studies (e.g. those on APP, PSEN1 and PSEN2 discussed above) were typically technologically and intellectually limited to isolating a specific gene (cause) and specific trait (effect) and investigating the relationships between them, perpetuating an assumption that a gene caused a trait, e.g. APP causes dementia. Over time, the idea that specific genes directly cause specific corresponding diseases has been replaced by the idea that collections of interacting genes, coupled with environmental influences, shape disease risk. From the mid-2000s onward, this more multifactorial approach has overtaken the single-gene-single-disease hypotheses of the 1990s.[36, 37] As with other developments in the dementia research economy, this shift has not occurred in a technological vacuum. The emergence of multifactorial models of genetic causation manifests the corresponding development of technologies capable of sequencing genomes. In response, genome-wide association studies (GWAS) have become increasingly popular in AD research. These studies sift through vast datasets to uncover constellations of genes that are collectively associated with increased AD susceptibility, often in combination with non-genetic factors. While around 40 potential candidates have been discovered via meta-analyses, none has yet emulated the influence of APOEε4.[35, 38]

Perhaps more than anything else, GWAS have re-emphasised the profound complexity of dementia. Increasing technological sophistication has generated aetiological conceptualisations of many different factors contributing to small increases and decreases in risk, as well as calling into question the pragmatic limits of causal typification. The past few decades of genetic research have highlighted the cross-fertilisation of technologies and onto-epistemologies, with our notions of disease cause and effect and our abilities to isolate those causes and effects, continuously reconfiguring one another. As the scope of technologies to collect and analyse complex datasets has become more expansive, e.g. progressing from genes to genomes, so the manner in which we are able to, and indeed seemingly have to, think about dementia as something that has a direct and isolatable cause(s) has become similarly expansive. Here, technological and aetiological sophistication are brought into dynamic relation, with the development and use of new technologies becoming integral to the nature of dementia itself. This amenability of dementia to techno-epistemic transformation is the focus of Chapter 5 because it has dramatic implications for contemporary trajectories of dementia research.

2.3 Complexity and Classification

As the complexity of post-1970s AD as a disease entity has become ever more apparent, the issue of disease classification, so influential throughout the history of dementia, has returned to the forefront of research. This issue has been fuelled by drug trial failures, with some commentators suggesting that those failures are due to study samples having too wide a range of AD subtypes. In response, some researchers have sought to break down AD into more specific types of dementia. As discussed, the conceptual coherence of types of dementia has historically been subject to considerable debate (e.g. presenile versus senile dementia). Similarly, critics have long questioned the conceptual coherence of AD, given the observation of substantial phenotypic heterogeneity within the diagnosis.[39] In this vein, researchers in 2019 described a new form of AD – *limbic-predominant age-related TDP-43 encephalopathy* – thankfully dubbed "LATE" for brevity.[40] LATE largely affects people aged over 80 and may account for around 17% of AD. The announcement was met with some cynicism, with one commentator stating that there were "only 849,999 more to go", referring to the commonly touted figure of there being 850,000 people with dementia in the UK. What is striking is that this sentiment would have resonated a century ago, highlighting the continuing difficulties of classifying dementias, especially those associated with later life. As Kraepelin and Alzheimer probably appreciated, the nebulousness of a neurocognitive entity, manifest via behavioural symptoms and reinterpreted via technological advances, lends itself to forms of iterative reclassification that characterise the internal political struggles of medical science.

Perhaps most indicative of contested processes of (re)classification is the recent turn to standard deviation in the *Diagnostic and Statistical Manual of Mental Disorders* (DSM). The DSM is a world-renowned publication by the American Psychiatric Association, which periodically sets out to provide a comprehensive overview of all contemporary psychiatric diagnoses. Since its first edition in 1952, the DSM has been influential in defining what things are considered psychiatric disorders and how they are approached in institutional psychiatry. The fifth edition was published in 2013. Notably, it replaced its previous category of "dementia, delirium, amnestic, and other cognitive disorders" with the new category of "neurocognitive disorders". This category contains three syndromes, "delirium", "major neurocognitive disorder" and "mild neurocognitive disorder", which themselves contain numerous aetiologies, including AD, vascular disease, Lewy body and other familiar dementias. Mild and major neurocognitive disorders are defined mathematically in reference to standard deviation from normative means. In practice, this means that a person's cognitive function is assessed against the average cognitive function of the wider population. If their cognition is a little below the average (specifically one to two standard deviations below), the person has mild neurocognitive disorder. If it is a lot below the average (more than two standard deviations), the person has major neurocognitive disorder. This turn to mathematical precision represents a fresh attempt to impose more clearly defined, and hence less contestable, categories on neurocognitive phenomena that can otherwise seem incomprehensibly messy.[41]

The DSM-5's new notion of mild neurocognitive disorder has warranted considerable attention because it captures the controversial diagnosis of "mild cognitive impairment" (MCI). MCI has become increasingly popular in clinical discourse and as a diagnostic category over recent years, as dementia has been pushed further back into the lifecourse.[10] Indeed, over the next decade, analysts anticipate a compound annual growth rate of 8.7% for the global MCI treatment market.[42] It represents not only the continuing evolution of classificatory regimes but also the concurrent conceptual problem of timescales, typically evident in ongoing discussions regarding ageing and the lifecourse. As drug trials have failed, aetiological hypotheses have increasingly emphasised that disease processes begin decades before symptoms and hence require early detection. The popularity of this elongated dementia, characterised by pathology rather than symptoms, is especially attributable to a paper from 2011 published on behalf of the NIA and the Alzheimer's Association, and is discussed in Chapter 5.[43] The push for earlier recognition, coupled with the publicising of dementia generally, has resulted in greater numbers of older adults with slight or possible cognitive decline seeking diagnoses. In response, the category of MCI has proliferated, aided by concurrent interest in dementia studies.[44] Though often thought of as a sort of prelude to dementia, the conversion rates of MCI to dementia are widely contested and are likely complicated by a number of interacting factors.[45] Beyond MCI, an additional category of subjective cognitive decline has been suggested for older adults who have no measurable cognitive decline but who, nonetheless, self-perceive some minor decline. Again, conversion to dementia is uncertain, echoing the wider heterogeneity of dementia prognoses generally.[46]

Overall, the development of neurocognitive dementia research has driven increasingly complex appreciations of cognitive decline in later life. Growing complexification at the micro level of gene mutations and protein misfolding means that the longstanding macro-level uncertainties regarding disease classification are probably as far from resolution as ever. A lot of the issues that remain central to this research economy have been salient for a long time. For instance, the turn to MCI and prodromal conceptualisations of dementia is the contemporary manifestation of the longstanding problem of dealing with ageing as both a process of physiological and psychological change, as well as simply the manner through which time is experienced by and writ large upon humans. The turn to standard deviation in the DSM-5, translated into major and minor categories, is but one attempt in a long line of classificatory battles seeking to institutionalise more concrete forms of later-life cognitive impairment in order to facilitate interventions.

Irrespective of fluctuating classifications, one idea has held continuous prominence since the 1970s – *Alzheimer's disease*. The savvy reader may have already noticed that this book, purportedly about "dementia" studies, has so far dedicated a lot of space to AD specifically. This warrants some consideration of Alzheimerisation. Alzheimerisation refers to the predominance of AD in the dementia research economy. As far back as the 1990s, critics observed that much of the public, political and scientific attention paid to dementia, and indeed ageing more generally, was dedicated to AD at the expense of all other considerations.[47] This reflects the NIA's development of AD as a catalyst for growth during the late 20th century (discussed in the previous chapter). AD has proved to be a remarkably powerful idea. While the symbolic dominance of AD has facilitated impressive growth in dementia research, for some scholars, it has also hindered the therapeutic effectiveness of the sector by obscuring the real-world complexities of dementia.[48] For better or worse, the story of the contemporary dementia research economy is very much the story of AD, and the story of AD is one of a quest for some coherence amidst the complexity.

2.4 (Bio)medicalisation and Selves

The intricate machinations of neurocognitive dementia research are not the principal focus of this book. However, some understanding is necessary if we are to more fully appreciate dementia studies and its relatedness (or lack thereof) to dementia research more broadly. In several ways, much dementia studies is a response to those machinations, both implicitly and explicitly, yet it can often be characterised by a sense of distance from them, as though such neurocognitive developments must be left alone by social scientists, or have relatively minor implications for us and our work. I will repeatedly argue against such distance in this book. Indeed, all that I have offered so far by way of introduction to both the AD movement and neurocognitive dementia research is intended to (1) make these machinations accessible and (2) emphasise the extent to which political processes can be traced throughout them. Contested institutional and personal approaches to ageing, nosology, aetiology, cognition, complexity, technoscience and classification saturate the historic and contemporary landscapes of neurocognitive dementia research. These phenomena are, I argue, the legitimate, if not the core, territory of a worthwhile dementia studies.

The term *dementia studies* describes a diverse collection of social science, humanities and arts scholarship and activity that centres on dementia as a political, economic, social, cultural and psychological phenomenon. As emphasised in previous volumes in this series,[49, 50] dementia studies is not a neat unified entity with a singular heritage (neither, for that matter, is neurocognitive research) but rather extends through a multitude of converging and diverging ideas and traditions, some of which can and do come into tension. My selective outline herein attends to some especially pertinent areas of dementia studies for my own argument. It should in no way be read as a definitive account, and to this end, those aforementioned texts in this series are far more instructive. That said, I would argue that there is sufficient coherence to the concept of dementia studies as an institutionalised intellectual and political pursuit that it makes sense for me to speak to it as my community of peers and hence my audience. I do so because I am convinced that much of that which I consider to be dementia studies is uniquely positioned to respond to the shortcomings of the contemporary dementia research economy. This book is a suggestion for how such a project might be realised.

Something resembling early dementia studies scholarship was evident in the late-1980s as social scientists responded to developments in the wider AD economy from the 1970s onward. As the AD movement succeeded in making dementia a household name, a diverse collection of scholars from different backgrounds and with distinct interests, e.g. Karen Lyman[51], John Bond[52] and Tom Kitwood,[53] separately adapted theories from medical sociology to develop critiques of what they saw as the (bio)medicalisation of dementia. Indeed, it speaks to the radical reconfiguration of dementia during the 1980s that these different writers offered similar arguments in isolation but almost simultaneously. The sociology of (bio)medicalisation has typically sought to unpack how human phenomena come to be understood as medical problems. The "bio" caveat denotes a creeping influence of the natural and computer sciences relative to traditional medicine, which different scholars engage with to greater or lesser extents. Historically, work in this tradition has been used to critique (bio)medicine, particularly regarding the creation of new diagnostic categories, which have been accused of transforming previously normal facets of human life into (bio)medical problems. Such analyses have been most substantively developed in relation to phenomena characterised by behaviours that deviate from established norms, particularly those falling under the rubric of mental illness.[54] Indeed, the conceptualisation and treatment of mental illness have been repeatedly critiqued in reference to (bio) medicalisation explicitly.[55–58]

Drawing on anti-(bio)medicalisation critiques, those early dementia studies scholars argued that the growing dementia research economy had transformed later-life cognitive decline, and to some extent later life generally, into a (bio)medical problem. A previously normal and non-medical part of human experience had been brought under the influence of (bio)medicine by reclassifying it as a disease. In a mundane sense, the observation was accurate. Before the 1970s, senile dementia had been largely normalised as a common feature of later life, and this approach was transformed to make dementia a more pronounced abnormality requiring (bio)medical attention. However, beyond simply identifying that this had happened, early dementia studies scholars were explicitly critical of the (bio)medicalisation of dementia, claiming that it was an intellectually underwhelming and morally questionable process. Kitwood[53] rejected the (bio)medical model of dementia as "faulty and deficient" and "far too negative and deterministic"; Bond[52] as "inadequate", "stigmatizing" and "extremely weak"; and Lyman[51] as "narrow, limited, and sometimes distorted in its ignorance". Kitwood even accused practitioners who accepted the (bio)medical model of "a good deal of 'doublethink'"[59]. It is important to recognise that this strong condemnation was emblematic of early anti-(bio)medicalisation critiques in the social sciences more generally, and such rhetoric has generally softened over time.

For them, the reclassification of dementia as a (bio)medical problem legitimised undue institutional control over the people diagnosed while simultaneously delegitimising those people by attributing their experiences and behaviours to a disease. In combination, these effects of (bio)medicalisation were accused of eroding the humanity of people diagnosed with dementia. For instance, Kitwood wrote of "banishment" whereby people with dementia were "removed from the human milieu"[53], while Herskovits argued that "the overwhelmingly dominant pernicious effect of the current Alzheimer's construct is the dehumanization or debasement of 'self'"[60]. Hence, while (bio)medicalisation was nominally the primary concern of early dementia studies, it was more specifically the corresponding dehumanisation of people with dementia that animated scholars. It was not so much the assumptions and activities of the AD movement per se that were critiqued as it was the downstream implications for the status of those diagnosed.

One of the earliest major areas of contemporary dementia studies to emerge from these anti-(bio)medicalisation critiques was a psychosocial tradition rooted in the work of social psychology scholars such as Tom Kitwood and Steven Sabat. These writers typically focussed on interpersonal interactions as a fundamental site in which the dehumanisation of (bio)medicalisation was manifest. This psychosocial approach cast the everyday interactions of dementia care as playing an essential role in determining the selves of the people involved. Specifically, interactions with the person with dementia under the influence of (bio)medical assumptions (i.e. that the person was lost to the disease) resulted in the degradation of that person as a social being because the person was not treated as a person. The work of Kitwood in this area became influential in the development of person-centred dementia care, an idea that remains prominent in contemporary dementia studies as well as care policy, albeit in a fairly bastardised form.[61] At the heart of this tradition is a reverence for the person's self, an argument that this self depends on it being respected by others, and an attempt to defend it from potentially harmful relationships.

Kitwood's version of this self was termed "personhood". While Kitwood appropriated the word from social psychology, his version encompassed social psychological, theological and ethical considerations.[62] From a psychological perspective, Kitwood argued that a person's self-esteem was dependent on one's position in relation to social groups, the associated roles that one performs, and the coherence of one's sense of self. Religiously, he observed an almost ubiquitous reverence for the sacredness of human life, and beyond this, he echoed Kantian philosophy in suggesting that humans must have an unqualified value for the social world to make sense.[63, 64] In synthesis, Kitwood defined this psycho-ethico-religious personhood as "a standing or status that is bestowed upon one human being, by others, in the context of relationship and social being. It implies recognition, respect and trust".[63] The oft-repeated quote has had significant influence across much dementia studies and related practice.

Kitwood progressed to argue that the personhood of people with dementia was too often eroded by "malignant social psychology" in everyday interactions. He typified these harmful relations into several forms that remain recognisable today. For instance, it is widely observed that people often talk about people with dementia as though they are not present. Mundane transgressions are common, such as asking a carer how the person with dementia sitting next to them is doing without first asking the person him/herself or speaking to the person like an infant. Kitwood argued that these forms of interaction, coloured by our (bio)medicalised assumptions about dementia, undermine the parts of personhood that are rooted in social recognition and are realised through interaction. In response, Kitwood, in collaboration with Kathleen Bredin[64, 65] drew on the work of Carl Rogers[66] to develop a model of person-centred care that would support the personhood of people with dementia by encouraging social recognition. While Kitwood's ideas regarding person-centredness have been somewhat misconstrued under the influence of individualism, person-centredness has become a key feature of much dementia care policy and practice, at least nominally.[61, 67, 68]

Around the same time as Kitwood's work exploring relationships as constraining the status of the person with dementia, Steven Sabat was developing concordant insights regarding "selfhood" in dementia.[69] Indeed, in 1992, he observed that Kitwood was "coming to similar conclusions".[70] He used the psychological philosophy of Rom Harré, which argued that the self was made up of several component selves.[71, 72] Sabat presented selfhood as a composite of three "manifestations", named Self-1, Self-2 and Self-3. Self-1 is articulated via personal pronouns (e.g. "me", "myself", etc.) and is akin to personal identity, manifest through our singular narrative experience of life. Self-2 encompasses our distinguishing personal characteristics, both physical and mental. Self-3 resembles the psychosocial component of personhood. It is the social personae comprised of the characters that we enact toward and are perceived by others.[73] As with personhood, some parts of selfhood can be relatively untouched by dementia. A singular experiential standpoint and physical characteristics will likely remain. However, Self-3 extends beyond the individual's innate attributes and is partially reliant on engagement with other people. Sabat observed that: "successful manifestations, or constructions, of Self 3 require, for their very existence, interpersonal interaction and the social recognition given by others".[69] Echoing malignant social psychology, Sabat decried "malignant positioning" whereby people acted in ways that were coloured by assumptions regarding dementia, and which therefore undermined the Self-3, and hence selfhood, of people with dementia.

In these early psychosocial versions of dementia studies, both authors argue that some essential attribute of the human is commonly undermined in dementia. However, they do not see this erosion of self as resulting directly from illness. Instead, the relational scaffolding that typically supports certain parts of personhood/selfhood is tainted by presumptions regarding dementia and the people diagnosed with it. Importantly, it is (bio)medicalised imaginings of dementia that are subject to critique here because they position people with dementia as erased under the conditions of disease and therefore undeserving of normal human interaction. People with dementia are hence somewhat socially disabled through dehumanisation under the symbolic influence of (bio)medicalisation. In response, Kitwood and Sabat argued for a sort of enabling rehumanisation of people with dementia through the cultivation of positive relationships and modes of interaction. These arguments were gaining some academic traction by the mid-1990s, laying firm intellectual foundations for dementia studies. Writing in 1995, Herskovits noted:

> There have been, especially since the mid-1980s, dissenting voices that have endeavored to restore dignity and resuscitate the humanity of individuals diagnosed with Alzheimer's.... In increasing numbers, social scientists have entered the fray, offering theories that reframe and reclaim the "self' in Alzheimer's. Most build on a social interactionist foundation.[60]

The arguments were also becoming more restrained in their critiques of the (bio)medical model, with both Kitwood and Sabat offering additive psychosocial approaches that could ameliorate some of the negative consequences of (bio)medicalisation without contesting those processes altogether. Especially in Kitwood's case, the critique seems to have evolved quickly, from strong rejections of (bio)medical aetiological claims in the 1980s[59, 74] to more consolatory appeals to complementary psychosocial considerations in the 1990s,[63, 64] with the latter work proving far more popular than the former. Hence, the psychosocial emerged as the legitimate territory for dementia studies, without the need to engage in debates regarding the neurocognitive. The early growth of these psychosocial, intersubjective and interpersonal scholarships remains influential today, with a substantial body of research still exploring the interacted nature of dementia and the ways in which relationships influence experiences of dementia.[75]

2.5 Sociopolitical Citizenship

While psychosocial self-focussed scholarship remains popular today, other approaches in dementia studies soon began to challenge psychosocial ideas and offer alternative insights. Perhaps most notable among these approaches have been the 21st-century works of scholars in critical[5] dementia studies. They have typically been interested in understanding and transforming the sociopolitical constitution of dementia. "Sociopolitical" here refers to the politics of social life, spanning traditional political concerns such as legislation and less obviously political considerations such as gender relations. Within this critical tradition, Ruth Bartlett and Deborah O'Connor developed several critiques of personhood in the 2000s, again in an additive manner, building on earlier scholarship. First, they argue that personhood disempowers people with dementia, who become passive beneficiaries of value that is conferred on them by others, with little recourse to actively forge their own value. Second, while notions of the self as intersubjective move past (bio)medical individualism to some extent, they transpose it onto individual interactions and ignore the importance of broader social locations such as class, gender and ethnicity. Third, focusing on the interpersonal intricacies of everyday interactions is problematically depoliticised because it ignores the sociopolitical constraints that shape all our interactions and in doing so, risks blaming individuals for circumstances over which they have little control.[76, 77] For instance, a carer might undermine the selfhood of a person with dementia by ignoring him/her during a care interaction, and a person-centred response might be to educate that carer to improve the interaction. However, critical scholars would situate that malignant social psychology within a highly pressurised working environment that offers little time for meaningful interaction, compounding the wider stresses of years spent working long hours for low pay amidst rising costs of living. Hence, much critical dementia studies seeks to pay attention to the bigger picture.

From this perspective, rather than targeting individual interactants, it is more fruitful to target the dehumanising sociopolitics of dementia. As with the dehumanising relationships that concern psychosocial dementia studies, these sociopolitics are attributed to (bio)medicalisation and for very similar reasons. The (bio)medicalisation of dementia undermines the value of those diagnosed because it labels them *de-mented* – literally *without mind* – and we typically consider our minds as integral to our very being. The person without mind can thus be viewed as lacking insight, rationality and experience and ultimately as being less than human and therefore less worthy of the status that we afford to other humans, be that status enshrined in our everyday actions toward others or in our legal system. Assumptions regarding the de-mented *ergo* de-minded *ergo* de-humanised *ergo* de-valued person inform the interpersonal relations that concerned Kitwood and the sociopolitical relations that concerned Bartlett and O'Connor.[77] Hence, while this critical tradition of dementia studies has critiqued psychosocial scholarship, the two are substantially aligned, with a sociopolitical sensibility adding another level of understanding to the insights of Kitwood, Sabat and their peers.

Just as psychosocial scholars have sought to push back against dehumanising interpersonal relations, so many critical scholars have offered means of resisting dehumanising sociopolitical relations. As one might expect, much of this scholarship has been more forthright in acknowledging and pursuing its political commitments to rehumanising people with dementia. An important example of these attempts is the *citizenship* tradition. Critical dementia studies scholars have been arguing for citizenship approaches to dementia since the early 2000s[76, 78, 79]. At a basic level, citizenship can be understood as encompassing the collection of rights and responsibilities that belong to members of a given society, be those in relation to other members, the populace generally or the state. Citizenship is a useful concept for dementia studies because it sustains the legacy of personhood as an appeal to the value that a person with dementia has (or at least *should* have), while also expanding the parameters of that value to encompass wider sociopolitical factors. It also provides some means for empowering people with dementia as sociopolitical agents who can actively manifest their own citizenship. This introduction of agency is a response to the aforementioned critique of psychosocial dementia studies, namely, that it renders people passively dependent on others for their status.[80]

Citizenship has a long history as a social scientific idea. It has been continuously popular since the work of Thomas Marshall in the 1950s, who wrote on citizenship in relation to social class. He defined citizenship simply as "a status bestowed on those who are full members of a community. All who possess the status are equal with respect to the rights and duties which the status bestows"[81]. One can see substantive parallels here with Kitwood's oft-repeated definition of personhood as relations of bestowal. As with all the versions of human status discussed so far, Marshall's citizenship was composite. It encompassed three types of rights: civil, political and social. Civil rights are enshrined in law and bestow personal liberty. Political rights are enshrined in enfranchisement and bestow democratic participation. Social rights are enshrined in welfare systems and bestow civilised life.

Taken together, this citizenship represents a type of value that is bestowed in relations with the state and its various institutions.

The development of citizenship in dementia studies is built on several earlier applications to related topics, including disability,[82] ageing,[83] care[84] and psychiatry.[85] Throughout these applications, a more postmodernist stance has developed (as opposed to Marshall's modernist position), emphasising complex diversity and action in everyday life. Modern citizenship tended to focus on the official legal and state apparatuses that restrict and enable people in various ways. For example, if I refuse to pay my taxes, I might be imprisoned. If I pay my taxes, I might expect access to healthcare if I become sick.[6] Postmodern citizenship retains an interest in these formal state-level relations, but it also attends to a range of other sociopolitical phenomena operating at various levels while simultaneously bringing in familiar concerns of personhood. Bartlett and O'Connor define this expansive postmodern citizenship as follows:

> A relationship, practice or status, in which a person with dementia is entitled to experience freedom from discrimination, and to have opportunities to grow and participate in life to the fullest extent possible. It involves justice, recognition of social positions and the upholding of personhood, rights and a fluid degree of responsibility for shaping events at a personal and societal level[77].

This notion of citizenship attempts to sustain the original insights of dementia studies regarding the intricacies of interpersonal relationships while introducing new considerations that exist at a larger and more general scale. Structure and agency, personal and political, micro and macro, are brought together. Rather than focusing on one or the other, Bartlett and O'Connor attempt to draw our attention to all these levels of the sociopolitics surrounding dementia:

> People with dementia are discriminated against at different levels and in different ways. On a macro level, discrimination can structure distress, disability and economic losses making it difficult for people to access health services and enjoy community activities… On a micro level, it can lead people with dementia to feel stigmatised and less worthy, and to be seen and treated by care workers and others as less than human.[76]

We can apply Bartlett and O'Connor's theoretical approach to my aforementioned example of a care interaction wherein a carer ignores a person with dementia. This interaction exemplifies the multi-layered nature of sociopolitical challenges to citizenship. The immediate act of ignoring is fundamentally political. It is situated within a care system that manifests (bio) medical values, performing tasks to satisfy bodies without minds and hence without humanity. Those tasks manifest a two-tier health–social welfare system, wherein cancer warrants free "health" care from highly qualified professionals with good standards of employment, but dementia warrants means-tested "social" care from poorly paid, unqualified staff working in poor conditions. Those employment conditions manifest gendered income inequality, with 80% of the UK's social care workforce being female, rising to 90% in lower-paid frontline roles.[86] Ultimately, the apparent mundanity of a particular interaction contains and conceals an array of potent sociopolitical considerations.

An attentiveness to these constraints on our experiences of dementia risks perpetuating the aforementioned problem of passivity in dementia studies, whereby people with dementia are cast as recipients of value and lacking in agency. This passive citizenship is important because it alerts us to the importance of our own actions toward people with dementia as well as the need for supportive welfare institutions. However, agency has proved similarly desirable for dementia studies scholars. Bartlett and O'Connor tackle the danger of pure passivity by making their concept of citizenship highly relative, whereby an individual can conceive of and pursue it however he/she likes. They also extend citizenship to include practices with public consequences. This is an expansive definition because "practices" entails doing something, and "public consequences" denotes any effect on any other person. From this perspective, something as seemingly mundane as a shake of the head can enact citizenship if it stirs some response in another person.

The expansive postmodernist approach to active citizenship has found substantive affinities with embodiment scholarship in dementia studies. The embodiment tradition of dementia studies has its own rich tradition and has only latterly joined up with citizenship. Indeed, it was initially much closer to Sabat's work on selfhood. Pia Kontos was instrumental in developing the embodiment tradition of dementia studies in the early 2000s.[87, 88] She rejected dualist philosophies that separated body and mind, and in their place, offered a model of embodied selfhood whereby selfhood is manifest in and enacted by the body, irrespective of cognition, mind and other psychic concepts. Embodied selfhood has pertinent implications for dementia because, as discussed, to be without mind has traditionally been conflated as to be without self, humanity, value, etc. While Kontos found merit in earlier psychosocial ideas of personhood and selfhood as fundamentally interactional, she also critiqued these approaches for perpetuating the separation of mind and body and then largely ignoring the latter.

As a solution to the lack of corporeality in psychosocial dementia studies, Kontos turned to classic anthropological and philosophical texts on unconscious internalisation and intentionality. She argued that we often act intentionally without needing to engage cognition or some underlying mental process. The innumerable actions of daily life – e.g. entering a bus, making a purchase in a shop – comprise various movements that require no foundational deliberation and yet convey agency, nonetheless. She also attended to the social character of bodily action, noting that we unconsciously internalise sociocultural behaviour simply by existing in any given context. Our mannerisms, postures, gestures, reflexes, etc. in amalgam constitute a personal manifestation of who we are as social beings. At first, Kontos aligned this bodily manifestation of the personal with the notion of selfhood as a valuable means of expressing one's humanity, irrespective of dementia. Writing in 2004, she documented the embodiment of class as a personal characteristic of two women with dementia:

> There was another contrast between the excessive swing of the hips in Edna's heavy stride and Molly's small and delicate walking steps. Molly's delicate manners were also apparent when she used a Kleenex tissue to softly wipe the tip of her nose while Edna, in contrast, covered her entire nose, clenched it tightly with the tissue and blew loudly. In these examples we see physical expressions of class distinctions.[88]

While initially intended as an example of personal distinction rendered in sociocultural particularities, it is easy to reappraise this example in light of citizenship scholarship to appreciate the sociopolitical nature of these embodied selfhoods. Hence, embodied selfhood has gradually morphed into embodied citizenship based on the recognition that our personal embodiments are sociopolitically constrained. Furthermore, there is evidently considerable scope for embodied active citizenship because corporeal manifestations of citizenship typically have an enactive quality, as in the example above. In a similar manner, Kontos and colleagues have presented examples of people with dementia living in care institutions actively embodying their sexualities despite repeated efforts by staff to prevent any sexual activity.[89] Beyond citizenship, such instances are increasingly framed in terms of human rights.[89, 90]

2.6 Humanism's Legacies

The trajectory toward a more actively politically engaged dementia studies has been most acutely realised in the emergence of a human rights tradition in recent years. Human rights represents one of the most direct avenues of resistance that dementia studies has offered to dehumanisation, not only intellectually but also practically in some ways. The application of human rights to dementia specifically stems from the idea that dementia is a disability and should be legally treated as such.[91, 92] This disability approach to dementia articulates a longstanding, albeit largely implicit, thread of social disability scholarship that runs throughout the history of dementia studies and again seeks to counter (bio)medicalisation, which is manifest in the "(bio)medical model".[93] Essentially, social models of disability contend that the human physiological and psychological attributes that we often consider to be disabilities are not inherently disabling. Instead, they become disabilities in disabling contexts.[94] The (bio)medical model blinds us to this context-dependency by essentialising the causative role of physiology (so the argument goes). As a simplistic example, when entering a building, a wheel-chair user is disabled by stairs and enabled by a ramp. These arguments have inspired significant progress toward rights for disabled people, but they have often focussed on physical impairments and have shied away from cognition. Proponents argue that aligning dementia studies with disability studies will lead to similar political outcomes for people with dementia.[95]

The most important legislative basis for the human rights tradition in dementia studies is the United Nations Convention on the Rights of Persons with Disabilities (UNCRPD). The UNCRPD is often invoked in human rights scholarship because, as its name suggests, it attends specifically to the protec-tion of human rights for disabled people. In doing so, it extends a collection of ethical-legal prescriptions to disabled people on the basis that they are fundamentally humans, like all other non-disabled people, and have inher-ent rights by virtue of their being humans.[96] Cahill defines these rights as "Universal (apply to everyone), indivisible (have equal status and cannot be placed in hierarchical order), inalienable (cannot be given or removed) and inabrogable (cannot be voluntarily relinquished or traded for other privi-leges)".[91] These attributes provide a foundation for relatively unqualified appeals to the inherent humanity of people with dementia. Human rights hence come to represent and reassert that which is potentially forfeit under (bio)medicalisation, as personhood and citizenship have similarly done.

Perhaps most influentially, the human rights tradition of dementia studies has inherited the more overtly activist stance of disability studies. At national and international levels, organisations such as the Dementia Engagement and Empowerment Project and Dementia Alliance International have rallied peo-ple with dementia to advocate for human rights. Through such active politi-cisation, some people diagnosed with dementia have come to enjoy a greater public platform,[92, 95] though it is important to remember that this has not necessarily extended to a wide range of sub-groups of people with dementia, e.g. those living in institutions. Dementia studies has hence expanded beyond a traditionally aloof academic pursuit to incorporate, to varying extents, a wider range of stakeholders and to become more explicitly involved in politi-cal activism. While a lot has changed, much of this effort remains dedicated to contesting the dehumanisation of people with dementia, echoing the early arguments of dementia studies scholars several decades ago.

Just as the psychosocial tradition remains alive and well, so work on citizen-ship, especially embodied and material citizenship, and human rights is still a major influence in dementia studies. In 2016, the journal *Dementia* dedicated a special issue to citizenship,[97] and there is even an international citizenship and dementia research group.[98] It is also important to acknowledge that, rather than one overriding the other, much critical dementia studies can seek to encompass work on personhood as an important consideration within a wider sociopolitical landscape. Indeed, Bartlett and O'Connor explicitly note the indebtedness of their work to the progress made by psychosocial scholars before them in refuting (bio)medicalisation:

This body of work highlighted the importance of shifting from a purely biomedical discourse to a more humanistic one… These reflections led to clearer standing and status for people with dementia, an important step towards recognising social citizenship.[77]

In this manner, various iterations of dementia studies, which emerge from critiques of other traditions, can be understood as a kind of sedimentation of understanding that, from a certain perspective at least, is remarkably harmonious – more additive than revolutionary. At first glance, this trajectory might have recently come under some pressure with the emergence of post-humanist dementia studies. As the name implies, this area of scholarship explicitly articulates itself in contrast to the humanist commitments that have characterised much dementia studies since its beginnings in the late 1980s, wielded in opposition to the dehumanising qualities of (bio)medicalisation. However, as I will suggest below, we should be cautious of any reactive appeals to a paradigmatic shift here.

Posthumanist dementia studies is essentially a response to a core tension within dementia studies generally. On the one hand, the discipline has long sought to challenge the dehumanisation of people with dementia by arguing for their value as humans, leading to very real gains in inclusion and empowerment. On the other hand, the belief that humans have some exceptional value generally grounds that value in cognitive capacities, positioning those without said capacities as valueless. Hence the dehumanising qualities of (bio)medicalisation are bound up with the dehumanising tendencies of humanism itself: de-mented *ergo* de-minded *ergo* de-humanised *ergo* de-valued. Nick Jenkins describes this as the "double-edged sword" of humanism in dementia studies.[99] Posthumanist dementia scholarship seeks to circumvent this tension by rejecting humanism outright. For instance, Jocey Quinn and Claudia Blandon argue that notions of human exceptionalism are a legacy of the 17th-century Enlightenment and are a fairly recent and unusual political development.[100] Rather than continuing in the tradition of trying to put people with dementia back into a special human category, posthumanists advocate taking all other people out of that category instead. The result is similar – nothing essential separates the value of people without dementia from the value of people with dementia. We take an alternative route to arrive at the same destination.

To achieve this, posthumanist dementia studies contests the existence of the person as an individually unified, rigidly demarcated and self-contained entity. That which we typically think of as the person is reconceived as a type of intellectual and material assemblage made up of various biological (e.g. viruses), physical (e.g. tattoos) and ideational (e.g. gender) components. As well as being composite, the person is also symbiotic, entailing profound interdependence with a range of other entities, human, animal, mechanical, digital and so on. To an extent, this represents a rearticulation of the relationality of early psychosocial dementia studies wherein that which we deem individual cannot be understood in isolation from its relations. However, that relationality becomes even more integral so that the very being of the component entities and any notions of agency attributed to them ultimately emanate from relations.

At first glance, posthumanist dementia studies might appear to be a radical rejection of the sub-traditions that preceded it. However, while positioning itself in contrast to an underlying humanism, posthumanist scholars generally do not seek to replace all that went before but rather to contribute new intellectual and political tools to the dementia studies canon.[100] Posthumanism should not be read as agreeing that people with dementia are worthless on the grounds that all humans are worthless. Instead, it argues that people with dementia have the worth of all humans who have the worth of all entities. This can feel rather relativist, though posthumanist dementia studies scholarship is typically normatively committed to advocating a high level of worth for all. Moreover, it does not contest the underlying argument, commonplace across dementia studies, that people with dementia are generally symbolically disadvantaged by popular conceptualisations of dementia. Instead, it extends that observation, suggesting that dementia studies might partially perpetuate that disadvantaging through overzealous commitments to humanism.

Hence, despite various discordances and occasionally direct criticisms, all approaches discussed here – personhood, selfhood, citizenship, embodiment, human rights and posthumanism – offer broad opposition to the dehumanising, or disadvantaging, effects of the (bio)medicalisation of dementia, wherein people diagnosed with dementia are rendered lesser by virtue of the conceptual and institutional power of that diagnosis. My contention is that this concern with the dehumanising effects of (bio)medicalisation has been a (if not *the*) core guiding intellectual commitment in the development of several major traditions of dementia studies scholarship. From this perspective, a meaningful intellectual heritage can be traced from contemporary arguments regarding human rights back to work in the 1980s, applying anti-(bio)medicalisation critiques to the emerging AD movement. This has produced some rich areas of dementia studies scholarship with positive implications for people affected by dementia. However, I will argue in the next chapter that it has also potentially distracted from the deeper consequences of the AD movement, particularly in terms of their corresponding biopolitics.

* * *

The first half of this chapter offered an overview of some major developments in neurocognitive research that have been facilitated by the success of the AD movement in generating a substantial dementia research economy. There, I highlighted many of the core contentions that have long dogged research – ageing, nosology, aetiology, technoscience and complexity – iteratively re-realised in new contemporary forms, from GWAS to MCI to LATE. Far from being some alien domain, neurocognitive dementia research manifests conceptual and practical problems that are familiar social scientific fodder. Beyond a dehumanising (bio)medical model, there is a lot of material here that warrants critical engagement. Nonetheless, much of the key theoretical development in dementia studies has centred on the dehumanising consequences of (bio)medicalisation, particularly regarding relational symbolisms. These scholarships argue that people with dementia are rendered lesser by the (bio)medical meaning that is ascribed to them, which then alters how individuals and institutions relate to them, typically for the worse. This scholarship has hence inadvertently diverged from other salient issues in the dementia research economy that might benefit from greater critical attention.

In the second half of the chapter, I attempted a similar characterisation of dementia studies, or at least particular examples of major conceptual flavours thereof. From a similar starting point – the late-20th-century political intensification of dementia – dementia studies has headed in a different direction, far less concerned with contesting onto-epistemologies of ageing and navigating complex typification schemas. Instead, it has developed social theory arguments relating to (bio)medicalisation and the social model of disability as a means of calling out and pushing back against the dehumanisation of people with dementia. To appropriate a phrase from Shakespeare, Zeilig and Mittler's seminal paper on dementia and disability, these two great traditions of studying dementia "seem like planets spinning on different axes, their inhabitants aware of each other's existence but apparently unable to communicate".[92] This relationship, I will argue, could be addressed to the betterment of dementia studies and the wider dementia research economy.

Overall, my aim in this chapter has been to show how dementia studies emerged in relation to the Alzheimer's movement at the end of the 1980s by cultivating anti-(bio)medicalisation arguments. Under the influence of that anti-(bio)medicalisation thought, particularly regarding dehumanisation, dementia studies has subsequently diverged from more mainstream neurocognitive research and some of the salient social scientific issues that have emerged in that research, e.g. the co-constitution of technologies and onto-epistemologies, the politics of classifying complexity and cause and effect. In this chapter, I have deliberately avoided criticising this relationship (or the lack thereof) or criticising anti-(bio)medicalisation dementia studies itself. Instead, I have sought to simply outline the divergent relationship between dementia studies and the wider dementia research economy. I have done so, firstly, because that relationship is the crucial context for the rest of the book, and secondly, because anti-(bio)medicalisation dementia studies scholarship has been a positive development in an immediate sense. Over several decades, it has repeatedly offered valuable counterpoints to the various pathogenic relations that can worsen the lives of people affected by dementia. From early psychosocial appeals to humanist care to contemporary activism groups, dementia studies has contributed to bettering the lives of many people affected by dementia.

That said, in the next chapter, I begin to highlight and deconstruct some of the potential problems that emerge from the heritage of anti-(bio)medicalisation thought in dementia studies. These are problems that are typically multifaceted, downstream, unintended and often unremarked. I will begin with the very notion of a (bio)medical model. Critique in dementia studies is still often aimed at a (bio)medical model that would be largely recognisable to scholars in the 1980s, albeit having steadily become a sort of Pandora's box of dementia studies, containing various nondescript evils. Given the fascinating developments outlined in the first half of this chapter, it is rather underwhelming, if not outright unjust, that this monolithic concept of a (bio) medical model continues to animate such criticism. In the next chapter, I offer several reasons for reconceptualising, at least in parts, that which has often fallen under the umbrella of (bio)medicalisation in dementia studies scholarship. In its place, I will suggest paying greater attention to "neuropsychiatric biopolitics" by re-engaging with medical sociology, which has itself built on a similar disposition toward (bio)medicalisation and nurtured more post-structuralist and sociopolitically astute forms of critique. Most importantly, I am not suggesting that dementia studies scholarship that implicitly or explicitly relies on anti-(bio)medicalisation critiques is bad, nor that it should be replaced. Instead, my argument is intended to provide a further set of intellectual tools, just as the different iterations of dementia studies discussed above have built on one another through both their frictions and their resonances.

Notes

1 The general lack of historical medical reference to dementia, or something similar, is notable and curious, perhaps partially owing to aforementioned abiotrophic sentiments and the relative youthfulness of pre–19th-century populations.
2 "Nosology" is the classification of disease in medical science.
3 It is worth noting that Frau Deter's delusions related to her husband having an affair with their neighbour, and historically many men sent their wives to asylums to facilitate new relationships.
4 PSEN2 is slightly less directly predictive of AD onset than APP and PSEN1, with some carriers surviving into later life without experiencing symptoms.
5 "Critical" is used here in the academic sense, outlined in detail in Chapter 3.
6 I appreciate that both these examples are naively idealised.

References

1. Robbert, R. (1989). *The Medicalization of Senile Dementia: From "Normality" to "Pathology"*. Western Michigan University.
2. Boller, F., and Forbes, M.M. (1998). History of dementia and dementia in history: An overview. *Journal of the Neurological Sciences 158*, 125–133. doi: 10.1016/S0022-510X(98)00128-2.
3. Albert, M.L., and Mildworf, B. (1989). The concept of dementia. *Journal of Neurolinguistics 4*, 301–308. doi: 10.1016/0911-6044(89)90022-5.

4. Fox, P. (1989). From senility to Alzheimer's disease: The rise of the Alzheimer's disease movement. *The Milbank Quarterly 67*, 58–102. doi: 10.2307/3350070.

5. Wilks, S. (1864). Clinical notes on atrophy of the brain. *Journal of Mental Science 10*, 381–392. doi: 10.1192/bjp.10.51.381.

6. Yang, H.D., Kim, D.H., Lee, S.B., and Young, L.D. (2016). History of Alzheimer's disease. *Dementia and Neurocognitive Disorders 15*, 115–121. doi: 10.12779/dnd.2016.15.4.115.

7. Dahm, R. (2006). Alzheimer's discovery. *Current Biology 16*, R906–R910. doi: 10.1016/j.cub.2006.09.056.

8. Fukui, T. (2015). Historical review of academic concepts of dementia in the world and Japan: With a short history of representative diseases. *Neurocase 21*, 369–376. doi: 10.1080/13554794.2014.894532.

9. Hippius, H., and Neundörfer, G. (2003). The discovery of Alzheimer's disease. *Dialogues in Clinical Neuroscience 5*, 101–108.

10. Beard, R.L. (2016). *Living with Alzheimer's: Managing Memory Loss, Identity, and Illness.* New York University Press.

11. Amaducci, L.A., Rocca, W.A., and Schoenberg, B.S. (1986). Origin of the distinction between Alzheimer's disease and senile dementia: How history can clarify nosology. *Neurology 36*, 1497–1497. doi: 10.1212/WNL.36.11.1497.

12. Barrett, A. (1913). A case of Alzheimer's disease with unusual neurological disturbances. *The Journal of Nervous and Mental Disease 40*, 361–374. doi: 10.1097/00005053-191306000-00001.

13. Fuller, S.C., and Klopp, H.I. (1912). Further observations on Alzheimer's disease. *American Journal of Insanity 69*, 17–29.

14. Assal, F. (2019). History of Dementia. *Frontiers of Neurology and Neuroscience 44*, 118–126. doi: 10.1159/000494959.

15. Fletcher, J.R. Black knowledges matter: How the suppression of non-white understandings of dementia harms us all and how we can combat it. *Sociology of Health & Illness*. doi: 10.1111/1467-9566.13280.

16. Terry, R.D. (1963). The fine structure of neurofibrillary tangles in Alzheimer's disease. *Journal of Neuropathology and Experimental Neurology 22*, 629–642. doi: 10.1097/00005072-196310000-00005.

17. Terry, R.D., Gonatas, N.K., and Weiss, M. (1964). Ultrastructural studies in Alzheimer's Presenile Dementia. *The American Journal of Pathology 44*, 269–297.

18. Wilson, D. (2017). Calculable people? Standardising assessment guidelines for Alzheimer's disease in 1980s Britain. *Medical History 61*, 500–524. doi: 10.1017/mdh.2017.56.

19. Hampel, H., Mesulam, M.-M., Cuello, A.C., Khachaturian, A.S., Vergallo, A., Farlow, M.R., Snyder, P.J., Giacobini, E., Khachaturian, Z.S., and Cholinergic System Working Group, and for the A.P.M.I. (APMI) (2019). Revisiting the cholinergic hypothesis in Alzheimer's disease: Emerging evidence from translational and clinical research. *The Journal of Prevention of Alzheimer's Disease 6*, 2–15. doi: 10.14283/jpad.2018.43.

20. Bowen, D.M., Smith, C.B., White, P., and Davison, A.N. (1976). Neurotransmitter-related enzymes and indices of hypoxia in senile dementia and other abiotrophies. *Brain 99*, 459–496. doi: 10.1093/brain/99.3.459.

21. Davies, P., and Maloney, A.J.F. (1976). Selective loss of central cholinergic neurons in Alzheimer's disease. *The Lancet 308*, 1403. doi: 10.1016/S0140-6736(76)91936-X.

22. Liu, P.-P., Xie, Y., Meng, X.-Y., and Kang, J.-S. (2019). History and progress of hypotheses and clinical trials for Alzheimer's disease. *Signal Transduction and Targeted Therapy 4*, 1–22. doi: 10.1038/s41392-019-0063-8.

23. Glenner, G.G., and Wong, C.W. (1984). Alzheimer's disease: Initial report of the purification and characterization of a novel cerebrovascular amyloid protein. *Biochemical and Biophysical Research Communications 120*, 885–890. doi: 10.1016/s0006-291x(84)80190-4.

24. Hardy, J.A., and Higgins, G.A. (1992). Alzheimer's disease: The amyloid cascade hypothesis. *Science 256*, 184–186.

25. Mehta, D., Jackson, R., Paul, G., Shi, J., and Sabbagh, M. (2017). Why do trials for Alzheimer's disease drugs keep failing? A discontinued drug perspective for 2010–2015. *Expert Opinion on Investigational Drugs 26*, 735–739. doi: 10.1080/13543784.2017.1323868.

26. Rubin, R. (2021). Recently approved Alzheimer drug raises questions that might never be answered. *JAMA 326*, 469–472. doi: 10.1001/jama.2021.11558.

27. Angelo, M., and Ward, L. (2021). Aducanumab fails to produce efficacy results yet obtains US Food and Drug Administration approval. *Population Health Management 24*, 638–639. doi: 10.1089/pop.2021.0189.

28. van Bokhoven, P., de Wilde, A., Vermunt, L., Leferink, P.S., Heetveld, S., Cummings, J., Scheltens, P., and Vijverberg, E.G.B. (2021). The Alzheimer's disease drug development landscape. *Alzheimer's Research & Therapy 13*, 186. doi: 10.1186/s13195-021-00927-z.

29. Daly, T., Houot, M., Barberousse, A., Petit, A., and Epelbaum, S. (2021). A proposal to make biomedical research into Alzheimer's disease more democratic following an International survey with researchers. *Journal of Alzheimer's Disease Reports 5*, 637–645. doi: 10.3233/ADR-210030.

30. Aschenbrenner, A.J., Gordon, B.A., Benzinger, T.L.S., Morris, J.C., and Hassenstab, J.J. (2018). Influence of tau PET, amyloid PET, and hippocampal volume on cognition in Alzheimer disease. *Neurology 91*, e859–e866. doi: 10.1212/WNL.0000000000006075.

31. Herrup, K. (2021). *How Not to Study a Disease: The Story of Alzheimer's*. MIT Press.

32. Lock, M. (2013). *The Alzheimer Conundrum: Entanglements of Dementia and Aging*. Princeton University Press.

33. Mullard, A. (2021). Failure of first anti-tau antibody in Alzheimer disease highlights risks of history repeating. *Nature Reviews Drug Discovery 20*, 3–5. doi: 10.1038/d41573-020-00217-7.

34. Bateman, R.J., Aisen, P.S., De Strooper, B., Fox, N.C., Lemere, C.A., Ringman, J.M., Salloway, S., Sperling, R.A., Windisch, M., and Xiong, C. (2011). Autosomal-dominant Alzheimer's disease: A review and proposal for the prevention of Alzheimer's disease. *Alzheimer's Research & Therapy 3*, 1. doi: 10.1186/alzrt59.

35. Van Cauwenberghe, C., Van Broeckhoven, C., and Sleegers, K. (2016). The genetic landscape of Alzheimer disease: Clinical implications and perspectives. *Genetics in Medicine 18*, 421–430. doi: 10.1038/gim.2015.117.

36. Mills, M.C., and Tropf, F.C. (2020). Sociology, genetics, and the coming of age of sociogenomics. *Annual Review of Sociology 46*, 553–581. doi: 10.1146/annurev-soc-121919-054756.

37. Heeney, C. (2021). Problems and promises: How to tell the story of a Genome Wide Association Study? *Studies in History and Philosophy of Science Part A* 89, 1–10. doi: 10.1016/j.shpsa.2021.06.003.

38. Ozaki, K., and Niida, S. (2019). Genetic background for Alzheimer's disease: Knowledge accumulated from AD GWAS. *Brain Nerve 71*, 1039–1051. doi: 10.11477/mf.1416201403.

39. Di Fede, G., Catania, M., Maderna, E., Ghidoni, R., Benussi, L., Tonoli, E., Giaccone, G., Moda, F., Paterlini, A., Campagnani, I., et al. (2018). Molecular subtypes of Alzheimer's disease. *Scientific Reports 8*, 3269. doi: 10.1038/s41598-018-21641-1.

40. Nelson, P.T., Dickson, D.W., Trojanowski, J.Q., Jack, C.R., Boyle, P.A., Arfanakis, K., Rademakers, R., Alafuzoff, I., Attems, J., Brayne, C., et al. (2019). Limbic-predominant age-related TDP-43 encephalopathy (LATE): Consensus working group report. *Brain 142*, 1503–1527. doi: 10.1093/brain/awz099.

41. Sachdev, P.S., Blacker, D., Blazer, D.G., Ganguli, M., Jeste, D.V., Paulsen, J.S., and Petersen, R.C. (2014). Classifying neurocognitive disorders: The DSM-5 approach. *Nature Reviews Neurology 10*, 634–642. doi: 1038/nrneurol.2014.181.

42. Data Bridge (2022). *Mild Cognitive Impairment (MCI) Treatment Market Analysis Report by 2029*. https://www.databridgemarketresearch.com/reports/global-mild-cognitive-impairment-mci-treatment-market.

43. Sperling, R.A., Aisen, P.S., Beckett, L.A., Bennett, D.A., Craft, S., Fagan, A.M., Iwatsubo, T., Jack, C.R., Kaye, J., Montine, T.J., et al. (2011). Toward defining the preclinical stages of Alzheimer's disease: Recommendations from the National Institute on Aging-Alzheimer's Association workgroups on diagnostic guidelines for Alzheimer's disease. *Alzheimer's & Dementia 7*, 280–292. doi: 10.1016/j.jalz.2011.03.003.

44. Yemm, H., Peel, E., and Brooker, D. (2022). Understandings of mild cognitive impairment (MCI): A survey study of public and professional perspectives. *Working with Older People*. doi: 10.1108/WWOP-08-2022-0035.

45. Oltra-Cucarella, J., Ferrer-Cascales, R., Alegret, M., Gasparini, R., Díaz-Ortiz, L.M., Ríos, R., Martínez-Nogueras, Á.L., Onandia, I., Pérez-Vicente, J.A., Cabello-Rodríguez, L., et al. (2018). Risk of progression to Alzheimer's disease for different neuropsychological Mild Cognitive Impairment subtypes: A hierarchical meta-analysis of longitudinal studies. *Psychology and Aging 33*, 1007–1021. doi: 10.1037/pag0000294.

46. Cheng, Y.-W., Chen, T.-F., and Chiu, M.-J. (2017). From mild cognitive impairment to subjective cognitive decline: Conceptual and methodological evolution. *Neuropsychiatric Disease and Treatment 13*, 491–498. doi: 10.2147/NDT.S123428.

47. Adelman, R.C. (1995). The Alzheimerization of Aging1. *The Gerontologist 35*, 526–532. doi: 10.1093/geront/35.4.526.

48. Mullane, K., and Williams, M. (2019). The de-Alzheimerization of age-related dementias: Implications for drug targets and approaches to effective therapeutics. *Current Opinion in Pharmacology 44*, 62–75. doi: 10.1016/j.coph.2019.01.004.

49. Fletcher, J.R., and Capstick, A. (2023). *A Critical History of Dementia Studies*. Routledge.

50. Ward, R., and Sandberg, L. (2023). *Critical Dementia Studies*. Routledge.

51. Lyman, K.A. (1989). Bringing the social back in: A critique of the biomedicalization of Dementia. *The Gerontologist 29*, 597–605. doi: 10.1093/geront/29.5.597.

52. Bond, J. (1992). The medicalization of dementia. *Journal of Aging Studies 6*, 397–403. doi: 10.1016/0890-4065(92)90020-7.

53. Kitwood, T. (1990). The dialectics of Dementia: With particular reference to Alzheimer's disease. *Ageing & Society 10*, 177–196. doi: 10.1017/S0144686X00008060.

54. Busfield, J. (2017). The concept of medicalisation reassessed. *Sociology of Health & Illness 39*, 759–774. doi: 10.1111/1467-9566.12538.

55. Cohen, C.I. (1993). The biomedicalization of psychiatry: A critical overview. *Community Mental Health Journal 29*, 509–521. doi: 10.1007/BF00754260.

56. Lang, C., and Jansen, E. (2013). Appropriating depression: Biomedicalizing ayurvedic psychiatry in Kerala, India. *Medical Anthropology 32*, 25–45. doi: 10.1080/01459740.2012.674584.

57. Kim, H.-S. (2014). From "medicalization" to "biomedicalization": The case of mental disorder. *Journal of Science and Technology Studies 14*, 3–33.

58. Watters, E. (2010). *Crazy Like Us: The Globalization of the American Psyche*. Free Press.

59. Kitwood, T. (1989). Brain, mind and Dementia: With particular reference to Alzheimer's disease. *Ageing & Society 9*, 1–15. doi: 10.1017/S0144686X00013337.

60. Herskovits, E. (1995). Struggling over subjectivity: Debates about the "self" and Alzheimer's disease. *Medical Anthropology Quarterly 9*, 146–164. doi: 10.1525/maq.1995.9.2.02a00030.

61. Fletcher, J.R. (2020). Renegotiating relationships: Theorising shared experiences of dementia within the dyadic career. *Dementia 19*, 708–720. doi: 10.1177/1471301218785511.

62. Kitwood, T.M. (1990). *Concern for Others: New Psychology of Conscience and Morality*. Routledge.

63. Kitwood, T.M. (1997). *Dementia Reconsidered: The Person Comes First*. Open University Press.

64. Kitwood, T., and Bredin, K. (1992). Towards a theory of Dementia care: Personhood and well-being. *Ageing & Society 12*, 269–287. doi: 10.1017/S0144686X0000502X.

65. Kitwood, T.M., and Bredin, K. (1992). *Person to Person: Guide to the Care of Those with Failing Mental Powers*, 2nd edition. Gale Centre Publications.

66. Rogers, C. (1951). *Client Centered Therapy*. Hachette UK.

67. Higgs, P., and Gilleard, C. (2016). Interrogating personhood and dementia. *Aging & Mental Health 20*, 773–780. doi: 10.1080/13607863.2015.1118012.

68. Hobson, P. (2019). *Enabling People with Dementia: Understanding and Implementing Person-Centred Care*. Springer Nature.

69. Sabat, S.R. (2001). *The Experience of Alzheimer's Disease: Life Through a Tangled Veil*. Wiley.

70. Sabat, S.R., and Harré, R. (1992). The construction and deconstruction of self in Alzheimer's disease. *Ageing & Society 12*, 443–461. doi: 10.1017/S0144686X00005262.

71. Harré, R. (1984). *Personal Being: A Theory for Individual Psychology*. Harvard University Press.

72. Harré, R. (1991). The discursive production of selves. *Theory & Psychology 1*, 51–63. doi: 10.1177/0959354391011004.
73. Sabat, S.R. (2002). Surviving manifestations of selfhood in Alzheimer's disease: A case study. *Dementia 1*, 25–36. doi: 10.1177/147130120200100101.
74. Kitwood, T. (1988). The technical, the personal, and the framing of dementia. *Social Behaviour 3*, 161–179.
75. Fletcher, J.R. (2020). Distributed selves: Shifting inequities of impression management in couples living with Dementia. *Symbolic Interaction 43*, 405–427. doi: 10.1002/symb.467.
76. Bartlett, R., and O'Connor, D. (2007). From personhood to citizenship: Broadening the lens for dementia practice and research. *Journal of Aging Studies 21*, 107–118. doi: 10.1016/j.jaging.2006.09.002.
77. Bartlett, R., and O'Connor, D. (2010). *Broadening the Dementia Debate: Towards Social Citizenship*. Policy Press.
78. Bartlett, R. (2003). *Meanings of Social Exclusion and Inclusion in Relation to Older People with Dementia in Care Homes*. Oxford Brookes University.
79. Hulko, W. (2004). *Dementia and Intersectionality: Exploring the Experiences of Older People with Dementia and Their Significant Others*. The University of Stirling.
80. Innes, A. (2009). *Dementia Studies: A Social Science Perspective*. SAGE.
81. Marshall, T.H. (1950). *Citizenship and Social Class*. Pluto Press.
82. Campbell, J., and Oliver, M. (1996). *Disability Politics: Understanding Our Past, Changing Our Future*. Routledge.
83. Gilleard, C.J., and Higgs, P. (2000). *Cultures of Ageing: Self, Citizen, and the Body*. Prentice Hall.
84. Barnes, D.M. (1997). *Care, Communities and Citizens*. Longman.
85. Sayce, L. (2000). *From Psychiatric Patient to Citizen: Overcoming Discrimination and Social Exclusion*. Macmillan Education UK.
86. The King's Fund (2022). Overview of the health and social care workforce. The King's Fund. https://www.kingsfund.org.uk/projects/time-think-differently /trends-workforce-overview.
87. Kontos, P.C. (2003). "The painterly hand": Embodied consciousness and Alzheimer's disease. *Journal of Aging Studies 17*, 151–170. doi: 10.1016/ S0890-4065(03)00006-9.
88. Kontos, P.C. (2004). Ethnographic reflections on selfhood, embodiment and Alzheimer's disease. *Ageing & Society 24*, 829–849. doi: 10.1017/ S0144686X04002375.
89. Kontos, P., Grigorovich, A., Kontos, A.P., and Miller, K.-L. (2016). Citizenship, human rights, and dementia: Towards a new embodied relational ethic of sexuality. *Dementia 15*, 315–329. doi: 10.1177/1471301216636258.
90. Peisah, C., Ayalon, L., Verbeek, H., Benbow, S.M., Wiskerke, E., Rabheru, K., and Sorinmade, O. (2021). Sexuality and the human rights of persons with Dementia. *The American Journal of Geriatric Psychiatry 29*, 1021–1026. doi: 10.1016/j.jagp.2021.05.016.
91. Suzanne, C. (2018). *Dementia and Human Rights*. Policy Press.
92. Shakespeare, T., Zeilig, H., and Mittler, P. (2019). Rights in mind: Thinking differently about Dementia and disability. *Dementia 18*, 1075–1088. doi: 10.1177/1471301217701506.

93. Fletcher, J.R. (2019). *A Problem Shared: The Interacted Experience of Dementia within Care*. King's College London.
94. Oliver, M. (1990). *Politics of Disablement*. Macmillan International Higher Education.
95. Thomas, C., and Milligan, C. (2018). Dementia, disability rights and disablism: Understanding the social position of people living with dementia. *Disability & Society 33*, 115–131. doi: 10.1080/09687599.2017.1379952.
96. Kelly, F., and Innes, A. (2013). Human rights, citizenship and dementia care nursing. *International Journal of Older People Nursing 8*, 61–70. doi: 10.1111/j.1748-3743.2011.00308.x.
97. O'Connor, D., and Nedlund, A.-C. (2016). Editorial introduction: Special issue on citizenship and Dementia. *Dementia 15*, 285–288. doi: 10.1177/1471301216647150.
98. Citizenship and Dementia: International Research Network.https://liu.se/en/research/citizenship-and-dementia-international-research-network.
99. Jenkins, N. (2017). No substitute for human touch? Towards a critically posthumanist approach to dementia care. *Ageing & Society 37*, 1484–1498. doi: 10.1017/S0144686X16000453.
100. Quinn, J., and Blandon, C. (2020). *Lifelong Learning and Dementia: A Posthumanist Perspective*. Springer Nature.

3 Anti-(bio)medical; Neuro-agnostic

Why Dementia Studies Needs Neurocritical Responses to the Biopolitics of Dementia

In this chapter, I argue that dementia studies should build on traditional critiques of the (bio)medical model, as outlined in the previous chapter, to develop a new focus on the *neuropsychiatric biopolitics of dementia*. I begin by outlining several reasons that a focus on a (bio)medical model is limited, both conceptually and in relation to the real-world circumstances of dementia and those affected by it. I then show how the neuropsychiatric biopolitics of dementia differs from (bio)medicalisation, contending that an alertness to those differences can lead us to engage with dementia research in newly productive ways. Central to this argument is the assertion that the neuropsychiatric biopolitics of dementia is fundamentally a political process, and while it relies on appeals to science as a means of legitimation, it is often at odds with basic science and should not be conflated with it. Importantly, I do not suggest that all dementia studies work relating to anti-(bio)medicalisation critiques should be abandoned as inadequate, but rather that we might build upon it.

Nonetheless, I go on to show that, with anti-(bio)medicalisation firmly embedded in its intellectual heartlands, much dementia studies has developed a "neuro-agnostic" disposition. By this, I mean that a lot of dementia studies scholarship too rarely addresses biopolitical claims head-on. An emphasis on humanist critiques of institutional medicine, a (bio)medical model and its symbolic effects on relationships, has failed to engage substantively with neurocognitive research, neuropsychiatric biopolitics and related normative prescriptions of dementia. I situate this lack of critical engagement within broader social scientific trends toward the acceptance of knowledge claims regarding neurocognitive science, or at least the dismissal of them as being somehow illegitimate subject matter for dementia studies. I argue that neuro-agnosticism not only fails to robustly challenge poor science and spurious associated claims but repeatedly aids its proliferation by reiterating its core assumptions as justifications for doing dementia studies.

In response, I suggest that the critical traditions of psychiatry and gerontology can provide us with the analytic tools to uncover and challenge the biopolitical reordering of dementia. I briefly introduce

DOI: 10.4324/9781003398523-3

some key tenets of critical psychiatry and critical gerontology. I highlight the longstanding deficit of critical psychiatric engagement with dementias in comparison with other psychiatric disorders and explicate contemporary work on the biopolitics of successful ageing. Together, these insights raise questions about how prescriptions of brain health and cognitive ableism in later life become publicly salient, the consequences of that salience and whose interests are at stake. I conclude that by combining critical psychiatry and critical gerontology, a critical dementia studies could engage more robustly with the neuropsychiatric biopolitics of dementia. However, this is not a matter of outright refutation but rather an attempt to constructively critique and strengthen those commitments that have proved fruitful in other areas.

3.1 The Case against (Bio)medicalisation

As discussed, much influential work in dementia studies has historically drawn on sociological critiques of (bio)medicalisation to offer some resistance to what is repeatedly identified as the (bio)medical model. At the most rudimentary level, this model lays out a particular ontology of dementia as brain disease(s). Drawing on Lyman's[1] aforementioned early anti-(bio)medicalisation work in dementia studies, Spector and Orrell offer the following definition:

> The medical model of dementia states that dementia is (a) pathological and individual, (b) organic in aetiology (caused by progressive deterioration of those parts of the brain that control cognitive and behavioral functioning), and (c) treated and managed according to medical authority.[2]

Traditionally, dementia studies scholars have criticised this conceptualisation of the (bio)medical model for (1) pathologising human circumstances that were previously considered normal,[3, 4] (2) dehumanisation,[5, 6] (3) substantiating the exertion of institutional power over (bio)medicalised people[7, 8] and (4) distracting from wider psychological, social, economic and political facets.[9, 10] Rather than contesting them outright, these arguments are justified to some extent, e.g. some institutions have deliberately sought to pathologise later-life cognitive impairment in explicit opposition to its widespread normalisation. Moreover, each has contributed to the strengthening of dementia studies as an intellectual pursuit and a project to improve the lives of people affected by dementia. Ultimately, much of the progress that has been made toward the better treatment of people with dementia, such as the popularity of person-centredness, has emerged from this tradition of critique. With this in mind, I am by no means suggesting that we abandon such work.

That said, traditional critiques of the (bio)medical model stem from mid-20th-century social theory and can only take us so far.[11, 12] They are rooted in decades-old arguments and, despite their significant strengths, have several limitations. Firstly, the (bio)medical model is often ascribed rather directly to professionals working within institutional medicine. This tendency to ascribe the model to professionals can be traced back to early psychosocial scholarship. Recall, for example, Kitwood's accusation of practitioner "doublethink" from the previous chapter.[13] Such conflations continue today. For instance, when recently advocating person-centredness, Venkatesan and Das argued, "due to the 'fix the patient' approach of the medical model of dementia, along with the health professionals' failure to revamp the model, the quality of life and well-being of dementia-afflicted individuals suffers."[14] Such arguments also extend into other sub-traditions of dementia studies. When arguing for a human rights approach, Cahill recently criticised the biomedical model's dominance in informing practitioners' treatment of people with dementia.[15] Hence, the ascription of a (bio)medical model to professionals remains prominent in dementia studies.

The conflation of medical staff with the (bio)medical model is something of a strawman mischaracterisation of those professions. The observation that a (bio)medical model reduces dementia, and potentially those diagnosed with it, to brain disease, does not mean that a nurse, psychiatrist or geriatrician does the same. In practice, medical professionals working with dementia typically have expansive and nuanced understandings of patients and their conditions[16] and are even explicitly critical of the (bio)medical model.[17, 18] Indeed, the best practice in geriatric psychiatry has relatively little to do with matters of organic aetiology and associated treatment. It is far more concerned with gaining a rounded view of people and their problems and helping them to achieve the goals that matter most to them.[19] Part of the problem here is that empirical observations of negative outcomes experienced by people with dementia can be misinterpreted as evidence of poor practitioner understanding as opposed to being caused by more pragmatic and material constraints on practice. For instance, a psychiatrist might have a rich appreciation of dementia but, in a dangerously understaffed care institution, might be faced with a binary decision of either prescribing antipsychotics or doing nothing at all. Similarly, reports of particularly bad experiences can be presented as evidencing a general inadequacy among staff. For instance, when advocating for her concept of "prescribed dis-engagement", Kate Swaffer argued, without citation: "Following a diagnosis of dementia, most health care professionals, including neurologists, geriatricians, physicians, general practitioners, and dementia service providers prescribe giving up a pre-diagnosis life".[20] While this clearly happened to her and has happened to some of the people with dementia that I work with, many others have not experienced such abjectly poor and disrespectful treatment by medical professionals.

Relatedly, much critique of the (bio)medical model attributes the model to medical professionals, their value commitments and their practices,[21] at the expense of an awareness of other stakeholders. As discussed in Chapter 1, historically, what is typically referred to as the (bio)medical model of dementia actually developed and proliferated under the stewardship of charities, activists, private enterprises, governments and other parties that collectively comprised the AD movement. The focus on institutional medicine distracts from the different roles and interests bound up with a neuropathological ontology of dementia. Indeed, from this perspective, medical professionals and institutional medicine more broadly are rather late entrants in the (bio)medical model's history and remain relatively peripheral. Nonetheless, healthcare practitioners have traditionally been subject to considerable scrutiny throughout the development of dementia studies, perhaps only comparable with family carers.

This leads neatly to another limitation, namely, that the (bio)medical model is too often depicted as the central conceptual basis of institutional medicine, from which medical practice takes its cues. As noted, while there are undoubtedly many individual instances, particularly historically, the idea that medical professionals typically view people with dementia as mindless disease entities, or in similar detrimental ways, is questionable, with surveys reporting positive humanistic attitudes.[22–26] Similarly, the conflation of institutional medicine with a (bio)medical model often relies on an epistemic mistake, whereby the practical outcomes of a system are interpreted as evidence of corresponding belief systems determining that system. Even if we take for granted that their practice, and medical intervention as a systemic whole, is unequivocally pathologising, dehumanising and simplistic, then a more pragmatic and structural social scientific interpretation of those observations might attend to the logistical and resource constraints on healthcare systems as much as any underlying conceptual model. Practical medical provision is often limited by a range of practical considerations that are directly at odds with (bio)medical conceptual commitments. Desirable traits such as respect, holism and affection can be impeded by pressurised circumstances. Hence, real-world instances of institutional medicine are, at best, adulterated manifestations of the conceptual model underpinning (bio)medicine and, therefore, cannot be interpreted as being strictly analogous to that model. For instance, as a British academic, I am sceptical of the UK's marketisation of higher education and financial exploitation of teenagers, yet I exist within that system and inevitably perpetuate it through my practice. My practical complicity does not necessarily reflect any conceptual agreement on my part, and at a macro level, the exploitative marketising effects of the institutional whole do not reflect an uncontested (or even widely accepted) underlying intellectual model.

Building on the recognition of real-world limitations to practice and the relations between the (bio)medical model and institutional medicine, it is also important to recognise that dementia is not really a (bio)medical concern in a pragmatic sense. Given the lack of effective treatments and the resource constraints that characterise care delivery, there is little that formal healthcare providers can do for people with dementia by way of traditional services. Indeed, in the UK and internationally, most people with dementia have little contact with institutional medicine by virtue of their dementias specifically, besides occasional interactions with general practitioners. Dementia has always been and continues to be, by and large, a non-institutional affair, medical or otherwise. It is dealt with by people themselves, their family members and friends.[27] The informal nature of dementia means that critiques targeting institutional (bio)medicine are limited with respect to the real-world situations that they are directly applicable to because so much of the experience of dementia plays out in isolation from formal services. Of course, it is widely recognised that the experience of formal diagnosis can be profoundly affecting, particularly when delivered badly[20] or leading to driving cessation,[28] but the lack of post-diagnostic infrastructure is repeatedly identified as a key shortcoming of institutional responses to dementia.[29, 30] In the UK, only 38% of people with a dementia diagnosis receive any related services.[31] Therefore, even if we accept that institutional medicine and medical professionals are fundamentally guided by a (bio)medical model and hence (bio)medicalising in nature, it is unclear to what degree those entities exert sustained influence over the lives of most people with dementia, who have little engagement with services.

Finally, the (bio)medical model of dementia has also been critiqued for having an exclusively curative focus at the expense of other important therapeutic components such as care, rehabilitation and palliation.[32, 33] However, given the rise of the dementia prevention agenda over the past decade,[34] which has partly positioned itself in contrast to curative efforts, this claim is increasingly difficult to sustain, even if we assume that it was once accurate. It is important to note that the preventative agenda as a substantive entity is relatively new and remains subject to varying articulations and ongoing adaptations. At its core, it may also manifest many of the same normative commitments as earlier curative work, an issue returned to below. Nonetheless, it is explicitly a major shift away from, or at least a thorough reimagining of, curative enterprises and has not been adequately accounted for in recent work regarding the (bio)medical model.[35] It opens up new territories of biopower in ways that complicate the (bio)medicalisation thesis, perhaps to the point of breaking it, and hence further underscores a need to extend our critical gaze beyond the (bio)medical model.

Ultimately, at the risk of sociological cliché, the development of dementia since the 1970s is far more complex than is typically implied by critiques of (bio)medicalisation. It is debatable to what extent a coherent (bio)medical model, in the traditional sense, exists beyond the critiques that invoke it. As noted, the suggestion that such a simplistic model guides medical professionals or medical institutions fails to acknowledge the intellectual sophistication and resource limitations that constrain real-world practice. Even after discounting these issues, the reality of dementia for most people is starkly (and perhaps regrettably) non-medicalised. Besides diagnosis, dementia is largely dealt with informally by families. Considering these limitations, I argue that the contemporary mainstream conceptualisation of dementia, which is often depicted as a (bio)medical model, is better understood as a tangle of moral, technoscientific and political economic phenomena that extends beyond the traditional terrain of (bio)medicalisation.

At this point, one might worry that an over-intellectualised concern with doing justice to the complexity of dementia and treatments thereof risks overlooking the power of a (bio)medical model in contrast to other approaches to dementia and perhaps forfeiting some of the laudable gains made by dementia studies. However, I am not suggesting that we abandon anti-(bio)medicalisation critiques outright. Rather, we might look to more recent social theory to open up distinctive and newly productive analyses of many of the same things that anti-(bio)medicalisation scholars have traditionally criticised. Collectively, I argue that tangle of moral, technoscientific and political economic phenomena can be more astutely interpreted as manifesting a neuropsychiatric biopolitics of dementia, with several important components and consequences that an anti-(bio)medicalisation approach alone cannot sufficiently deconstruct. Principally, far from being an unwarranted institutional transgression into previously normal aspects of human existence, I argue that dementia is better addressed as more pervasively and sociopolitically transformative, affecting our relations with our brains, minds and ultimately the nature of ourselves.

3.2 The Case for Biopolitics

In making the argument for turning our attention to a biopolitical understanding of dementia, I am influenced by the work of sociologist Nikolas Rose. Rose has, like me, criticised social scholarship that focuses on (bio)medicalisation. Writing on the proliferation of neuropsychiatric meaning in public life, he has suggested that "medicalisation, implying the extension of medical authority beyond a legitimate boundary, is not much help in understanding how, why, or with what consequences these mutations have occurred."[36] He is not alone in this observation. Williams, Kats and Martins have argued that we must look "beyond medicalisation ... to find new ways to critically understand the ideas about life and health as they travel, translate or migrate from (neuro)scientific and clinical spheres to cultural life."[37] It is precisely this looking beyond (bio)medicalisation that I wish to pursue here as an appeal for dementia studies to critically engage with the ways in which dementia is manifest as a political and cultural entity.

"Biopolitics" describes the governance of human life via the proliferation of ideas that guide personal conduct in ways that are conducive to certain political projects. This is not the physical implementation of governance but rather the "art of governance."[38] It is the subtle ordering of life through the generation of conceptual schemas that constrain our experiences. This ordering of our seemingly personal and intrinsic experience is realised through the imposition of a select normativity. We are unconsciously beholden to these normative schemas, and our lives play out accordingly. Importantly, this taken-for-granted quality of existence is what critical theory seeks to reveal and challenge, as I will outline below. Biopolitical scholarship has documented the biological and historical plasticity of public and personal life, the conditions under which we are made responsible for ensuring our compliance with health norms, and even the pursuit of enhancement, seeking to become the best versions of us that we can be through correct conduct[39, 40] With this in mind, a biopolitical sensibility draws our attention to the spread of particular political conceptualisations of dementia into public life in a manner that shapes our perceptions, experiences and enactments of dementia.

I argue that the contemporary biopolitics of dementia largely relies on and rearticulates a *neuropsychiatric* biopolitics. The term "neuropsychiatry" itself requires qualification because it is a widespread but often obscure concept.[41] I begin with Berrios and Marková's observation that neuropsychiatry is best understood in relation to its core contention: "mental disorders are disorders of the brain."[42] This is a useful starting point, but there is little here to distinguish a neuropsychiatric biopolitics from the aforementioned (bio)medical model. Elaborating further, I depict the vital tenets of a neuropsychiatric biopolitics of dementia as follows:

A syndrome of cognitive decline caused by discrete neuropathologies that are distinct from ageing, and … not enough people are aware of this. Furthermore, because dementia is caused by disease, and biomedical sciences have cured some diseases, dementia is a technoscientific challenge that will be solved through technoscientific endeavours.[43]

These are biopolitical in as much as they are not simple truth claims. Rather, they appeal to scientist aesthetics as a means of persuading people to nurture certain knowledges and, more importantly, to act in certain ways according to those knowledges. In the next chapter, I will attend in more detail to three component claims of this neuropsychiatric biopolitics: (1) that dementias are caused by discrete diseases of the brain, (2) that dementia is not a normal part of ageing and (3) that research will discover a cure. Before doing so, it is helpful to clarify and contextualise the nature of contemporary neuropsychiatric biopolitics beyond dementia specifically. This is important because the neuropsychiatric biopolitics of dementia do not exist in a biopolitical vacuum and, in many ways, can be understood as echoing a broader set of circumstances.

Historically, neuropsychiatry can be traced back in some form to the 17th century,[42] and variations of neuropsychiatry and dementia have a longstanding relationship. As discussed in Chapter 1, this book primarily speaks to a biopolitics that has developed since the 1970s under the influence of the AD movement. However, as outlined in Chapter 2, different notions of dementia were subject to neuroscientific and psychiatric attention long before this period. For instance, Samuel Wilks first presented his account of brain atrophy in the mid-19th century,[44] and the pathologist Solomon Carter Fuller published detailed accounts of his painstaking investigations into dementia-related neuropathologies in the early 20th century.[45, 46] Hence, biogenic (i.e. fundamentally biologically generated) conceptualisations of dementia in a manner that seem remarkably conducive to contemporary neuropsychiatric biopolitics, and have traditionally featured in (bio)medical characterisations, can be traced back well over a century.

Of more direct importance to our current circumstances is the 1960s emergence of the neurosciences in a form recognisable today as an amalgam of initiatives that were previously distinguished into neuroscientific and psychiatric styles. Rose and Abi-Rached have documented an epistemic transition whereby matters such as behaviour, emotion, thought, beliefs and cognition were all reimagined as essentially neuromolecular in nature.[47] Whether worrying, despairing or forgetting, publics came to intuitively comprehend and express psychogenic phenomena in terms of disease and the brain.[48] This shift motivated and assembled a diverse array of stakeholders beyond scientific researchers themselves, including charities and governments, and most importantly publics, in relation to specific imaginings of the brain as a molecular entity that contained the answers to human life. Today, these neuromolecular sensibilities pervade public experience. An endless procession of media, from newspapers to pop songs, reiterates the centrality of our brains in simultaneously determining our deepest interior lives and the ebb and flow of society broadly. The brain has become a defining precondition of self and society,[49, 50] with a corresponding potential for providing solutions to a vast array of social problems. Williams, Higgs and Katz cast this infiltration into public life in terms of "neuroculture":

> Neuroculture is not simply a question of the power or persuasive appeal of the neurosciences within the laboratory or clinic, but of their wider social, cultural, political and economic salience and significance about the future of humanity.[51]

Neuroculture hence translates piecemeal neuroscientific observations into a schema of existential implications for being both ill and well.[52] Notions of neuroplasticity[1] suggest that all this brain stuff is amenable to intervention, meaning that the savvy citizen (or consumer) can enhance his or her neuronal existence through appropriate personal conduct. Neuroplasticity softens biological determinism by reassuring us that, while our brains may dictate our destinies, those brains can be crafted deliberatively.[53] Sociological work in this area has largely attended to more orthodox mental illnesses such as schizophrenia, anxiety and depression.[48, 54] However, the post-1970s neuropsychiatric biopolitics of dementia can also be read within this wider context of neuropsychiatry's recent history.

It is also important to recognise that neuropsychiatry is not an institutional or professional denomination in the clear-cut manner that "psychiatry" is. For example, the AD movement,[55, 56] discussed in Chapter 1, refined and propagated contemporary neuropsychiatric ideas about dementia, yet this movement has never been confined to, nor even strictly centred on, professional neuroscientists and psychiatrists specifically. Key stakeholders in the neuropsychiatric biopolitics of dementia have included researchers, governments, charities, businesses and activists. Many researchers with expertise well outside of the neurosciences predicate their work on neuropsychiatric claims as a means of norm-compliant justification, e.g. health economics, cognitive sociology and medical anthropology. Charities are similar in this respect. Many third-sector organisations rely on, and therefore promote, neuropsychiatric biopolitics in their activities. The two stakeholder groups are heavily entwined, with charities appealing to research findings to emphasise the importance of dementia as a problem and hence argue for resource donations, a large portion of which is then reallocated to the researchers producing the requisite evidence. A range of activists and advocates, again far removed from institutional neuroscience and psychiatry, are also important. For instance, high-profile celebrities and people diagnosed with dementia play an important role in fronting various related initiatives.

Governments are also integral because the neuropsychiatric biopolitics of dementia speaks directly to issues of political economy, especially regarding the demographic ageing of welfare states.[57] In the early 2010s, British prime minister David Cameron introduced financial incentives for dementia diagnoses, while the later Prime Minister Boris Johnson pledged to double dementia research funding in his 2019 election manifesto. The pharmaceutical industry is another key player in neuropsychiatric biopolitics, providing significant funding for associated research. Indeed, several commentators have attributed the aducanumab debacle, whereby an ineffective and harmful drug received regulatory approval (discussed at length in Chapter 5), to inappropriately close relationships between the Alzheimer's Association and its advocates, the FDA, the pharmaceutical company Biogen and the US government. Considering the roles played by each of these groups, it is apparent that neuropsychiatry is far from a discrete expert, professional and institutional concern. It is reliant on a broad and eclectic mix of stakeholders.

Ultimately, a neuropsychiatric biopolitics of dementia is distinct from a (bio)medical model by virtue of its all-pervading cultural and political power to generate the available terrains of public and personal experience and action. To this end, shrewd actors seem to have an intuitive appreciation of the biopolitical power that dementia can catalyse. In the 1900s, Kraepelin needed to realise AD as a distinct disease to distinguish his lab from competitors, in much the same way that the NIA's founding fathers did in the 1970s to strengthen its funding claims against competing agencies. Disease is capital and brain disease is even more so. Paying attention to neuropsychiatric biopolitics takes us far beyond questions relating to the exertion of symbolic and institutional (bio)medical control over people who are illegitimately recast as patients and hence dehumanised. Instead, it speaks to the very conditions of life itself and how publics come to conduct certain forms of life.[58]

3.3 Neuro-agnosticism

So far, I have argued that dementia in its contemporary form could be more fruitfully analysed if we attended to it as biopolitical in nature, moving beyond traditional preoccupations with the (bio)medical model. Many of the shortcomings of the latter conceptualisation can be somewhat resolved by the comparable strengths of the former, sensitising us to dementia as a political entity negotiated by diverse stakeholders and manifest in personal and public life. The two approaches, and their comparative influences in dementia studies, are intimately bound up with one another. The inattentiveness of much dementia studies scholarship to biopolitics is, at least in part, attributable to a corresponding over-attentiveness to (bio)medicalisation as a sort of disciplinary bogeyman. As Gallacher and Burns put it, "from this approach, all other sins seemed to proceed."[59] Particularly obstructive is the tendency to focus on (bio)medicalisation as a problem because of its symbolic contributions to dehumanisation. This risks limiting the negative circumstances of people affected by dementia to the (bio)medical model and hence doing something of an injustice to the many challenges that people can face. Core biopolitical claims, especially those purporting neurocognitive absolutes, typically receive little comparable critical engagement amid more humanistic concerns. This tendency to shy away from the purportedly neurocognitive, and thereby failing to attend to its biopolitical nature, is what I term the "neuro-agnosticism" of too much dementia studies scholarship.

Of course, it would be inaccurate to say that all dementia studies is somehow entirely naïve to the questionable neurocognitive truth claims that characterise the biopolitics of dementia. As mentioned in the previous chapter, Kitwood's earlier publications strongly rejected what he then referred to as the "standard paradigm" of dementia, citing contradictory neuropathological evidence and questionable cognitivist assumptions regarding mind–brain relations.[13, 60] However, this work seemingly passed largely unnoticed, and by the time of his more popular writing, his criticisms had softened and moved onto more additive psychosocial concerns. Nonetheless, influential works in the field, including Kitwood's, do contain at least some fleeting reference to such issues. For example, though primarily focussing on challenges to personhood, in his seminal monograph, Kitwood does, in one instance, attend to some other shortcomings with what for him is a medical model:

> Medical approaches in psychiatry have, however, brought their own problems, as we have already seen: simplistic views of organicity, research led not so much by theory as by available technique, and exaggerated hopes that science will deliver wonder-cures.[61]

Similarly, while not their main concern, Bartlett and O'Connor briefly note that mainstream neurocognitive claims are flawed on their own terms:

Neurodegenerative changes alone do not always adequately account for the trajectory of the dementia path. There is no doubt that changes in the brain do matter, but separating neuropathology out as the only relevant factor is increasingly challenged as overly simplistic in terms of its explanatory power.[62]

In this manner, significant scholarships spanning different sub-traditions of dementia studies seem to have at least some inkling that there are other problems besides dehumanisation inherent in what they have traditionally conceptualised as the (bio)medical model. However, such mentions are relatively fleeting. My contention is that such suspicion, and explicit articulation of it, is problematically underdeveloped in a lot of dementia studies work because of a certain degree of neuro-agnosticism that pervades much of the field.

By *neuro-agnosticism*, I am demarcating a kind of uncritical (semi-)acceptance of, or at least an inattentiveness to, aspects of what has traditionally been attributed to the (bio)medical model of dementia, in as much as it denotes a conceptualisation of dementia as principally neuropathological and therefore prospectively amenable to chemical intervention. At face value, the appeal to brain disease(s) is important because it determines the ontological nature of dementia, the very entity to which dementia studies is dedicated. One might assume that the ontological nature of dementia would be a paramount concern in dementia studies. However, it is often unremarked upon. Much dementia studies simply takes the diseased brain for granted or does not speak to it at all, so that it has inadvertently become a significant normative commitment. My observation here is not innovative. In 1998, the anthropologist Lawrence Cohen argued that much social science that self-identified as attending to "dementia" was perpetuating a particular neuropsychiatric configuration of cognitive decline in later life.[63] His observation remains salient 25 years later.

It is understandable that a social scientific field might be hesitant in its engagements with knowledge claims that purport to neurocognitive absolutes. At a basic level, most social scientists have far less expertise in natural scientific matters than their natural scientific peers, which is not to suggest that I view cognitive science as an obvious member of the natural sciences. However, robust engagement with phenomena that social scholars might intuitively disregard as belonging to (bio)medicine is imperative to the development of sophisticated social scientific work on health and illness generally, and dementia is no exception. This means that any dementia studies scholarship that identifies as critical must pursue some corresponding critical engagement with the most fundamental ontological commitments regarding dementia. To sidestep this is to be neuro-agnostic. To be neuro-agnostic, as I will argue throughout this book, is, at best, to be complicit, and frequently slides into cheerleading for the normative commitments that much dementia studies purportedly sets out to challenge. Ultimately, it entails an inadvertent depoliticisation of dementia, naturalising that which is biopolitical and hence rendering it invulnerable to challenge or change.

The critique of (bio)medicalisation as dehumanising essentially defines the problem as being the symbolic positioning of people with dementia as less than human, as well as the various ramifications that stem from that symbolism. There is a troublesome implication here that if we could address the offending symbolism, then (bio)medicalisation would be far less problematic for dementia and those affected by it. As I will argue throughout the rest of this book, I do not think that (bio)medical dehumanisation is the major problem faced by people affected by dementia. Not even close. Of course, there are strong arguments that dehumanisation is a substantial failing, or at least a regrettable side-effect, of (bio)medicalisation as it is traditionally construed. A great deal of dementia studies has done much to counter this, and admirably so. However, the dehumanising capacities of (bio)medicalisation are not the only associated problems that should animate dementia studies. The risk is that attending to dehumanisation with such zeal distracts from other concerns that I will explicate throughout this book, e.g. the marketing of harmful drugs, the exploitation of dementia as an investment market and the racialisation of health inequalities. This is one reason why dehumanisation critiques can become inadvertently complicit in perpetuating the very model that they are intended to contest. Such critiques risk leveraging so much of our attention toward (bio)medical dehumanisation that they distract from other issues. This, however, is a minor problem compared with the more pervasive complicity of much dementia studies in perpetuating a neuropsychiatric biopolitics of dementia.

As noted in the previous chapters, to some extent, the existence of dementia studies is indebted to the AD movement and its intensification of the neuropsychiatric biopolitics of dementia. Hence, it is unsurprising that much dementia studies work complicitly leans into that biopolitics explicitly as a form of existential scaffolding. As a rudimentary example of this complicity, we can consider the pervasiveness of formulaic introductory conventions in dementia studies publications. Many papers in dementia studies begin with appeals to select biopolitical claims regarding dementia, providing cliché introductions to a diverse array of scholarship. At the time of writing, the current issue of *Dementia* contains 19 papers. Of these, five open with neuropathological definitions of dementia.[64–68] A further four open with appeals to disease incidence predictions.[69–72] Such invocations are intriguing given that this is perhaps the premier dementia studies journal. If nothing else, authors can reasonably assume that the readership has a definitional knowledge of dementia. Nonetheless, statements regarding the neuropathological and epidemiological gravity of dementia are common introductory tropes in dementia studies. The repeated use of neuropsychiatric biopolitical claims as an opening gambit in dementia studies is not accidental. It performs precisely the same function as the arguments made by the various AD movement stakeholders discussed in the first chapter. By positioning dementia as a

major disease entity, work across dementia studies can justify its own existence as warranted by the troubling nature of the problem that it seeks to
address. Bluntly, diseases are surmountable problems that warrant our attention, expertise and resources.

I am not going to say much more about depictions of dementia in the
introductions of dementia studies publications. I use that example here as an
albeit simplistic provocation to begin to think critically about forms of neuro-
agnosticism in dementia studies that beget biopolitical complicity. My point
is that we should be more mindful of seemingly mundane and inconsequential
conventions in our work. Even small acts matter. Guilty authors reading this
could perhaps re-evaluate their opening passages. Those lines can likely be
used to say something of more value than "dementia is caused by more than
100 neurodegenerative diseases" or "X million people will have dementia by
20XX". Ultimately, little of the biopolitical complicity that concerns me is
this explicit or basic. Much of this book is dedicated to unpacking far more
grandiose, complicated, subtle and damaging forms of neuro-agnosticism
that have wider-reaching consequences. These consequences extend through
drug discovery to ethnic inequalities, and from cryptocurrency forums to
celebrity appeals, all of which are rooted in the cultivation of neuro-agnostic
dispositions toward the biopolitics of dementia.

Ultimately, the continued salience in dementia studies of the (bio)medical
model and its consequent dehumanisation is itself a manifestation of neuro-
agnosticism. Anti-(bio)medicalisation work can inadvertently facilitate that
which much dementia studies has traditionally pertained to critique by
obscuring the extent to which dementia is biopolitical. Hence, a truly critical – or rather, a *neurocritical* – dementia studies would benefit from reconceptualising some of what has too often been lumped into the (bio)medical
model as instead owing to a neuropsychiatric biopolitics of dementia. This
is not an attempt to refute and replace (bio)medicalisation scholarship outright but rather to progress it into the 21st century and expand its range of
critique. Nonetheless, developing apt biopolitical critiques will require some
challenging of orthodox intellectual commitments across a lot of dementia
studies. This can be achieved by drawing on resonant forms of critical theory.
In particular, a neurocritical dementia studies has much to gain from greater
engagement with critical psychiatry and critical gerontology, two distinct
traditions of social scholarship that are surprisingly untapped by dementia
studies despite considerable affinities.

3.4 Critical Psychiatry

I characterise my argument in this book as a form of *critical* dementia studies. By this, I do not mean that I take a dim view of dementia studies. Instead,
I use "critical" in the sociological sense to indicate that I am concerned with
deconstructing the politics of some dementia studies. In doing so, I am particularly indebted to critical psychiatry and critical gerontology. Together,

these areas of scholarship provide a collection of conceptual tools that help me to unpack some of the political commitments within dementia studies. It is worth noting here that I do not mean to suggest that dementia studies has a specific political stance in a colloquial sense – dementia studies is not a member of a political party; it is not on the voting register. Rather, I mean that some work in dementia studies (far too much, I argue) implicitly perpetuates a certain set of ideas about what dementia is like. Critical theory can shed some light on those ideas. Both critical psychiatry and critical gerontology are yet to be fully utilised in dementia studies. Hence, as well as my stated aim of exploring the politics of dementia, it is my secondary aim that this text acts as a more implicit argument for the greater application of critical psychiatry and critical gerontology across dementia studies.

As noted, the term "critical" should be read with a specific theoretical meaning rather than in the everyday sense of being disparaging about something. Critical theory is a broad social scientific tradition primarily associated with the Frankfurt School of social and philosophical thought, which was founded in early 20th-century Germany. Its progenitors were interested in furthering Marxist theory and socialism. Much of their work attended to the question of why Marx's predicted socialist revolutions had largely failed to materialise. One answer was that social ideology helped to normalise, conceal and sustain problematic social relations. With this in mind, the philosopher and sociologist Max Horkheimer outlined critical theory as a means of deconstructing ideology and pursuing political emancipation.[73] Critical theory focuses on the often obscure political circumstances that sustain societal status quo. Rather than attempting to study these phenomena in a detached manner, critical theory actively pursues political transformation. Researchers in this tradition are not merely concerned with understanding but also with enacting change. Today, critical theory exerts considerable influence over a great deal of social scientific thought. It draws our attention to that which we assume to be normal, encouraging us to reflect on why our normality is normal, what the effects of that normality are and how we might transform the normal in pursuit of positive ends. This book echoes that tradition. I want to draw attention to assumptions in dementia studies and directly challenge them. The core tenets of critical theory have inspired distinct sub-traditions of psychiatry and gerontology, each of which I will now outline.

Psychiatry, as a medical speciality, has long courted controversy, and so it is perhaps unsurprising that it has inspired a good deal of critical reflection. Much well-justified criticism stems from the historical imprisonment and abuse of people deemed to have psychiatric disorders by those charged with their care. Until the 19th century, people with mental illnesses were typically dealt with under poor laws, being sent to workhouses or prisons. From the mid-19th century, these people could be locked away in lunatic asylums, kept in poor conditions and subjected to inhumane treatments. Though originally well-intentioned, asylums became involuntary warehouses for the socially undesirable. For various reasons, a programme of deinstitutionalisation from the 1960s onward led to the closing down of the asylums, purportedly replaced by community-based care.[74] Today, inpatient mental health care is relatively rare. However, the Social Care Institute for Excellence estimates that around 80% of care home residents have a dementia.[75] Hence, dementia remains entwined with institutionalisation even after processes of deinstitutionalisation in the 20th century.

Beyond institutionalisation and mistreatment, criticism of psychiatry has also targeted classifications of mental disorder. Historically, many people deemed socially problematic by more powerful groups have been treated as suffering from mental illnesses and, therefore, in need of psychiatric intervention. Today, many historic diagnostic categories seem farcical, if not deeply problematic. For example, in the 19th century, non-compliant women were diagnosed with hysteria,[76] while it was hypothesised that escaped slaves were suffering from drapetomania.[77] Understandably, such "illnesses" have been held up as examples of psychiatry's function as a means of social oppression. Today, we recognise that these diagnoses more accurately reflected bigotry than any real medical condition. Hence, psychiatric disorder has sometimes functioned as an institutionally legitimate means of transforming, controlling or concealing peoples deemed problematic by more privileged groups. Our first reaction may be to baulk at the thought that the American Psychiatric Association classified homosexuality as a mental illness until 1973[78, 79] and to be thankful that such things are confined to history. However, we must beware of slipping into self-congratulatory naivety, as future generations will almost certainly cast a similarly disdainful eye over our contemporary classification and treatment of mental illness.

Criticism of historic injustices is largely warranted and generally accepted. More challenging are arguments related to contemporary classifications of psychiatric disorder and associated treatments. To this end, my concern throughout the book is not with the dramatic institutional abuses of historic psychiatry but rather with the conceptual tenets of contemporary psychiatric disorder. That said, we must stay alert to the continuation of institutional abuse. It is important to recognise that high-profile abuse scandals in care homes are not indicative of the sector as a whole. However, they are painful reminders that people with psychiatric disorders can still be subjected to sustained and systemic abuse within institutions charged with their care. Another major cause for concern is the overuse of antipsychotics to manage the behaviour of people diagnosed with dementia in institutional settings.[80] Indeed, this has increased significantly in recent years.[81] Although beyond the scope of this text, such instances represent a continuation of historic abuses. They deserve our sustained attention and condemnation, but we should be cautious of tarring psychiatry per se with this brush, which risks encouraging unhelpful animosities.

In the 1960s, an intellectual tradition of anti-psychiatry began to question the very notion of mental illness upon which institutional psychiatry relied. At its extremes, anti-psychiatry argued that mental illness was a myth perpetuated by psychiatry to grant it undue power over people judged to be undesirable. In response, some advocated the abolition of psychiatric practice altogether. Figureheads such as R.D. Laing[82] and Franco Basaglia[83] gained notoriety for their outspoken and often outlandish refutations of institutional psychiatry. The proponents of "anti-psychiatry" never subscribed to that label. They were categorised as such by others. Beyond their basic rejection of psychiatry, these critics were highly distinct in their approaches and beliefs. For instance, David Cooper[84] contended that insanity was a sane response to an insane world, whereas Thomas Szasz[85] argued that mental illness was a fabrication. Ultimately, the better-known mid-20th-century anti-psychiatrists were often intellectually vague and seemed to be purposefully abrasive, to an extent that risked obscuring the merit of certain arguments. This is the jumping-off point for critical psychiatry, which attempts to develop those worthwhile arguments in more robust and less combative ways. It questions the conceptual nature of mental illness and associated interventions, particularly regarding their political facets, but pursues a reformist agenda regarding psychiatric practice. Critical psychiatrists typically acknowledge that people suffer from qualitatively real mental problems and generally believe that we should devise responses to help those people.[86]

The first major depiction of a "critical" psychiatry, explicitly drawing on the Frankfurt School, was David Ingleby's 1980 text *Critical Psychiatry: The Politics of Mental Health*.[87] In it, Ingleby argues that anti-psychiatry ultimately failed to transform psychiatry because it was intellectually weak and politically detached, echoing the general faux-revolutionary culture of the time. In response, he seeks a robust conceptual critique of psychiatry. He targets psychiatry's positivism – the belief that mental illness is knowable via objective scientific observations. In its place, he offers interpretivism – the belief that mental illnesses are personally meaningful responses to specific situations. For Ingleby, we can only appreciate mental states (e.g. a person feeling angry) by drawing on our innate interpretive understanding of human life and applying it to the idiosyncrasies of a particular individual in a particular context. There can be no entirely objective, valid and generalisable measurement and description of something like anger. Hence, psychiatric efforts to systematise mental phenomena as a means of emulating certain ideas of what the natural sciences are like are ultimately somewhat irreconcilable with the phenomena in question. Such systematisation persists because it performs a political function of individualising mental health and rendering it a technical problem with technical solutions (e.g. pharmaceutical intervention). This obscures potential societal constituents of psychiatric disorder that might warrant social, economic or political reform.

Building on Ingleby's text, Duncan Double sets out his application of critical theory to psychiatry as a means of contesting the notion that natural science (or, again, certain ideas thereof) is the sole vehicle of progress.[88] For him, this opens up questions regarding the widespread normalisation of biogenic accounts of mental phenomena. He suggests that "the message of critical psychiatry is that it is possible to practice psychiatry without the justification of postulating brain pathology as the basis for mental illness". It is, therefore, unsurprising that the first of his core critical psychiatric principles is that neurobiology is no more important than social, cultural, economic and political context in psychiatric aetiology and intervention. It is perhaps worth adding here, by way of mediation, that it is not necessarily less important either. Moving beyond neurophysiology alone entails an ethical requirement to engage with the person's perspectives and the sociopolitical circumstances that constitute their experience.

Unfortunately, at least from our perspective, given its characteristic scepticism of classificatory systems, critical psychiatry has tended to focus on mental disorders collectively and broadly conceived. Where scholarship has been more targeted at particular diagnoses, the entities in question have been those relatively familiar phenomena that we might colloquially deem to be mental illnesses, such as schizophrenia,[89] anxiety[90] and depression.[88] While I have argued that the post-1970s neuropsychiatric biopolitics of dementia is emblematic of the wider context of recent neuropsychiatric history, critical psychiatry has tended to shy away from the age-associated dementias as being a distinct type of thing. My first experience of this tendency occurred as an undergraduate when I sought to apply critical psychiatry to dementia in my thesis.[2] My supervisor dismissed the idea on the grounds that dementia is a different type of thing. Many years later, at a book launch of a high-profile scholar, I asked why his text explicitly discounted the age-associated dementias from his otherwise generalised critical approach to psychiatric disorder. Again, I was told that dementia is a different type of thing. In this manner, it seems that critical psychiatry has largely steered clear of engaging with dementia out of a sense that it is poignantly distinct from all else that might readily be subsumed into categories such as "psychiatric disorder" or "mental illness", historically compartmentalised by notions of functional and organic disease.

Nonetheless, in this book, I draw heavily on ideas from critical psychiatry, hopefully emphasising their applicability to dementia studies. In summary, critical psychiatry requires us to question dominant values in contemporary circumstances of psychiatric disorder and institutional responses to it.[86] It draws our attention to the social, cultural, political and economic facets of attempts to systematise mental illness, particularly those that privilege neurophysiology and generalisation over context and subjective experience. It requires us to reflect on the social implications of psychiatric political commitments, especially the pursuit of biochemical interventions in the sick individual rather than social, cultural, economic and political intervention in the sick society. In response, it is the critical psychiatrist's task to explore alternative therapeutic politics. As a simplistic example, post traumatic stress disorder (PTSD) in veterans might be treated by discovering the neural mechanics of PTSD and developing corresponding pharmaceutical interventions. It might also be treated by the prevention of war. Neither is easy, and neither is problem-free. Ultimately, critical psychiatry cautions that our mental normalities and abnormalities are not inherent, and are hence demarcated as such, usually in line with particular interests. I find this a useful way of thinking about disorder in as much as it is additive; that is, it expands our suite of tools for helping people. Critical psychiatry becomes less helpful when it is exclusive. However, the so-called critical psychiatrists who argue that sociopolitical determinants and interventions are the only legitimate causes of and responses to psychiatric disorder might be better conceived of as reflecting a more abrasive and extremist anti-psychiatry.

3.5 Critical Gerontology

Besides critical psychiatry, the other key theoretical foundation of this book is critical gerontology. Gerontology can be broadly defined as the study of ageing, encompassing a wide range of traditional academic disciplines. In the UK, social scientific ageing research can be traced back to the late-19th-century work of Charles Booth on pauperism.[91] He raised awareness of later-life poverty and stimulated social reform around pensions, but scholarly interest in ageing per se remained relatively sparse. In the mid-20th century, Talcott Parsons made a case for treating age as social structure,[92] and C. Wright Mills dedicated a chapter of *The Sociological Imagination* to the importance of considering history and biography together,[93] an observation that would become central to gerontology. Still, the social scientific study of ageing remained rather niche. It was not until the 1960s that gerontology became formalised through debates regarding whether old age should be a period of disengagement or activity.[94, 95] The latter approach, pursuing ideals of active later life, continues to inspire a great deal of gerontological research.

The emergence of gerontology as a research field is intimately bound up with the phenomena that it studies. Demographic transformation during the 19th and 20th centuries meant that older age and older people were increasingly socially, politically and economically salient issues. A number of things combined to make ageing a hot topic. The population aged amidst declining fertility and increasing longevity.[96] In rapidly urbanising contexts, impoverished older people made up a growing proportion of the pauper population at the same time as states were taking on new welfare responsibilities toward their populaces.[97] The expanding lifecourse became increasingly institutionalised. Kids went to school, adults worked, older people retired.[98] Again, the state was drawn into these lifecourse stages. In the UK, compulsory state education was legislated in the late 19th century, followed by state pensions in the early 20th century. Improved record keeping also meant that people knew their own ages and states knew the ages of their populaces.[99] Hence, the agedness of a population became an influential administrative consideration.[100] As age gained new types of importance, gerontology flourished.

For much of its history, gerontology has largely been a functionalist affair. By this, I mean that research has tended to take ageing for granted as a natural and universal phenomenon. For instance, early theories of old age as a period of disengagement assumed that everybody got older, declined physically and mentally and retired from society in preparation for death. In this predominant view, ageing happens, and the individual responds accordingly. In the 1970s, critical gerontology began to question the assumed naturalness of ageing and agedness. At that time, global economic crises led to international retrenchments of state welfare. The ageing population became increasingly politicised in economic terms that are familiar to us today – as a burden on public finances. These developments drew the attention of critical gerontologists toward the ways in which political and economic systems influenced experiences of ageing and later life. For instance, scholars noted that older people were often made dependent on welfare by exclusion from labour markets (e.g. mandatory retirement), that this removed their citizenship in countries where it was heavily tied to participation in the labour market, that the gendering of the historic labour market meant that many women entered later life almost entirely dependent on a pension via marriage, etc.[101, 102] Today, we even have an emerging appreciation of the effects of social determinants such as race or poverty on the biology of ageing.[103] Social inequalities can hence age us at a molecular level. Critical gerontology has driven recognition of the potential for institutional arrangements and social norms to exert considerable influence over ageing and older people, challenging the idea that ageing is merely natural.

While early critical gerontology was markedly structural, focussing on political economies of ageing in terms of public policies and institutions, more recent hermeneutic work has turned to the impact of social norms on later life and associated questions of meaning. Old functionalist theories of ageing had pronounced normative commitments, offering narrow cultural prescriptions of what constituted a good later life. These typically reflected the values of the white middle-class scholars who developed them – leisure activities, church membership, retirement communities, etc. Normative prescriptions of ageing can be subtly ubiquitous. If I ask you to imagine an 85-year-old woman, you will likely conjure a particular imagery replete with appropriate appearance, clothing, setting, mannerisms, activity, etc. This woman, formed in your imagination, might be far more likely to be knitting than swiping through Tinder or moderating a Discord server. Similarly, consider how statements such as "she had children late" or "he married young" can be reflexively meaningful to us. In this sense, we each unconsciously inhabit and maintain the normative parameters of age. Indeed, the great paradox of critical gerontology is that it is dedicated to deconstructing the normalisation of old age as a distinct type of thing, yet in doing so, it simultaneously positions older people as a distinct category. The age system is so pervasive that it is difficult to escape its gravitational pull.[104]

The structural (economics, policies, institutions, etc.) and hermeneutic (norms and values, meanings, interpretations, etc.) traditions of ageing research form two halves of critical gerontology.[105] In practice, they are intimately entwined with one another. For instance, policies on retirement age are predicated on and reinforce an assumption that age demarcates the appropriateness of a person for participation in the labour market. Thanks to critical gerontological insights, we now recognise that later life is massively diverse in the real world. Older people often have little more in common than their decades of birth.[106] At the same time, social structures such as age-based eligibility criteria impose artificial homogeneities on later life, albeit homogeneities that some people are better able to navigate than others. Attempts to describe ageing, agedness and aged people as singular types of thing are hence deeply suspect. In this respect, critical gerontology asks us to be sceptical of claims regarding "normal" or "natural" ageing. As with all critical theoretical traditions, we must ask what political interests are at stake when aspects of age and ageing are normalised in this way.[107]

Critical gerontology has a long heritage of generating its own forms of biopolitical critique, centring on concerns regarding the biopolitics of successful ageing.[108] As far back as the 1990s, Stephen Katz sought to deconstruct the roles of gerontology and geriatrics as disciplining ageing and agedness; as mediums of the art of governance.[109] Today, the biopolitics of successful ageing is conceptualised as generating notions of ageing as individual decline toward greater dependencies (or at least the risk thereof). This risk should be staved off by good citizens through appropriate personal actions, safeguarding the body and the mind against ageing, often via dedicated forms of consumption.[103] Dementia can be, and has been, read as an influential component of the biopolitics of successful ageing. It functions as a cautionary tale – the ultimate evil that may be exacted upon us if we fail to take responsibility for our ageing selves. The biopolitical function of this dementia is perhaps most pointedly realised in Paul Higgs and Chris Gilleard's theorisation of the social imaginary of the fourth age, wherein fears of dementia provide an impetus for patterns of lifestyle consumption that promise to stave off agedness.[110–112] Nonetheless, there is more that critical dementia studies can feed back into critical gerontology. For instance, the contemporary turn to notions of "brain health" and the prevention agenda's reimagining of dementia as a lifecourse process are both emblematic of a biopolitics of successful ageing.[103, 113]

Hopefully, you will now have at least some sense of the two major theoretical inspirations behind this text and the ways in which they overlap via their indebtedness to critical theory. Put simply, critical psychiatry questions the political commitments that shape "mental illness", while critical gerontology questions the political commitments that shape "old age". Both issues manifest a politics that is often obscured by normalisation, i.e. the notion that mental illness and old age are simply things that exist *out there*, irrespective of how we approach them. As I will argue in this text, the intuitive naturalness of disease and the intuitive naturalness of ageing come together in the naturalisation of dementia. The effects are predictable: the political contingencies of dementia are obscured. Using critical psychiatry and critical gerontology, I will argue that dementia studies should challenge that obfuscation by questioning prescriptions of normality. I do not suggest this because of some moral commitment to truth. Rather, I argue that an inattentiveness to the biopolitics of dementia has a range of damaging implications for dementia studies and its relations with people affected by dementia. This matters a lot because if dementia is afflicted by sociopolitical problems, then dementia studies is likely best placed to address them.

Before progressing, it is worth pausing to clarify an ontological issue that inevitably emerges from the application of critical scholarships to dementia. Indeed, given the aforementioned ill feeling that anti-psychiatry once stirred, coupled with a tendency for critical gerontology to be somewhat dismissive of physiology, such clarification seems paramount. The story of the post-1970s development of dementia can easily be read as a moral panic.[114] Certain stakeholders have acted as moral entrepreneurs, stoking public and political alarm as a means of furthering their interests, particularly financial. For example, in personal communications reproduced by Patrick Fox, NIA director Robert Butler stated:

> I decided that we had to make it [Alzheimer's] a household word. And the reason I felt that, is that's how the pieces get identified as a national priority. And I call it the health politics of anguish.[55]

In this context, one might reasonably assume that I am going to, in line with much traditional medical sociology (or at least a popular caricature of it), question the validity of dementia as a disease entity or collection thereof. I might suggest that dementia was "constructed" to satisfy particular social, political and economic interests. Nothing could be further from the truth. Dementia is manifestly real. Moreover, it is manifestly problematic. While some contemporary dementia scholarship is cautious of the potentially offensive language of "burden" and "suffering", a great many people do suffer as they, or their family members, experience cognitive decline to an extent that markedly worsens their lives. For many people, to claim that they are no different to anybody else implies a disregard for the harsh realities of their struggle. We must also be cautious of downplaying the suffering that dementia can cause for practical reasons. For instance, in cases where state welfare provision might be tightly governed by punitive official judgements regarding disability-based deservedness, the suggestion that people do not suffer by virtue of a given condition might have disastrous ramifications. With all this in mind, I am distinctly realist when it comes to the often-grim consequences of cognitive impairment.

Where I am sceptical of specific claims regarding dementia, I am so explicitly, and always from a basic recognition of the harsh reality of cognitive decline and its effects, coupled with a respect for robust natural science. Epistemic arguments against particular imaginings of dementia should not be misconstrued as ontological arguments against dementia-as-cognitive-impairment per se. Too often, the political aspects of a phenomenon are used as evidence to undermine the entire existence of the phenomenon. We should be wary of such arguments, which misleadingly conflate political and ontological claims. Yes, in recent decades, dementia has been reimagined and promoted because of its expediency to various political interests. That does not change the fact that dementia is a source of considerable suffering for many people. Both observations can exist together and are, in fact, a likely constellation of circumstances.

* * *

The central argument of this chapter is that much dementia studies scholarship could move beyond foundational critiques of (bio)medicalisation and pay more attention to the neuropsychiatric biopolitics of dementia. Scholarship relating to (bio)medicalisation risks criticising a strawman caricature of institutional medicine, extending its authority over previously normal human experiences in a manner that is somehow illegitimate. By attending explicitly and/or implicitly to the dehumanising consequences of (bio)medicalisation as a symbolic project, dementia studies has too often fallen into a trap of neuro-agnosticism. By this, I mean that various traditions have attended to the interpersonal and institutional relational politics of dementia after the (bio)medical fact. This has come at the expense of deconstructing the biopolitical nature of dementia as it is manifest in personal and public life, shaped by a heterogeneous collection of stakeholders, potentially at odds with evidence from the natural sciences, promoting schemas of what is (ab)normal and making promises about the future, all to serve particular interests. These ideas are unpacked in depth in the next chapter.

To return to the above definition of biopolitics, it is a proliferation of conceptual schemas that subtly guide personal conduct and order human life in ways that are conducive to certain political projects. It is an artful governance of what is natural, normal and moral. It entails the cultivation of publics that know and act accordingly. In the case of dementia, a select range of core claims – (1) discrete pathogeneses, (2) normal ageing, (3) techno-curative futures (all deconstructed in Chapter 4) – are repeatedly articulated in this manner, each demarcated as an irrevocable natural kind. We can see the confluence of such disciplining naturalisation in the following statement given by Hilary Evans, Chief Executive of ARUK:

> Our #ShareTheOrange campaign will help bring global attention to an important truth – that dementia is not an inevitability of age, but is caused by diseases that we can fight. The condition has been blighted by misconceptions for generations, and it's now time to turn our fatalism into hope, and research holds the key to overcoming the diseases that drive the symptoms.[115]

We might note the irony of the phrase "blighted by misconceptions", but that accusatory approach quickly leads us down something of a blind alley. It is not the absolute rightness or wrongness of (mis)conceptions that is crucial here so much as the ways that different conceptions are generated and spread, by whom, for whom, under what influences and with what consequences. The claims that typify the neuropsychiatric biopolitics of dementia are not simply truth-telling for truth-telling's sake. This biopolitics is fundamentally motivated by particular interests and desired futures. As I will show in the next chapter, these interests entail the accrual of resources through donations and grants, the improvement of particular forms of knowledge and practice, the greater public profile of dementia and associated initiatives, or the ultimate annihilation of dementia altogether. Hence, many specific normative commitments are at stake within the overarching biopolitics. As I will keep reiterating, it is not that biopolitical commitments are good or bad per se. Indeed, they are so complexly intertwined that it is almost impossible to describe them as such, even before we deal with the question of (mal)intention. Rather, I am interested in the generation of conceptualisations that come to appear inevitable or natural and, by extension, the naturalisation of their consequences.

This is where a critical approach encourages and enables us to respond to dementia by challenging the normative determinants of it, with the ultimate aim of transforming it. Critical psychiatry and critical gerontology reveal to us how the classifications and circumstances of mental disorder and ageing are normatively inscribed, often serving particular interests at the expense of others. Political constitution can be concealed behind naturalisation and normalisation, and it is the task of critical theory to make those things explicit. With this in mind, critical dementia studies could adopt a familiar public health stance by attending to the environmental determinants of dementia. However, in this instance, the environment in question is neuropsychiatric biopolitics. Just as public health seeks to optimise environments, my aim in this text is not to do away with biopolitics altogether but rather to consider the potential for a more salutogenic biopolitics or perhaps a sociopolitics. This is not an obvious task. As noted, the good and the bad are deeply enmeshed under biopolitics. For instance, a greater attentiveness to ethnic inequalities has come hand in hand with a sensationalisation and exploitation of ethnicity, sometimes at the expense of minoritised ethnic people (an issue returned to in Chapter 7). Similarly, the heightened public profile of dementia has generated mass sympathies, donations and initiatives, yet dementia has simultaneously moved from obscurity to one of our most feared conditions.[103] Hence, the neuropsychiatric biopolitics of dementia blends good and bad effects.

My immediate focus here is bringing critical psychiatry and critical gerontology to bear in critical dementia studies. That said, critical dementia studies also has much to offer in return, and new forms of trans-disciplinary engagement can potentially further the projects of critical psychiatry and critical gerontology. As noted, critical psychiatry has largely attended to conventional mental illnesses such as schizophrenia,[89] anxiety[90] and depression,[88] or more commonly to mental disorders broadly conceived. While I argue that the post-1970s neuropsychiatric biopolitics of dementia is emblematic of recent neuropsychiatric history more generally, critical scholars have tended to shy away from the age-associated dementias. A neurocritical dementia studies could offer critical psychiatry a route toward meaningful engagements with dementia. The influence of dementia studies on critical gerontology is far more established. Indeed, this unidirectional relationship is perhaps the best developed between any of the three traditions. Critical gerontologists have repeatedly pointed to imaginings of dementia and their effects on people's experiences as exemplifying a biopolitics of successful ageing. As noted, Paul Higgs and Chris Gilleard identify fears regarding dementia as central to their theory of the fourth age.[110, 111] As another example, Amanda Grenier and Chris Phillipson consider dementia a powerful manifestation of later-life precarity.[116, 117] Hence, a gerontology-informed critical dementia studies will undoubtedly continue to feed back into and invigorate critical gerontology, especially as dementia becomes increasingly financialised (discussed in Chapter 8).

Overall, this chapter has made a rather big-picture argument for cultivating critical approaches to the neuropsychiatric biopolitics of dementia. With that in mind, it is worthwhile considering in more minute detail some of the particular components of that biopolitics. To reiterate, I have briefly characterised neuropsychiatric biopolitics as positioning dementia as:

> A syndrome of cognitive decline caused by discrete neuropathologies that are distinct from ageing, and … not enough people are aware of this. Furthermore, because dementia is caused by disease, and biomedical sciences have cured some diseases, dementia is a technoscientific challenge that will be solved through technoscientific endeavours.[43]

In the next chapter, I will deconstruct, in detail, three core claims that have become especially influential and diversely problematic across much dementia studies, as well as the dementia research economy more broadly. These claims are (1) dementia is caused by diseases of the brain, (2) dementia is not a normal part of ageing and (3) research will discover a cure. Taken together, these commonplace proclamations comprise something akin to the three neuropsychiatric commandments. Hence, they warrant more substantive critical exploration, a task to which I will now turn.

Notes

1 "Neuroplasticity" is the idea that neurophysiology can be altered by experience. It is another concept with a long heritage but which intensified into its contemporary form during the 1970s and 1980s.
2 If the book has an origin story, then perhaps it is this.

References

1. Lyman, K.A. (1989). Bringing the social back in: A critique of the biomedicalization of Dementia. *The Gerontologist 29*, 597–605. doi: 10.1093/geront/29.5.597.
2. Spector, A., and Orrell, M. (2010). Using a biopsychosocial model of dementia as a tool to guide clinical practice. *International Psychogeriatrics 22*, 957–965. doi: 10.1017/S1041610210000840.
3. Fletcher, J.R. (2020). Mythical dementia and Alzheimerised senility: Discrepant and intersecting representations of cognitive decline in later life. *Social Theory & Health 18*, 50–65. doi: 10.1057/s41285-019-00117-w.
4. Whitehouse, P.J., and George, D.R. (2008). *The Myth of Alzheimer's: What You Aren't Being Told About Today's Most Dreaded Diagnosis*. St. Martin's Griffin.
5. Wigg, J.M. (2010). Liberating the wanderers: Using technology to unlock doors for those living with dementia. *Sociology of Health & Illness 32*, 288–303. doi: 10.1111/j.1467-9566.2009.01221.x.
6. Camp, C.J. (2019). Denial of human rights: We must change the paradigm of Dementia care. *Clinical Gerontologist 42*, 221–223. doi: 10.1080/07317115.2019.1591056.
7. Bond, J., Corner, L., Lilley, A., and Ellwood, C. (2002). Medicalization of insight and Caregivers' responses to risk in Dementia. *Dementia 1*, 313–328. doi: 10.1177/147130120200100304.
8. Ronch, J.L. (2004). Changing institutional culture. *Journal of Gerontological Social Work 43*, 61–82. doi: 10.1300/J083v43n01_06.
9. Fletcher, J.R. (2018). A symbolic interactionism of dementia: A tangle in 'the Alzheimer Conundrum.' *Social Theory & Health 16*, 172–187. doi: 10.1057/s41285-017-0050-5.
10. Harris, P.B. (2010). Dementia and Dementia care: The contributions of a psychosocial perspective. *Sociology Compass 4*, 249–262. doi: 10.1111/j.1751-9020.2010.00276.x.
11. Conrad, P. (1975). The discovery of hyperkinesis: Notes on the medicalization of deviant behavior. *Social Problems 23*, 12–21. doi: 10.2307/799624.
12. Zola, I.K. (1972). Medicine as an institution of social control. *The Sociological Review 20*, 487–504. doi: 10.1111/j.1467-954X.1972.tb00220.x.
13. Kitwood, T. (1989). Brain, mind and Dementia: With particular reference to Alzheimer's disease. *Ageing & Society 9*, 1–15. doi: 10.1017/S0144686X00013337.
14. Venkatesan, S., and Das, L. (2022). Person-centered care, dementia and graphic medicine. *Journal of Visual Communication in Medicine 45*, 263–271. doi: 10.1080/17453054.2022.2097060.
15. Cahill, S. (2022). New analytical tools and frameworks to understand Dementia: What can a human rights lens offer? *Ageing & Society 42*, 1489–1498. doi: 10.1017/S0144686X20001506.
16. Gawande, A. (2015). *Being Mortal: Illness, Medicine and What Matters in the End*. Profile Books Ltd.
17. Roe, J., Coulson, S., Ockerby, C., and Hutchinson, A.M. (2020). Staff perceptions of caring for people exhibiting behavioural and psychological symptoms of dementia in residential aged care: A cross-sectional survey. *Australasian Journal on Ageing 39*, 237–243. doi: 10.1111/ajag.12734.

18. Hector, M. (2023). Is Dementia a disease? *Caring for the Ages 24*, 11. doi: 10.1016/j.carage.2023.03.016.
19. Pollock, L. (2021). *The Book About Getting Older*. Michael Joseph.
20. Swaffer, K. (2015). Dementia and prescribed dis-engagement. *Dementia 14*, 3–6. doi: 10.1177/1471301214548136.
21. Andrews, J. (2011). We need to talk about dementia. *Journal of Research in Nursing 16*, 397–399. doi: 10.1177/1744987111414851.
22. Norbergh, K.-G., Helin, Y., Dahl, A., Hellzén, O., and Asplund, K. (2006). Nurses' attitudes towards people with Dementia: The semantic differential technique. *Nurs Ethics 13*, 264–274. doi: 10.1191/0969733006ne863oa.
23. de Vries, K., Drury-Ruddlesden, J., and McGill, G. (2020). Investigation into attitudes towards older people with dementia in acute hospital using the approaches to Dementia questionnaire. *Dementia 19*, 2761–2779. doi: 10.1177/1471301219857577.
24. Beer, C., Horner, B., Almeida, O.P., Scherer, S., Lautenschlager, N.T., Bretland, N., Flett, P., Schaper, F., and Flicker, L. (2009). Current experiences and educational preferences of general practitioners and staff caring for people with dementia living in residential facilities. *BMC Geriatr 9*, 36. doi: 10.1186/1471-2318-9-36.
25. Livingston, G., Pitfield, C., Morris, J., Manela, M., Lewis-Holmes, E., and Jacobs, H. (2012). Care at the end of life for people with dementia living in a care home: A qualitative study of staff experience and attitudes. *International Journal of Geriatric Psychiatry 27*, 643–650. doi: 10.1002/gps.2772.
26. Pulsford, D., Duxbury, J.A., and Hadi, M. (2011). A survey of staff attitudes and responses to people with dementia who are aggressive in residential care settings. *Journal of Psychiatric and Mental Health Nursing 18*, 97–104. doi: 10.1111/j.1365-2850.2010.01646.x.
27. Fletcher, J.R. (2019). *A Problem Shared: The Interacted Experience of Dementia within Care*. King's College London.
28. Liddle, J., Tan, A., Liang, P., Bennett, S., Allen, S., Lie, D.C., and Pachana, N.A. (2016). "The biggest problem we've ever had to face": How families manage driving cessation with people with dementia. *International Psychogeriatrics 28*, 109–122. doi: 10.1017/S1041610215001441.
29. Frost, R., Walters, K., Wilcock, J., Robinson, L., Harrison Dening, K., Knapp, M., Allan, L., and Rait, G. (2020). Mapping post-diagnostic dementia care in England: An e-survey. *Journal of Integrated Care 29*, 22–36. doi: 10.1108/JICA-02-2020-0005.
30. Hevink, M., Wolfs, C., Ponds, R., Doucet, S., McAiney, C., Vedel, I., Maćkowiak, M., Rymaszewska, J., Rait, G., Robinson, L., et al. (2023). Experiences of people with dementia and informal caregivers with post-diagnostic support: Data from the international COGNISANCE study. *International Journal of Geriatric Psychiatry 38*, e5916. doi: 10.1002/gps.5916.
31. Alzheimer's Society (2022). *Left Alone to Cope: The Unmet support Needs After a Dementia Diagnosis*. Alzheimer's Society.
32. Chaufan, C., Hollister, B., Nazareno, J., and Fox, P. (2012). Medical ideology as a double-edged sword: The politics of cure and care in the making of Alzheimer's disease. *Social Science & Medicine 74*, 788–795. doi: 10.1016/j.socscimed.2011.10.033.

33. Manthorpe, J., and Iliffe, S. *The dialectics of dementia*. Social Care Workforce Research Unit.

34. Leibing, A., and Schicktanz, S. eds. (2020). *Preventing Dementia?: Critical Perspectives on a New Paradigm of Preparing for Old Age*. Berghahn Books.

35. Fahey, M., Tinker, A., and Fletcher, J.R. (2023). Dementia's preventative futures: Researcher perspectives on prospective developments in the UK. *Working with Older People*. doi: 10.1108/WWOP-10-2022-0049.

36. Rose, N. (2007). Beyond medicalisation. *Lancet 369*, 700–702. doi: 10.1016/S0140-6736(07)60319-5.

37. Williams, S.J., Katz, S., and Martin, P. (2011). Neuroscience and Medicalisation: Sociological Reflections on Memory, Medicine and the Brain. In: M. Pickersgill and I. Van Keulen (eds.), *Sociological Reflections on the Neurosciences Advances in Medical Sociology*. Emerald Group Publishing Limited, pp. 231–254. doi: 10.1108/S1057-6290(2011)0000013014.

38. Foucault, M. (2010). *The Birth of Biopolitics: Lectures at the Collège de France, 1978–1979*. Palgrave Macmillan.

39. Goodley, D. (2018). Understanding disability: Biopsychology, biopolitics, and an in-between-all politics. *Adapted Physical Activity Quarterly 35*, 308–319. doi: 10.1123/apaq.2017-0092.

40. Mitchell, D.T., and Snyder, S.L. (2015). *The Biopolitics of Disability: Neoliberalism, Ablenationalism, and Peripheral Embodiment*. University of Michigan Press.

41. Sachdev, P.S., and Mohan, A. (2013). Neuropsychiatry: Where are we and where do we go from here? *Mens Sana Monographs 11*, 4–15. doi: 10.4103/0973-1229.109282.

42. Berrios, G.E., and Marková, I.S. (2002). The concept of neuropsychiatry: A historical overview. *Journal of Psychosomatic Research 53*, 629–638. doi: 10.1016/S0022-3999(02)00427-0.

43. Fletcher, J.R., and Maddock, C. (2021). Dissonant dementia: Neuropsychiatry, awareness, and contradictions in cognitive decline. *Humanities and Social Sciences Communications 8*, 1–11. doi: 10.1057/s41599-021-01004-4.

44. Wilks, S. (1864). Clinical Notes on Atrophy of the Brain. *Journal of Mental Science 10*, 381–392. doi: 10.1192/bjp.10.51.381.

45. Fuller, S.C. (1911). A study of the miliary plaques found in brains of the aged. *American Journal of Psychiatry 68*, 147–220–16. doi: 10.1176/ajp.68.2.147.

46. Fuller, S.C. (1912). Alzheimer's Disease (Senium Præcox): The Report of a Case and Review of Published Cases. *The Journal of Nervous and Mental Disease 39*, 440–455.

47. Rose, N., and Abi-Rached, J.M. (2013). *Neuro: The New Brain Sciences and the Management of the Mind*. Princeton University Press.

48. Rose, N. (2018). *Our Psychiatric Future*. Polity.

49. Pickersgill, M. (2013). The social life of the brain: Neuroscience in society. *Current Sociology 61*, 322–340. doi: 10.1177/0011392113476464.

50. Vidal, F., and Ortega, F. (2017). *Being Brains: Making the Cerebral Subject*. Fordham University Press.

51. Williams, S.J., Higgs, P., and Katz, S. (2012). Neuroculture, active ageing and the 'older brain': Problems, promises and prospects. *Sociology of Health & Illness 34*, 64–78. doi: 10.1111/j.1467-9566.2011.01364.x.

52. Williams, S.J., Katz, S., and Martin, P. (2011). The neuro-complex: Some comments and convergences. *MediaTropes 3*, 135–146.
53. Pitts-Taylor, V. (2010). The plastic brain: Neoliberalism and the neuronal self. *Health 14*, 635–652. doi: 10.1177/1363459309360796.
54. Manning, N. (2019). Sociology, biology and mechanisms in urban mental health. *Social Theory & Health 17*, 1–22. doi: 10.1057/s41285-018-00085-7.
55. Fox, P. (1989). From senility to Alzheimer's disease: The rise of the Alzheimer's disease movement. *The Milbank Quarterly*, 58–102.
56. Lock, M. (2013). *The Alzheimer Conundrum: Entanglements of Dementia and Aging*. Princeton University Press.
57. Innes, A. (2009). *Dementia Studies: A Social Science Perspective*. SAGE. doi: 10.4135/9781446213599.
58. Rose, N. (2009). Normality and pathology in a biomedical age. *The Sociological Review 57*, 66–83. doi: 10.1111/j.1467-954X.2010.01886.x.
59. Gallacher, J., and Burns, A. (2021). Social prescribing for dementia. *The Lancet Neurology 20*, 707–708. doi: 10.1016/S1474-4422(21)00208-8.
60. Kitwood, T. (1988). The technical, the personal, and the framing of dementia. *Social Behaviour 3*, 161–179.
61. Kitwood, T.M. (1997). *Dementia Reconsidered: The Person Comes First*. Open University Press.
62. Bartlett, R., and O'Connor, D. (2010). *Broadening the Dementia Debate: Towards Social Citizenship*. Policy Press.
63. Cohen, L. (2000). *No Aging in India: Alzheimer's, The Bad Family, and Other Modern Things*. University of California Press.
64. Grunberg, V.A., Bannon, S.M., Reichman, M., Popok, P.J., and Vranceanu, A.-M. (2022). Psychosocial treatment preferences of persons living with young-onset dementia and their partners. *Dementia 21*, 41–60. doi: 10.1177/14713012211027007.
65. Killen, A., Flynn, D., O'Brien, N., and Taylor, J.-P. (2022). The feasibility and acceptability of a psychosocial intervention to support people with dementia with Lewy bodies and family care partners. *Dementia 21*, 77–93. doi: 10.1177/14713012211028501.
66. Saragosa, M., Jeffs, L., Okrainec, K., and Kuluski, K. (2022). Using meta-ethnography to understand the care transition experience of people with dementia and their caregivers. *Dementia 21*, 153–180. doi: 10.1177/14713012211031779.
67. Harel, D., Band-Winterstein, T., and Goldblatt, H. (2022). Between sexual assault and compassion: The experience of living with a spouse's dementia-related hypersexuality—A narrative case-study. *Dementia 21*, 181–195. doi: 10.1177/14713012211032068.
68. Armstrong, M.J., Alliance, S., Corsentino, P., Lunde, A., and Taylor, A. (2022). Informal caregiver experiences at the end-of-life of individuals living with dementia with Lewy bodies: An interview study. *Dementia 21*, 287–303. doi: 10.1177/14713012211038428.
69. Breuer, E., Comas-Herrera, A., Freeman, E., Albanese, E., Alladi, S., Amour, R., Evans-Lacko, S., Ferri, C.P., Govia, I., Iveth Astudillo García, C., et al. (2022). Beyond the project: Building a strategic theory of change to address dementia care, treatment and support gaps across seven middle-income countries. *Dementia 21*, 114–135. doi: 10.1177/14713012211029105.

70. Rajagopalan, J., Arshad, F., Hoskeri, R.M., Nair, V.S., Hurzuk, S., Annam, H., Varghese, F., BR, R., Dhiren, S.R., Ganeshbhai, P.V., et al. (2022). Experiences of people with dementia and their caregivers during the COVID-19 pandemic in India: A mixed-methods study. *Dementia 21*, 214–235. doi: 10.1177/14713012211035371.

71. Hanna, K., Giebel, C., Butchard, S., Tetlow, H., Ward, K., Shenton, J., Cannon, J., Komuravelli, A., Gaughan, A., Eley, R., et al. (2022). Resilience and supporting people living with dementia during the time of COVID-19; A qualitative study. *Dementia 21*, 250–269. doi: 10.1177/1471301221 1036601.

72. Skov, S.S., Nielsen, M.B.D., Krølner, R.F., Øksnebjerg, L., and Rønbøl Lauridsen, S.M. (2022). A multicomponent psychosocial intervention among people with early-stage dementia involving physical exercise, cognitive stimulation therapy, psychoeducation and counselling: Results from a mixed-methods study. *Dementia 21*, 316–334. doi: 10.1177/14713012211040683.

73. Horkheimer, M. (1972). *Critical Theory: Selected Essays*. A&C Black.

74. Barham, P. (1997). *Closing the Asylum: The Mental Patient in Modern Society*, 2nd edition. Penguin.

75. Prince, M., Knapp, M., Guerchet, M., McCrone, P., Prina, M., Comas-Herrera, A., and Wittenberg, R. (2014). *Dementia UK: Update*, 2nd edition. Alzheimer's Society.

76. Ussher, J.M. (2013). Diagnosing difficult women and pathologising femininity: Gender bias in psychiatric nosology. *Feminism & Psychology 23*, 63–69. doi: 10.1177/0959353512467968.

77. Hogarth, R.A. (2017). *Medicalizing Blackness: Making Racial Difference in the Atlantic World, 1780–1840*. UNC Press Books.

78. Drescher, J. (2015). Out of DSM: Depathologizing homosexuality. *Behavioral Sciences 5*, 565–575. doi: 10.3390/bs5040565.

79. Rosenberg, C.E. (2006). Contested Boundaries: Psychiatry, disease, and diagnosis. *Perspectives in Biology and Medicine 49*, 407–424. doi: 10.1353/pbm.2006. 0046.

80. Ralph, S.J., and Espinet, A.J. (2018). Increased all-cause mortality by antipsychotic drugs: Updated review and meta-analysis in Dementia and general mental health care. *Journal of Alzheimer's Disease Reports 2*, 1–26. doi: 10.3233/ADR-170042.

81. Howard, R., Burns, A., and Schneider, L. (2020). Antipsychotic prescribing to people with dementia during COVID-19. *The Lancet Neurology 19*, 892. doi: 10.1016/S1474-4422(20)30370-7.

82. Laing, R. (1960). *The Divided Self: An Existential Study in Sanity and Madness*. Penguin UK.

83. Foot, J. (2015). *The Man Who Closed the Asylums: Franco Basaglia and the Revolution in Mental Health Care*. Verso Books.

84. Cooper, D. (1967). *Psychiatry and Anti-Psychiatry*. Routledge.

85. Szasz, T.S. (1972). *The Myth of Mental Illness*. HarperCollins.

86. Steingard, S. (2018). *Critical Psychiatry: Controversies and Clinical Implications*. Springer.

87. Ingleby, D. (1981). *Critical Psychiatry: The Politics of Mental Health*. Penguin.

88. Double, D. (2006). *Critical Psychiatry: The Limits of Madness*. Springer.

89. Moncrieff, J., and Middleton, H. (2015). Schizophrenia: A critical psychiatry perspective. *Current Opinion in Psychiatry 28*, 264. doi: 10.1097/ YCO.0000000000000151.
90. Cutler, E.S. (2019). Listening to those with lived experience. In: S. Steingard, (ed.), *Critical Psychiatry: Controversies and Clinical Implications*. Springer International Publishing, pp. 179–206. doi: 10.1007/978-3-030-02732-2_8.
91. Booth, C. (1892). *Pauperism, a Picture: And The Endowment of Old Age, an Argument*. Macmillan and Company.
92. Parsons, T. (1942). Age and sex in the social structure of the United States. *American Sociological Review 7*, 604–616. doi: 10.2307/2085686.
93. Mills, C.W. (1959). *The Sociological Imagination*. Oxford University Press.
94. Cumming, E., and Henry, W.E. (1961). *Growing Old: Process of Disengagement*. Basic Books.
95. Havighurst, R.J. (1961). Successful aging. *The Gerontologist 1*, 8–13. doi: 10.1093/geront/1.1.8.
96. Bloom, D.E., and Luca, D.L. (2016). The global demography of aging: Facts, explanations, future. In: J. Piggott and A. Woodland (eds.), *Handbook of the Economics of Population Aging*. North-Holland, pp. 3–56. doi: 10.1016/bs .hespa.2016.06.002.
97. Davenport, R.J. (2020). Urbanization and mortality in Britain, c. 1800–50. *The Economic History Review 73*, 455–485. doi: 10.1111/ehr.12964.
98. Anderson, M. (1985). The emergence of the modern life cycle in Britain. *Social History 10*, 69–87. doi: 10.1080/03071028508567611.
99. Bytheway, B. (2005). Ageism and age categorization. *Journal of Social Issues 61*, 361–374. doi: 10.1111/j.1540-4560.2005.00410.x.
100. Hacking, I. (1990). *The Taming of Chance*. Cambridge University Press.
101. Townsend, P. (1981). The structured dependency of the elderly: A creation of social policy in the twentieth century. *Ageing & Society 1*, 5–28. doi: 10.1017/ S0144686X81000020.
102. Walker, A. (1981). Towards a political economy of old age. *Ageing & Society 1*, 73–94. doi: 10.1017/S0144686X81000056.
103. Fletcher, J.R. (2020). Anti-aging technoscience & the biologization of cumulative inequality: Affinities in the biopolitics of successful aging. *Journal of Aging Studies 55*. doi: 10.1016/j.jaging.2020.100899.
104. Pickard, S. (2016). *Age Studies: A Sociological Examination of How We Age and are Aged Through the Life Course*. SAGE.
105. Dannefer, D., and Lin, J. (2013). Commentary: Contingent ageing, naturalisation and some rays of intellectual hope. In: J. Baars, J. Dohmen, A. Grenier, and C. Phillipson (eds.), *Ageing, Meaning and Social Structure*. Policy Press. doi: 10.13 32/policypress/9781447300908.003.0010.
106. Dannefer, D. (1987). Aging as intracohort differentiation: Accentuation, the Matthew effect, and the life course. *Sociological Forum 2*, 211–236. doi: 10.1007/BF01124164.
107. Wellin, C. ed. (2018). *Critical Gerontology Comes of Age: Advances in Research and Theory for a New Century*. Routledge. doi: 10.4324/9781315209371.
108. Bülow, M.H., and Söderqvist, T. (2014). Successful ageing: A historical overview and critical analysis of a successful concept. *Journal of Aging Studies 31*, 139–149. doi: 10.1016/j.jaging.2014.08.009.

109. Katz, S. (2002). *Disciplining Old Age: The Formation of Gerontological Knowledge*. University of Virginia Press.
110. Gilleard, C., and Higgs, P. (2010). Aging without agency: Theorizing the fourth age. *Aging & Mental Health 14*, 121–128. doi: 10.1080/13607860903228762.
111. Gilleard, C., and Higgs, P. (2014). Studying dementia: The relevance of the fourth age. *Quality in Ageing and Older Adults 15*, 241–243. doi: 10.1108/QAOA-10-2014-0027.
112. Higgs, P., and Gilleard, C. (2017). Ageing, dementia and the social mind: Past, present and future perspectives. *Sociology of Health & Illness 39*, 175–181. doi: 10.1111/1467-9566.12536.
113. Latimer, J. (2018). Repelling neoliberal world-making? How the ageing–dementia relation is reassembling the social. *The Sociological Review 66*, 832–856. doi: 10.1177/0038026118777422.
114. Cohen, S. (2002). *Folk Devils and Moral Panics: The Creation of the Mods and Rockers*. Psychology Press.
115. ARUK (2018). Bryan Cranston confronts misunderstanding of dementia…using an orange. Alzheimer's Research UK. https://www.alzheimersresearchuk.org/bryan-cranston-confronts-misunderstanding-dementiausing-orange/.
116. Grenier, A., Lloyd, L., and Phillipson, C. (2017). Precarity in late life: Rethinking dementia as a 'frailed' old age. *Sociology of Health & Illness 39*, 318–330. doi: 10.1111/1467-9566.12476.
117. Grenier, A., and Phillipson, C. (2023). Precarity and dementia. In: R. Ward and L. Sandberg (eds.), *Critical Dementia Studies*. Routledge.

4 Deconstructing Biopolitical Commitments

A Neurocritical Analysis of Biogenic Disease, Normal Ageing and Promissory Futures

In this chapter, I begin to sketch a neurocritical dementia studies analysis of the biopolitics of dementia. Drawing on critical psychiatry and critical gerontology, I deconstruct three core tenets of neuropsychiatric biopolitics, regarding disease, ageing and the future. I specifically alight on these three facets because of their centrality and commonality to notable biopolitical endeavours, as well as having traditionally been subsumed within the (bio)medical bogeyman. First, I investigate the claim that dementia is caused by discrete diseases of the brain and the underlying idea that specific molecular occurrences lead to cognitive impairment. From a critical psychiatric standpoint, I consider the development of this view in relation to the efforts of key stakeholders and their underpinning rationales, attending to how different conceptualisations of dementia serve different interests. I also consider some of the evidence to the contrary, including longstanding questions regarding purported associations between neuropathology and cognitive impairment, and cognitive science scholarships on distributed cognition and cognitive reserve.

Second, I explore the claim that dementia is not a normal part of ageing. I contextualise this idea as emerging from the late 20th-century rejection of senility and show that it has become an important knowledge claim across several neuropsychiatric initiatives. I critique the concept of "normal" ageing from a critical gerontological perspective, drawing on Alexander Comfort's notion of ageing in terms of senescence and Georges Canguilhem's sociology of the normal and the pathological. While we might intuitively have our own personal ideas about what normal and abnormal ageing and agedness are like, at the level of population health, it becomes remarkably challenging to develop robust operationalisations of *normal ageing* versus *abnormal disease*. Moreover, critical gerontology has long revealed that normative schemas regarding ageing typically serve the interests of their progenitors, from patriarchal ideas about family roles in 1950s gerontology to contemporary consumption-based ideas about third-age lifestyles.

Finally, I turn to the claim that dementia research will discover a cure. I draw on the sociology of science and technology and associated

DOI: 10.4324/9781003398523-4

work on promissory science communication to analyse the ways in which neuropsychiatric endeavours colonise the future. I show that the fight for the future matters because it has substantial repercussions for our present, particularly in terms of where resources coalesce and what types of initiative gain support. Overall, this chapter builds on the previous one by tracing a neuropsychiatric biopolitics of dementia more specifically, to demarcate its particular divergences from a (bio)medical model and facilitate critical engagement with its core components. Rather than contesting or refuting this biopolitics per se, I instead show that, as with politics broadly, it is fundamentally a matter of normative commitments, the politics of which are semi-concealed behind a scientistic aesthetic. This means that it is open to deconstruction and transformation across numerous fronts (e.g. how might drug regulation for age-related disease be reconfigured if we were to abandon notions of "normal ageing"? Or how might investment structures shift if our biopolitics of dementia focussed on the present rather than the future?), with potentially profound implications for our experiences of dementia, and therefore should not be uncritically accepted.

* * *

The previous chapter sought to crudely distinguish a neuropsychiatric biopolitics of dementia, which I argue deserves far greater critical attention in dementia studies, from a (bio)medical model of dementia, which has traditionally been the focus of a great deal of critique in dementia studies. This chapter will go much further in pinpointing some specific characteristics. Scholarship relating to (bio)medicalisation has centred on institutional impositions onto previously normal aspects of human life, with the consequence that people experiencing those things are dehumanised. While there are several meaningful affinities between the two (e.g. a privileging of biogenic neuropathology), biopolitics differs markedly in its cultural and political pervasiveness and in its multifaceted cultivation of modes of public and personal life. As I have argued, various notable figures throughout the history of dementia appear to have had some sense of the biopolitics of dementia as a transformative project. Kraepelin used AD to strengthen his lab; Butler used AD to strengthen the NIA. In both instances, the gambit paid considerable dividends. Hence, an alertness to biopolitics means that we are now analysing the conditions of life itself, the ways in which publics and persons are (self-)disciplined, and the artful governance of our seemingly introspective relationships with ourselves. We can do so, I have argued, by turning to the resonant yet largely untapped traditions of critical psychiatry and critical gerontology. Together, these scholarships offer some potential for addressing the effects of neuro-agnosticism in dementia studies, thereby fostering a neurocritical dementia studies.

Having provided some theoretical and historical context to the nature of the neuropsychiatric biopolitics of dementia, I will attend more closely to some core components of this biopolitics. In doing so, I will attempt to practically exemplify the doing of neurocritical dementia studies. As noted, the three areas that I will cover are often articulated via the following claims: (1) dementia is caused by diseases of the brain, (2) dementia is not a normal part of ageing and (3) research will discover a cure. Taken together, these commonplace proclamations comprise something akin to three fundamental neuropsychiatric principles. Moreover, as will become evident through this book, they are the claims through which a great deal of combative, and potentially harmful, biopolitics comes to be done in the world. Hence, they warrant substantive critical exploration as a means of empowering dementia studies to contest that biopolitics, particularly when it becomes deleterious to people affected by dementia, and perhaps older people more broadly.[1]

4.1 "Dementia Is Caused by Diseases of the Brain"

The first[1] core message of the neuropsychiatric biopolitics of dementia – that dementia is caused by diseases of the brain – is perhaps the most familiar, obvious and long critiqued. It is what Berrios and Marková[2] have identified as the foundational claim of neuropsychiatry and has been equally fundamental to the (bio)medical model of dementia. Evidence of its dominance is widespread because stakeholder assertions of "brain disease" are a mainstay of neuropsychiatric biopolitics. Such assertions often combine two ideas: (1) that dementia is caused by physiological phenomena (typically brain-based) and (2) that these phenomena can be differentiated into discrete disease entities. Consider the following:

> *Alzheimer's Society (major charity)*: Dementia can be caused by many different diseases. These diseases affect the brain in different ways, resulting in different types of dementia.[3]
>
> *David Cameron (former UK prime minister)*: We know now that dementia is caused by diseases of the brain, such as Alzheimer's.[4]
>
> *Daily Mail (major newspaper)*: Dementia is an umbrella term used to describe a range of progressive neurological disorders (those affecting the brain) which impact memory, thinking and behaviour.[5]
>
> *Bryan Cranston (actor)*: It all starts and ends with the brain. Dementia is caused by diseases, most commonly Alzheimer's. It physically destroys cells.[6]

These claims are made by the same broad and eclectic collection of stakeholders described in Chapter 3. In these examples, a charity, newspaper, former prime minister and actor are united in a singular biogenic message. Their involvement is interesting because it is questionable to what extent celebrities, politicians and journalists are able to appraise hypothesised aetiologies of cognitive decline. However, it is important to remember that what is at stake here is not necessarily the intricacies of robust scientific research but rather the neuropsychiatric biopolitics of dementia. Hence, we are dealing with broad claims that seek to set out authoritative ontological (what dementia is), epistemological (how and what we know about it) and normative (how and why it is bad) schemas surrounding dementia. Moreover, they are doing material work, operating as rallying cries for action and donation, a point I will return to shortly.

Neuropsychiatric appeals to neurogenic dementia aetiologies are emblematic of a broader idea that the validity of an illness or diagnosis should be predicated on that category having a dedicated pathophysiological manifestation. This belief was popularised during the 19th century as the medical sciences turned away from a reliance on the clinical observation of symptoms in favour of generalisable physiological definitions of distinct diseases.[7] These universal ailments were characterised by specific molecular mechanisms that corresponded with specific clinical signs. Under this system, clinical observation, which was previously the essence of medical practice, was relegated to a means of generating presumptions of disease that could then be properly legitimated in relation to appropriate pathophysiological characteristics.[8] These pathophysiologies are essentially physical bits of the body that are somehow different from what a physician would normally expect or desire, and that can be observed in some manner. So, for example, if a child falls from a tree and visits a hospital crying about leg pain, we might suspect a fractured tibia and therefore perform procedures to observe pathophysiological evidence that confirms/disproves our suspicions, in this case, an X-ray to generate an image of the bone. Such pathophysiological legitimation was, and still is, facilitated by the development of new measurement technologies to capture those pathophysiologies, an issue discussed further in Chapter 5.

The turn to pathophysiology as a form of legitimacy is essentially an attempt to make the classification of disease value-neutral by removing the human interpretation of symptoms.[8] In the case of mental disorder, such interpretation can be particularly subjective and hence vulnerable to human error because diagnosis is often heavily reliant on personal, emotional and behavioural factors, as well as institutional pressures.[9] Such diagnoses can become dependent on the personal predilections of a particular practitioner. I once observed this for myself during a cognitive battery in a memory clinic. It was evident that the person being tested fell below the threshold for dementia if one was to apply the test strictly. However, the practitioner was clearly not inclined to pursue a dementia diagnosis. She first prompted the person to reconsider wrong answers, then suggested correct answers, and eventually completed certain items herself. The result was a respectable test score indicating no dementia. I did not ask the practitioner why she had done this, but I assume it was because she decided that a dementia diagnosis would probably worsen the final months of this person's life without offering any benefits.

The purported subjectivity, be that unconscious or deliberate, of diagnosing psychiatric disorder has historically stirred controversy. For instance, the question of whether homosexuality should remain in the DSM was ultimately decided by vote, conducted in the context of lobbying and protests. Many physicians were dismayed that the existence of a disease entity could be determined in this manner, as opposed to some more rigorous, objective and altogether scientific approach.[8] Responding to such concerns, pathophysiology can seem to represent a more scientifically legitimate, and hence satisfying, means of disease classification than lobbying, protesting, voting and the like. The basic empiricist premise at play here is that seeing is believing.[10] If we can reliably observe a distinct molecular thing, then the associated disease must exist in some tangible, and intuitively real, sense. Dementia, alongside mental disorder generally, causes particular tensions here because we have no direct means of observing it. We cannot objectively capture psychic phenomena and must instead rely on downstream effects, e.g. functional magnetic resonance imaging (fMRI) scans, behaviour observation, questionnaires, the exact relationship of which with cognition we can never realistically know.[11] Such issues can trouble empiricists. Of course, many would argue that such nit-picking is troublingly far removed from the poignant everyday problems faced by people affected by cognitive impairment. To some extent, this is entirely the point – to do away with mental qualia and lived experience so as to make diagnoses more robust.

An interesting implication of the physiological turn, which remains particularly evident in neuropsychiatric biopolitics today, is the existence of discrete disease entities.[12] Herein, the specificity of the affliction is attributed to the nature of the somatic mechanism rather than the nature of the patient and his/her circumstances. By extension, that specific affliction can occur in an almost identical manner in many separate and dissimilar individuals. The continued influence of nosological specificity regarding dementia is evident in contemporary arguments that drug trials have failed because study populations were not defined carefully enough to capture discrete diseases. Such arguments suggest, often explicitly, that we can only successfully address dementias if we tightly specify discrete pathophysiologies. Again, such approaches are often in tension with experiential realities. I have often found in my own research that people affected by dementia can account for their experiences as evolutions or exaggerations of longstanding personality traits. The person with aphasia has always found it difficult to maintain a conversation. The disinhibited person has always been a risk taker.[13] The forgetful husband has never listened properly to his wife. In this manner, personally flexible notions of dementia persist beyond neuropsychiatric prescriptions.

The legitimacy of a particular disease is not simply a conceptual matter of satisfying notions of scientific objectivity for their own sake; it is a means of capital accumulation. Perceived legitimacy has important practical consequences because public and political sympathies, and by extension resources, have traditionally been more forthcoming for physiologically established problems, like cancer, than physiologically contested problems, like depression. As an example of physiology's fiscal utility, since 2009, the National Institute of Mental Health has requested that funded research focus on four objectives, three of which are expressly pathophysiological.[14] Psychiatrist Mona Gupta has argued that researcher and funder preoccupations with pathophysiology in psychiatric disorder are co-reinforcing. Researchers are incentivised to discover pathophysiology to garner funding, and funders are incentivised to fund pathophysiological research because its legitimacy suggests the probable production of straightforward and potentially profitable physiological solutions.[15] Societal responses are also entwined with personal rationales for pursuing biogenic legitimacy. Conditions such as chronic fatigue syndrome and irritable bowel syndrome reveal the potential for social dismissal of illness experiences that are not substantiated by accepted pathophysiologies and the extent to which people affected can passionately resist psychogenic aetiological hypotheses (let alone sociogenic) in favour of biogenesis.[16] This issue of personal status is returned to in Chapter 6.

Focusing on dementia specifically, we find that its story sits neatly within the wider turn to pathophysiological legitimacy. The neuropathological biogenic hypothesis, that dementia is caused by diseases of the brain, has animated researchers since at least the nosological turn of the mid-19th century.[17] It is no coincidence that Wilks first depicted dementia-associated brain atrophy at this time. However, dementia nosology garnered far greater scientific interest following Alois Alzheimer's anatomical studies on the brain of Auguste Deter and his resulting characterisation of the hallmark neurofibrillary tangles and amyloid plaques of AD. As discussed, Alzheimer's hypothesis was popularised by Emil Kraepelin in the early 20th century, despite both men having misgivings, and fed into a taxonomical arms race, with rival laboratories competing to discover new disease classifications. Over the following decades, there was significant debate over the nature of Alzheimer's hypothesis, much of which centred on the uncertain causative and correlative relations between the described neuropathology and symptomology. By the late 1920s, a collection of discrepant observations was already casting doubt on the notion that dementia stemmed directly from toxic protein aggregation.[18] Hence, contemporary uncertainties regarding the relationships between Aβ and cognitive impairment, which have been magnified by the failure of anti-Aβ therapies to meaningfully influence cognition, actually stem back almost as far as the hypothesis itself.

Nonetheless, under the conditions of nosological legitimacy and the corresponding politics of funding allocation, the post-1970s AD movement has leant heavily into the notion that dementia is caused by discrete neuropathological diseases, with a particular reliance on Aβ causing AD. Contemporary neuropsychiatric proclamations of the type offered by David Cameron and Bryan Cranston (at the beginning of this section) represent a continuation of the struggle for molecular legitimacy, both the general struggle to legitimise disease categories – especially regarding mental disorder – and the specific struggle that characterised the early years of the AD movement. As outlined in Chapter 1, the promotion of AD as a leading cause of death stemmed from the attribution of cognitive symptoms to specific neuropathologies via new electron microscopy techniques.[17] Here, new observational technologies provided a tangible means of empirically substantiating the disease classification. This development offered the possibility of observing the real (corporeal) essence of dementia, echoing the wider neuropsychiatric promise that by looking into the brain, we will discover the secrets of our lives, our minds, our selves.

Today, the naturalisation of biogenesis in dementia, and the concurrent movement away from psychic phenomena that evade direct physical observation, continues apace in various forms. For example, the aforementioned DSM-5 reclassification of dementia moved from "cognitive disorders" to "*neuro*cognitive disorders", better capturing the centrality of the brain.[19, 20] The joint Alzheimer Scotland and Scottish government public health campaign entitled "Brain Health Scotland" focuses on the brain with such dedication that one could be forgiven for forgetting that this is a programme to address dementia.[21] It is the world of biomarkers that most strongly manifests the deep importance of biogenesis to contemporary neuropsychiatric biopolitics. Substantial efforts have been dedicated to robustly measuring in-vivo Aβ via various technologies, with the intention of more precisely differentiating diseases.[22-24] Indeed, the NIA and Alzheimer's Association have recommended a greater focus on discovering and refining dementia biomarkers.[25] In the next chapter, I will discuss in more detail the complex arguments surrounding the contemporary gold rush for biomarkers. For now, suffice it to say that this mainstay of neuropsychiatric biopolitics is emblematic of commitments to positioning dementia as a consequence of discrete brain diseases.

The symbolic, cultural and political pursuit of discrete physiopathology has been incredibly successful. Today, the idea that dementia is a brain thing is utterly unremarkable, echoing the wider proliferation of neuroculture and brain-centric conceptions of self and society discussed in Chapter 3. In my own research with people affected by dementia, I have often been struck by how intuitively people can weave mentions of brain disease into their personal accounts of dementia. Indeed, even people who are sceptical of neuropsychiatric claims can fleetingly, almost unconsciously, appeal to a symbolism of brain disease alongside their favoured conceptualisations of dementia, be that in terms of morality, psychology, personality and/or ageing.[13] Indicative of this general pervasiveness, I once asked a renowned medical social scientist why dementia seemed to be ignored in the sociology of mental illness. This scholar, who has dedicated several decades to critiquing biogenic fervour, answered that dementia was distinct because it was fundamentally neurological in nature. This instance is telling of the extent to which a neuropsychiatric biopolitics of dementia has succeeded in winning the most unlikely hearts and minds.

Despite considerable symbolic accomplishment, scientifically, the biogenic quest has proved to be more challenging. One problem is the long-recognised discrepancy between physiopathology and symptomology. Some people diagnosed with AD lack Aβ, while some with Aβ are cognitively intact.[26–37] Moreover, several drug trials have now successfully cleared Aβ without halting cognitive decline.[38] We must also be wary of appeals to molecules such as Aβ as though they simply exist and are observed as such. In practice, Aβ is a heterogeneous entity that can be difficult to isolate and measure, especially in brains[39]. The general physiological messiness of ageing brains is another impediment to isolating discrete disease entities,[40] which I will return to below. Briefly, at least two-thirds of people aged above 80 have non-AD neuropathologies that likely influence cognition,[41] and both cerebral atrophy and Aβ aggregation are common in later life.[42, 43] Aβ is also fairly ubiquitous in the human brain more generally. In 2011, one study of the brains of 2,332 people aged between 1 and 100 discovered that only 10 people did not have evidence of Aβ.[44]

These problems have been recognised for a long time. Indeed, the microscope work that Robert Katzman based his assertions on explicitly reflected these ambiguities and did not really support his claims at all. It revealed the familiar complicated picture of neuropathology and symptoms not neatly aligning. Only 50% of the senile dementia cases studied satisfied AD criteria, and there were no pathophysiologies in the dementia group that could not be found in the control group. The research made no causal claims and did not single out Aβ from other pathophysiologies as in any way special.[45, 46] Overall, research suggests that later-life neurodegeneration and associated cognitive decline are characterised by pronounced heterogeneity.[29] In this context, the pursuit of discrete pathophysiologies is extremely difficult. Annette Leibing has noted that, despite decades of research, conventional dementia biomarkers today remain largely identical to those suggested in the 1990s.[47]

Neuropsychiatric devotion to biogenesis has long animated a crude antipsychiatric scholarship. In extreme instances, critics have pointed to the lack of robustly established neuropathology across various mental disorders to justify their arguments that such disorders are, in some sense, not real, perhaps mythic. The famous work of Thomas Szasz, provocatively titled *The Myth of Mental Illness*, exemplifies this approach.[48] Such arguments can be deeply problematic in their reiteration of the belief that pathophysiology is the singular legitimate form of disease. Of course, there is no real reason that the validity or severity of an illness should depend on the parallel existence of accompanying molecular phenomena. Few people would suggest that suicidal ideation stems from a discrete neural mechanism[2], but its reality, severity and consequences are blatantly obvious. In principle, whether or not a person experiencing progressive cognitive impairment has a particular neuropathology associated with that impairment does not inherently (un)substantiate the reality and gravity of his/her experiences. Nonetheless, in practice, a particular cultural commitment to the specificity of physiological disease entities partially constrains dementia's status as a serious problem warranting proper attention. This question – of the legitimacy of a problem and corresponding efforts to address the problem – underpins the second major neuropsychiatric claim that I wish to explore: dementia is not a normal part of ageing.

4.2 "Dementia Is Not a Normal Part of Ageing"

As with the notion of discrete disease, the claim that dementia is not a normal part of ageing is integral to the neuropsychiatric biopolitics of dementia. It is, by extension, relatively ubiquitous in related outputs, authoritatively reiterated by an eclectic mix of actors. Consider the following examples:

> *Alzheimer's Society*: Dementia is not a natural part of ageing. We all forget a name or a face sometimes. Especially as we get older. But dementia is something different.[51]
>
> *David Cameron*: So many people just think, well, dementia it's just part of ageing; it's just a natural thing that happens. It isn't.[52]
>
> *Daily Mail*: Dementia ISN'T just part of old age.[53]
>
> *Bryan Cranston*: Too many people still believe that dementia is just a natural part of ageing.[54]

The Alzheimer's Society actually has a page dedicated to helping people distinguish between dementia and normal ageing, including a comparative reference chart.[55] The effort that stakeholders dedicate to expounding the conceptual differentiation of ageing and dementia can be considerable. This provokes questions regarding why such differentiation is so important to some actors and what is at stake in the acceptance or rejection of a dementia–ageing binary. As it turns out, the answers to these questions are integral to understanding the neuropsychiatric biopolitics of dementia.

The first thing to note here is that, as indicated in the previous section, ageing and dementia are deeply entangled not only in a conceptual sense but also at epidemiological and physiological scales. The greatest risk factor for AD is age.[56] Epidemiologically, AD incidence increases exponentially with advancing age, though it is difficult to measure in the oldest old due to the small sample sizes and the idiosyncrasies of survivor effects that typify the extremely old.[57] In the US, AD affects 3% of people aged 65–74, 17% aged 75–84 and 32% aged over 85.[58] Hence, the positive correlation with age is stark. Furthermore, the importance of age as a risk factor increases with age, so that in the oldest old, age is the only significant risk factor for AD.[57] However, as noted, research on this population must be read with considerable caveats.

Beyond epidemiology, the molecular entanglements of ageing and dementia are similarly deep rooted. An ageing process of physiological deterioration seems to occur in all humans. This can broadly be accounted for in terms of "senescence", that is, progressive physiological degeneration and functional decline, whereby homeostasis is increasingly imperilled.[59] At a foundational level, senescence is characterised by decreasing DNA repair and increasing mutation, and the accumulation of damaged proteins.[60, 61] That said, the fundamental nature of the ageing process is not fully understood, being subject to ongoing debate.[60, 62] The effects of this ageing process are manifest in many familiar forms – tooth enamel wears away, arteries harden, and bone density diminishes, to name but a few.[63] In particular, it appears that a threshold is typically reached after the age of 60 at which the overall senescent load is implicated in the acceleration of chronic disease and various syndromes.[61]

The brain is not immune from the deterioration of age. Neurological research on senescence is less developed than that on senescence more broadly, but that which has been conducted generally suggests that similar processes occur in the brain. The characteristic inflammation, oxidative stress and protein aggregation of senescence have all been shown to occur in the ageing brain,[64] which typically atrophies in later life, losing around 20% of its mass.[43] At a practical level, the ageing brain is typically characterised by functional deterioration, as with the ageing body in general. This is especially evident in broad cognitive decline from around the age of 30 onwards, clinically deemed normal age-related cognitive impairment.[65] However, it is important to be cautious of such cognitive observations because cognition is typically conceptualised as comprising various different domains, all of which age in different ways. Moreover, conceptualising, operationalising, measuring and interpreting cognition is challenging and subject to different perspectives. However, different strands of neurological and cognitive research paint a picture in which ageing can seem remarkably pathological in nature.

Many biochemists note that while age-related conditions are typically approached as distinct diseases with discrete aetiologies at a clinical level, the molecular evidence suggests that they could be rooted in senescence.[61, 66] The pathobiological pathways of several neurodegenerative conditions, such as Parkinson's, Huntington's and AD, share considerable similarities that can be traced back to senescent processes, including protein aggregation and DNA dysfunction.[67] However, caution is required. While there is a substantial body of evidence supporting associations between senescence and various age-related conditions, the mechanisms involved are too poorly understood to enable researchers to make causal claims with confidence. In particular, uncertainties persist regarding whether the types of quasi-pathophysiological phenomena seen in ageing brains are pathogenic or pathognomonic (or perhaps even neuroprotective), that is, whether they cause dementia, result from it or are an attempt to limit damage.[68–70, 41] Indeed, following Alzheimer's initial publication, many physicians suspected that plaques were a downstream effect.[71] The physiological messiness of ageing means that it is difficult to isolate discrete processes of ageing and/or disease.[40] As noted, at least two-thirds of people aged above 80 have non-AD pathologies that likely affect cognition.[41]

When it comes to dementia, the picture is complicated further by a lack of understanding of the brain and neurodegenerative disorders in general. Ageing introduces further complications because it entails an assortment of molecular changes, such as neuron loss and synapse weakening, that are also implicated in dementia.[43] The physiology of normal brain ageing (to the limited extent that such a concept makes sense) is under-researched due to a focus on neurodegenerative conditions,[72] but the basic intractable messiness of the aged brain has been recognised for a long time. Twenty years ago, the Medical Research Council Cognitive Function and Ageing Study found that the majority of a sample of 209 deceased older people showed patho-physiological signs of mixed dementias.[73] Moreover, the authors concluded that there was no pathological threshold for dementia. A recent study of 75 people diagnosed with Alzheimer's disease found that 38 had an additional dementia-related pathology at post-mortem.[74] One should not read too much into these results because several similar studies have produced widely different estimates. Collectively, the evidence points toward substantial pathological heterogeneity, but even the measurement of pathology is varied.[29] These findings are also in line with one of the most significant puzzles in dementia research, that some people with symptoms do not have the associated pathology, while some people with pathology do not experience symptoms.[75] Intriguingly, the latter group is variably classified as "pathological ageing" and "preclinical Alzheimer's disease".[41]

In practice, the aged brain is typically characterised by a complex amalgamation of age-related pathologies.[41, 76] While the diagnosis of a single type of dementia is common in living patients, at post-mortem, most affected brains are found to have a mixture of interrelated pathologies and features of age-related deterioration.[28, 77] There are two major interpretations of this molecular heterogeneity. Some commentators support a spectrum model of ageing and dementia, encompassing broad physiological and functional decline,[78–80] while others argue that contemporary classifications such as AD currently encompass several different diseases and require further deconstruction and more sophisticated diagnosis.[81, 82] None of this proves that dementia is or is not caused by ageing. Ultimately, our understandings of the ageing brain and associated disorders are far too rudimentary to inform causal claims or neat disease classifications that are sanitised of ageing. What it does provide us with is a means of distinguishing neurological and cognitive science and clinical realities from neuropsychiatric biopolitics. The former openly engages with real-world complexities in an effort to better understand them, while the latter conceals them behind mantras. This observation leads us neatly into the conceptual entanglements of ageing and dementia.

For much of human history, cognitive impairment has been an expected component of later life. In 2000 BC, Ancient Egyptians wrote of the memory problems that accompanied old age, while in 500 BC, Ancient Greek law made allowances for mental impairment in later life.[83] In the Middle Ages, religious leaders portrayed the mental decline of old age as stemming from original sin,[84] and William Shakespeare's description of old age as a second childishness in *As You Like It* is typically used to represent perceptions in the 16th and 17th centuries. However, depictions of senility or dementia are largely notable by their historic absence, with cognitive decline in later life having likely received little attention for much of human history.[83] The prevailing view was likely one of senility – that cognitive decline was a natural condition of growing old. "Dementia", often misattributed to renowned French physician Philippe Pinel in the 19th century, was evident in some early psychiatric writings throughout the 16th and 17th centuries, though it was generally used as a catch-all phrase for insanity and foolishness.[85]

The first serious attempts to classify "dementia" as a distinct category came in the 19th century, first through Pinel and subsequently his student Jean-Étienne Esquirol. Each applied the term dementia to a group of people characterised by "insanity", "incompetence" and "incapacity", partly caused by old age.[83, 84] While both Pinel and Esquirol deemed those with dementia to be suffering from a problem of the emotions as much as any disease, their delineations of a distinct category of people with dementia were subsequently transformed during the mid-19th-century popularisation of separate nosologies as localised disease entities,[17] most notably by Wilkes, as discussed above. Importantly, the nosological turn was similarly influential in transforming conceptualisations of ageing. Mid-19th-century research into age-associated cell degeneration supported the idea of senescence, positioning ageing as a process of broad physiological deterioration which led to various diseases.[17] In this context, Binswanger and Alzheimer introduced the term "presenile dementia", differentiating those aged below 60 from those aged above 60, who had "senile dementia" attributed to ageing.[86] The dementia age distinction was grounded in abiotrophy, the notion that a certain range of physiological deterioration is normal as people age, but when this senescence occurs prematurely it is pathological.[17]

As discussed above, Alzheimer brought this conceptual distinction to bear on AD, which he classified as a discrete disease, distinct from senility, because it only occurred in people aged below 60. Here then, age itself became the means of distinguishing dementia from ageing. The distinction between AD and senility was immediately subject to debate.[87, 88] During the early 20th century, studies revealed that neurofibrillary tangles and amyloid plaques were present in many conditions that caused dementia symptoms and were sometimes not present in those otherwise deemed to have AD. As such, many of the contemporary problems with AD as a disease entity were documented soon after the condition was first publicised.

However, the notion of AD as a specific condition affecting people aged below 60 continued as a clinical entity throughout the mid-20th century, while senility remained the popular clinical and public explanation for similar symptoms in older people. As noted in Chapter 1, the removal of age distinctions in dementia was integral to the post-1970s flourishing of the AD movement and our contemporary biopolitics of dementia. This was realised in Robert Katzman's work showing that senile dementia echoed AD pathophysiology.[89] Here, Katzman redefined the relationship between AD, ageing and senility. In his schema, senility was incorporated into dementia, with all cases being caused by disease irrespective of age. Notions of senility were abandoned, and ageing was disassociated from cognitive impairment. Hence, in transforming AD, the social movement behind this transition also transformed ageing and its relationship with dementia.

The major implication of Katzman's work is that there exists a binary of normal ageing and abnormal dementia, and the two phenomena are entirely distinct. This is an intriguing imagining of ageing and dementia because it catalyses longstanding and deeply institutionalised uncertainties relating to ageing, senescence, disease and the corresponding parameters of the normal, the abnormal and the pathological. As far back as the beginning of the 20th century, Ignatz Nascher, who coined the term "geriatrics", noted that physicians tended to ignore the complexities of ageing and agedness because they could not distinguish the normal from the pathological in older patients.[90] Such questions are especially applicable to geriatric syndromes because many are typified by a slow and insidious slide from normal states of being toward states that can cause problems (or, less normatively inscribed, from states that we take for granted toward states that provoke concern).

Consider, for instance, osteoporosis, a common condition experienced by older women in particular, whereby bones become brittle and prone to fracture. In the context of senescence, the lessening resilience of bone is a gradual process, beginning without notice but culminating after many years in a substantially heightened risk of fracture. How are we to determine the moment at which a specific bone density is pathological? In practice, the most problematic aspect of low bone density is fracture, and fracture is highly environmentally determined. You are probably much less likely to break a bone sitting still in an armchair than you are while mountaineering. Nonetheless, osteoporosis as a condition is assessed in relation to the bone itself rather than the breaking of it. In practice, the designation of a pathological boundary is achieved mathematically via standard deviations from average values.[91] This approach is very similar to the new DSM definitions of major and minor neurocognitive disorder, discussed in Chapter 2, and indicates the importance of quantified normalities in age-associated conditions.

The philosopher and physician Georges Canguilhem described the modern concept of disease as being founded on the idea of spectrums of quantified normality and abnormality. Pathology is an extreme variation of a possible range of physiology, deviating from a healthy average. Canguilhem contended that biomedicine promotes the quantified notion of disease but that this is fundamentally flawed because health is not an average state, varying widely from person to person. He suggested that this quantified notion of pathology is an attempt to claim value-neutrality but that deeming any human condition normal or abnormal cannot be neutral. By definition, non-normative ab/normality is logically impossible. The rationale underpinning human efforts to distinguish the pathological from the normal is a desire to derive therapeutics to restore the suffering individual to a preferable state, as espoused by contemporary neuropsychiatric biopolitics. This is fundamentally a value-laden endeavour, with resulting notions of objective disease based on quantified normality and abnormality being intrinsically suspect.[92]

The DSM's major and minor neurocognitive disorder categories exemplify the difficulty of defining what counts as a pathology, as opposed to a normality, and where its boundaries lie. These categories are far from the first attempts to quantify the abnormality of dementia. A range of numerical cognition scales in old age psychiatry emerged in late 20th-century Britain as a means of designating age-related dementias as a psychiatric territory.[93, 94] Today, many dementia diagnoses still rely on a numerical score derived from cognitive tests. For instance, on the 30-point Mini Mental State Examination, 20–24 indicates mild dementia, 13–20 indicates moderate dementia and <12 indicates severe dementia. Normality is, hence, 24–30. As exemplified in my earlier story of witnessing a rigged cognitive test, cognition is measured through subjectively interpreted proxies and is ultimately inaccessible in a strictly objective sense, no matter the extent to which we apply numerical scales. Ultimately, as Canguilhem observed, we cannot truly escape some form of normative commitment when distinguishing normality.

The presentation of AD's status as a disease and not ageing speaks to many of the issues discussed by Canguilhem in relation to positioning disease in relation to a value-laden average. Ageing problematises physiological quantification because of its inherent variability. It is often characterised as life's great leveller, but this could not be further from the truth. Critical gerontology teaches us that, if ageing is anything, then it is a powerful medium of heterogeneity. Since the late 20th century, critical gerontological research on cumulative inequality has revealed substantial "aged heterogeneity"[95, 96]. Herein, inequality across diverse domains is positively correlated with time, so inequality overall is greatest among older people, simply by virtue of them having lived so long. Over 80 years, small differences between any two people – be that biological, psychological or social – can develop into huge differences through processes of cumulative inequality.[97] Research is even showing that aged heterogeneity is increasing in the 21st century, so that the diversity of later life is ever more difficult to fold into an idea of *normal ageing*, particularly in the wake of COVID.[98, 99]

The difference-driving force of time undermines the imposition of a concept of averageness onto later life across almost all meaningful domains. We see aged heterogeneity borne out in the molecular nature of older brains and the psychic phenomena of older minds, which are diversely messy owing to lifetimes of idiosyncratic physiological and psychological occurrences. With this in mind, it becomes difficult to define the average neurocognitive state of an older person with any degree of specificity. Any average must be fairly broad to account for a multitude of factors. To meaningfully apply to ageing per se, "normal" ageing has to contain a lot of stuff, and in doing so, struggles to represent any particular person all that well. Turning to neurocognitive characteristics specifically, the required breadth hinders a binary normal/abnormal distinction because a broad average of ageing overlaps with a broad average of dementia. Therefore, one logical endpoint of a disease account of dementia based on quantified abnormality is that the category will unwittingly encompass a lot of ageing, while a corresponding notion of ageing as quantified normality will inadvertently overlap a lot of dementia.

Given that the differentiation of dementia and ageing is so empirically and conceptually problematic, the question inevitably arises of why a neuropsychiatric biopolitics of dementia remains so committed to it. At a practical level, the very fact that stakeholders are moved to reiterate the message indicates that the opposite belief – the conflation of dementia and ageing – is problematically prolific. As discussed above, for much of human history, a view that we might call "senility" has been relatively commonplace. Senility is the notion that cognitive decline is a natural experience of growing older. Of course, this basic belief is concurrent with much contemporary cognitive science. Where senility differs significantly is in its tendency to not differentiate ageing-related cognitive decline into normal and abnormal subcategories. Decline, in its varied manifestations, is broadly cast as a feature of ageing.

Such conceptualisations of cognitive ageing seem to be relatively common among people affected by dementia, as well as the public more broadly, and are often labelled "lay beliefs". Several studies have shown that large proportions of the general population believe that dementia is caused by ageing, though exact figures vary widely.[100–104] Similarly, I have often encountered senility beliefs when interviewing people affected by dementia about their experiences. However, the claim that people simply attribute dementia to ageing OR disease OR something else entirely misrepresents the complex and oftentimes seemingly contradictory composite understandings that I have found in my own research.[13] In practice, people can experience dementia as a confluence of ageing, disease, exposures, emotions and even psychological continuation. Nonetheless, a sizeable body of research characterises the public as subscribing to variations of senility. Neuropsychiatric appeals to normal ageing can hence be understood as a response to this observation.

Even if we take for granted a simplistic view that senility beliefs are widespread, we might still wonder why neuropsychiatric biopolitics offers such resistance. As discussed above, attributing phenomena to a discrete disease entity can legitimise those phenomena as a particular problem, catalysing action and resource accumulation. Looking back to the 1970s, Patrick Fox has attributed the NIA's promotion of a disease model to status and funding accrual. By centring on a disease, the NIA was able to fashion powerful alliances between researchers, government, advocates, the media and the public, which, as documented in Chapter 1, quickly facilitated an exponential increase in status and funding.[105] While a disease focus has proved successful in this sense, it is doubtful whether a more holistic, and therefore nebulous, ageing-based approach could have supported similar development.

Whether cognitive impairment is caused by a disease or ageing has intertwined conceptual and practical implications for research initiatives. Conceptually, people are generally more ambivalent toward the idea of seeking to treat or cure ageing.[106] Ageing-based initiatives could be hampered by sentiments that seeking to combat ageing is inappropriate, foolish or even outright dangerous. The conceptual issue of intervening in ageing feeds into institutional governance. Practically, the European Medicines Agency (EMA) and the FDA do not sanction research that does not target approved indications. Ageing is not recognised as such an indication due to the aforementioned uncertainties surrounding its quasi-disease status and broader ethical misgivings.[107, 108] Hence, significant sociopolitical considerations underpin the biopolitical differentiation of dementia and ageing. As historian Jesse Ballenger puts it: "Government funds research for dread disease, not for discovering the fountain of youth".[79] Ultimately, we can see the effectiveness of this strategy realised in the flourishing dementia economy that has emerged following the removal of age differentiation from AD. The importance of separating *abnormal* dementia from *normal* ageing provides a conceptual, ethical and administrative foundation for pursuing technical intervention. This leads us to a third claim at the heart of the neuropsychiatric biopolitics of dementia, the assertion that research will discover a cure.

4.3 "Research Will Discover a Cure"

The claim that research will eventually result in the development of cures for dementia is commonplace among the usual collection of stakeholders. It builds on the presentation of dementia as abnormal disease, as opposed to normal ageing. The former claims having established the logicalness, feasibility and rightfulness of pursuing technical interventions in dementia, promissory curative claims then shore up the prospects of such interventions. Appeals to future cures can be found across a familiar mix of voices:

> *Alzheimer's Society*: One day, research will cure dementia.[109]
> *David Cameron*: The aim of trying to find a cure or disease-halting therapy by 2025 by a big collective boost to research funding is within our grasp.[110]
> *Daily Mail*: Continued investment in research … will allow us to keep searching for ways to better treat and care for people with dementia today and, ultimately, find a cure for tomorrow.[111]
> *Bryan Cranston*: Research has already made great breakthroughs in other diseases, like cancer and AIDS, and with your support, Alzheimer's Research UK will break through against dementia.[6]

Such assertions are perhaps the most obviously questionable conceptual component of neuropsychiatric biopolitics. By explicitly appealing to a future that will be different from the present, the aura of scientific factuality is somewhat imperilled. We can perhaps accept that these stakeholders know disease and ageing in a definitive manner, but intuitively, it seems more of a stretch to accept that they know the future as well. Nonetheless, the assertion of particular futures is a mainstay of neuropsychiatric biopolitics. It is here, amidst the inevitability of scientific and technological progress, that dementia becomes a matter of promissory technoscience.

Notions of progress, whereby the future will be better than the present, are an important cultural conception. Indeed, abstract ideas of progress are often as publicly venerated as notions of justice, democracy and freedom.[112] Economic growth, computational speed, algorithm sophistication, medical precision, battery capacity – we are surrounded by depictions of progress and the futures that it is leading toward. Crucially, the idea of progress, and our exposure to it, is materially influential. The sociology of expectation has long revealed the power of the future to shape our presents.[112, 113] If a future is convincing enough, it can act as a lightning rod for resources dedicated to the realisation of that future. Contemporary tech investment is emblematic of the potential for faith in the future to catalyse resources. Well-known companies such as Airbnb, Dropbox and Uber have attained multi-billion-dollar valuations despite making huge losses, simply because investors believe that those losses will eventually be more than offset by major profits in the future. Hence, claims about the future, and belief in its progressive trajectory, are themselves the very means to arrive at that future.[114]

The coalescence of resources around a particular future has two major effects. It increases the likelihood of that future, and it decreases the likelihood of alternative futures. In particular, sociological studies of science and technology have documented the tendency for promissory technoscience to present possibilities in a manner that effectively colonises the future.[115] The possible becomes probable; the probable becomes predestined. A good example of this is the early-21st-century fascination with self-driving cars, which are repeatedly presented as a question of *when* rather than *if*.[116–119] The small autonomous vehicle is hence inevitable in many depictions. The continued reiteration of that particular inevitability can preclude alternative futures, futures that are perhaps more feasible and desirable, such as improved public transport. Conceptual investment in a future begets material investment in that future. The likelihood of Airbnb superseding regular B&Bs and Uber superseding regular taxis becomes more probable by virtue of the belief that it will happen, sometimes even at odds with the evidence. The colonisation of the future hence blends conceptual and material processes.

The colonisation of the future is not inherently a harmful phenomenon. Our subscription to the promise of brighter futures, irrespective of their actual feasibility, can be a major boon to our everyday lives and sustained societal cohesion. Many people invest great efforts in the development of children in the belief that this will pay dividends in the future. The opposite is also true. A lack of future promise can become a social problem in itself.

For example, pessimism about climate change prospects is repeatedly cited as contributing toward declining fertility, which itself endangers future societal prosperity.[120] In this manner, a lack of faith in the goodness of the future can lead to a damaging lack of investment in that future today, begetting a self-fulfilling prophecy. Many dementia studies scholars will be familiar with the notion of prescribed disengagement,[121] whereby nihilistic dementia diagnoses can rob people of their futures, leading them to prematurely shut down much of their lives (e.g. retiring and forfeiting driving licences), hastening a sort of social death. Hence, while hype is often misleading and warrants scepticism, disillusionment can also be costly.[113]

The promise of technoscientific solutions is a powerful normative ideal across many aspects of human life. In enforcing a particular schema onto a given phenomenon, such an ideal can effectively shut down alternatives. Sometimes this shutting down can be rendered visible through explicit contestation and active resistance. For instance, cochlear implants are often cast as a remarkable technoscientific fix for hearing impairment, which is hence demarcated as a problem to be solved. However, cochlear implants have angered some in the hearing-impaired and Deaf communities, for whom deafness is not a problem to be fixed but a different mode of existence.[115] Such tensions are explored in the film *Sound and Fury*, which documents the difficulties experienced by deaf parents when deciding whether to pursue cochlear implants for their deaf children. Here, we find a powerful example of how simplistic problem–solution narratives that typify promissory technoscience rely on peculiar normative commitments that are not inherently moral, natural or universal.

The tensions evident in *Sound and Fury* can be roughly transposed onto dementia and longstanding debates regarding the relations between care and cure, and the claim that a focus on curative futures impedes the realisation of caring presents. Such debates extend back to the beginnings of contemporary neuropsychiatric biopolitics in the 1970s. One of the earliest areas of contention in the fledgling AD movement concerned the extent to which their efforts should be distributed between cure-focused and care-focused endeavours. Key founding figures such as Robert Katzman and Robert Butler argued for a focus on basic science research to inform drug development. However, the movement was somewhat beholden to carer advocacy groups, who argued that resources should be focused on providing support and assistance. The future and the present were hence brought into tension. This conflict led to the withdrawal of grassroots groups during the early 1980s, leaving the movement to pursue a cure-focused strategy.[105]. Later that decade, when critiquing (bio)medicalisation, Karen Lyman bemoaned the lack of attention paid to care amidst the general emphasis on finding a cure, a criticism that remains common in dementia studies.[122] Today, of over 30,000 projects registered in the International Alzheimer's Disease Research Portfolio database, only 5% attend to care, compared with 45% on pathophysiology and drug discovery.[123]

Critics of the curative focus argue that vast resources have been squandered on pathogenic research and drug development based on poor and often disproven aetiological hypotheses, which has ultimately resulted in predictably high failure rates.[124] Those resources could have instead been dedicated to care provision, potentially making a significant material difference to the well-being of many people affected by dementia today. Such arguments can be enticing in hindsight. However, we should be wary of pursuing a zero-sum analysis of resource distribution, whereby curative funding would simply be redirected to care. In practice, as shown, promissory futures have material consequences for the present. They catalyse and, indeed, generate resources. It is likely that, without the appeal of future cures and the campaigns built around that future, dementia as a whole would not have gained the pronounced public profile and resource investment that it has enjoyed over recent decades. Hence, we cannot simply dismiss promissory biopolitics as folly or as somehow stealing resources that would otherwise be distributed elsewhere.

It is not uncommon for different stories about the future to compete in a promissory ecosystem in which one story comes to dominate. This promissory survival of the fittest incentivises optimistic exaggeration. To win over the popular imagination, the story must be as appealing as possible within the bounds of perceived feasibility.[113] In this manner, care can resemble public transport – dreary, boring and undesirable – while cure is the self-driving car – exciting, enticing and inevitable. A particular normative schema is at stake here, wherein problems are made material, and by extension amenable to technoscientific examination, intervention and optimisation.[115] A certain pseudo-religiosity is palpable: fund research to solve problems; make sacrifices to deliver us from evil. I do not mean this to be read as a simple argument for increasing care research at the expense of cure research or that cure research is in some way especially *bad* in this respect. Much care research is similarly promissory, albeit less financially successful, because research is by its very nature a material, intellectual and emotional appeal to future advancement. Rather, it simply exemplifies the normative commitments that underpin the promissory neuropsychiatric biopolitics of dementia, revealing that these normativities are doing real work and have material consequences for our present.

One particularly intriguing aspect of the futures invoked by the neuropsychiatric biopolitics of dementia, as with promissory technoscience more broadly, is that experience tells us that these futures often fail to live up to their promises, yet technoscientific expectations continue to colonise the future nonetheless.[113] For instance, the promise of anti-Aβ monoclonal antibodies that will cure dementia remains powerful despite decades of failure. Various expert and popular publications frequently celebrate the prospects of the latest research breakthrough,[125] but the developments in question are often slight variations on interventions with a long history of early promise and ultimate disappointment. In this manner, the successful cure of AD in mice[3] is repeatedly achieved in research projects and subsequently publicised as an important breakthrough, but curative successes in animal dementias have long been commonplace and have never been emulated in humans. This observation is too often overlooked in articles detailing the latest supposed breakthroughs. There is some risk in this strategy because the consistent failure of promises to materialise can eventually lead to disillusionment or scepticism, undermining the power of such promises. Hence, promissory biopolitics is always walking a time-limited tightrope when colonising the future.[113] Claim too much too loudly, and the future may hold you to account.

Social scientists often fail to reflect on their inadvertent complicity in colonising the future when they work on promissory technoscience.[114] This is equally evident in some dementia studies engagements with neuropsychiatric futures. For example, consider the publication of bioethical assessments of the pros and cons of developing early diagnosis technologies based on biomarkers.[126, 127] Though not intended as such, the publication of these works, which aim to assess a possible future, lends credibility to the idea that such tests will be developed and implemented. Indeed, this implicit enhancement of credibility is somewhat integral to the success of the papers themselves. A paper that evaluates a future that seems probable (e.g. pre-symptomatic dementia screening programmes) is more likely to prosper in the competitive ecosystem of academic publication and citation than a paper that evaluates a seemingly farfetched future (e.g. aliens visit the earth and cure all dementia instantly). Ultimately, the normative commitments of neuropsychiatric biopolitics are far less likely to be deconstructed and challenged if a neuroagnostic dementia studies is repeatedly complicit in perpetuating them.

None of this is to refute the prospects of dementia research to result in advances in quality of life. Instead, it is useful to consider promissory biopolitics in terms of proportionality.[113] Given our experience to date, in terms of dementia research specifically and age-associated morbidities generally, it seems highly unlikely that hard "silver bullet" claims – "research will discover a cure" – will be fully realised in practice.[128] Nonetheless, it does seem reasonable to assume that dementia research will lead to some improvements in some form. To this end, some critics argue that dementia research requires a recentring of clinically meaningful effect as a headline ambition.[129] By putting simplistic notions of a breakthrough cure to one side, we can pragmatically hope for gradual improvements in condition management, onset delay, tailored support, etc. That hope is important because, as discussed, expectation shapes the present, and by extension, the future. This is where the colonisation of the future is most problematic, because its shutting down of alternative futures can become an active impediment to realistic progress. Promissory technoscience does not steal money from care research as much as it positions care research as futile, weakening its abilities to generate its own promissory capacities. Hence, the concept of proportionality can offer a worthwhile foundation for neurocritical dementia studies as it engages with the contemporary hypes and frustrations of neuropsychiatric biopolitics.

Proportionality is also an important concept for considering what we actually want to achieve through our appeals to the future. Promissory technoscience can be misleading and feed into the squandering of resources on false promises at the expense of alternatives to some extent. However, as we have seen, the promise of brighter futures, even when perhaps unrealistic, can be integral to future prosperity itself. The neuropsychiatric biopolitics of dementia manifests this tension. Since the 1970s, vast resources have been dedicated to as-yet unrealised promises of curative therapeutics. However, dementia research as a whole is probably substantially more developed today than it would have been without an exaggerated and misleading biopolitics. While undoubtedly wasteful in some respects, it is not unlikely that some positives will emerge from the overall development of dementia research. For instance, while seemingly unrelated, it is questionable whether contemporary gains in rights for people with dementia[130] would have been as forthcoming without the publicity that dementia has attained, thanks to cure-focused disease-based lobbying by the NIA.

One ethically dubious feature of promissory neuropsychiatric biopolitics that is yet to be discussed but which certainly requires considerable reflection in terms of proportionality is the use of people's personal experiences as fodder for advocacy and advertisement. It is common for promissory biotechnologies generally to employ the personal illness stories of people affected by the condition that the technology promises to address. By emphasising the suffering caused by a certain condition, stakeholders can develop powerful moral rationales for the development of interventions.[113] Indeed, the NIA's successful promotion of AD was greatly aided by the publication of an emotive account of caring for a family member with dementia in a national newspaper in 1980. This piece prompted more than 30,000 letters of response and a groundswell of support for dementia research.[105] The approach remains powerful today. When the FDA advisory panel voted against aducanumab in 2020, the Alzheimer's Association organised a "listening event" based on the personal testimonials of several people affected by dementia. Many commentators believe that this event was influential in persuading the FDA to approve aducanumab in spite of the contrary expert panel advice (discussed at length in the next chapter).

Another interesting example of the use of personal stories to support promissory biopolitics can be found in ARUK's "Dementia Uncovered" webpage. This resource intersperses a series of short videos documenting personal accounts of dementia and scientists advocating the need for research into future cures.[131] The first video features a woman tearfully relaying the "heart-breaking" and "tragic" story of her mother's dementia, ending with the claim that "further research could stop this happening to other families". The second video features a doctor who believes that future treatments will be uncovered by research. His belief is spurred on by personal family experience of dementia and a desire for his 17-month-old daughter to live in a dementia-free world. The page's video clips continue in this manner, juxtaposing tragic presents and promissory futures from the individual's perspective.

Such activities are contentious. The presentation of traumatic personal experiences can be read as a form of exploitation whereby the lives of disadvantaged people are made amenable to the desires of powerful stakeholders. There is potentially an injustice in that the people whose stories are used will not benefit directly because the resources elicited are largely dedicated to future cures rather than present support. Dramatic and apocalyptic presentations of these experiences also risk exacerbating negative perceptions of the conditions in question and the people affected by them. Indeed, rising public fear of dementia has coincided with the proliferation of neuropsychiatric biopolitics.[132] This is an issue returned to at length in Chapter 6. However, again, while we might bemoan the exploitation of suffering for biopolitical purposes and the potential exacerbation of negative sentiment, it is equally probable that progress has been and will be made across diverse aspects of dementia because of these occurrences. In this manner, disparate facets of the dementia economy, however good or bad, are intricately entwined with one another. Guided by an appreciation of proportionality, critical dementia studies could seek to emphasise the good and minimise the bad, recognising that both are, to some extent, necessary.

* * *

One of the capacities that is most vital if a neurocritical dementia studies is to succeed in deconstructing and transforming the biopolitics of dementia is for us to fashion better relations with basic science and medical practice so as to be better able to robustly engage with biopolitics. This is difficult because, while it is somewhat distinct from and often at odds with basic science and clinical practice, biopolitics relies on and is good at fashioning a scientific and (bio)medical aura because biopolitics is an integral part of science and medicine to varying extents. We cannot simply divide the two. In this chapter, I have attempted to dissolve some of that aura. From a basic neuroscientific perspective, it is difficult to argue that most dementia is attributable to discrete disease, and the idea that ageing can be divided into normal and abnormal categories is untenable. Clinically, recognition of and engagement with the diversity of ageing is at the heart of good geriatric practice, while promises of future treatments are largely inconsequential to ensuring patient wellbeing today. Across science and medicine, researchers and clinicians hold and act upon a wide variety of definitions of dementia. The neuropsychiatric biopolitics of dementia – wherein dementia is caused by discrete diseases of the brain, is not a part of normal ageing and will be cured through research – is something altogether different. To return to the above definition, it is a proliferation of conceptual schemas that subtly guide personal conduct and order human life in ways that are conducive to certain political projects and interest groups.

Each of the claims discussed in this chapter is doing particular types of work. They have strong normative stakes. The claim that dementia is caused by discrete diseases of the brain works to emphasise its badness, drawing on the established normative schema of disease as bad.[133] It also indicates the probable amenability of that badness to technical interventions because other diseases have historically been addressed in a similar manner. The claim that dementia is not a normal part of ageing pushes back against the traditional normalisation of cognitive decline in later life, thereby demarcating dementia as deserving of intervention. It also resonates with the biopolitics of successful ageing, perpetuating moral imperatives for good citizens to take personal responsibility in crafting desirable forms of ageing based on consumption rather than welfare. The claim that research will discover a cure builds on the previous two claims and fosters a scientistic aesthetic to substantiate a route toward overcoming the badness of dementia and thereby ensure a successful, i.e. normal, later life. That route relies on resource accumulation by key stakeholders within the dementia research economy, who are hence incentivised to further the neuropsychiatric biopolitics of dementia.

Collectively, the claims covered in this chapter generate circumstances that are conducive to the interests of biopolitical stakeholders. Perhaps the most obvious instance of this conductivity can be found in the biomarker and drug development sectors, and it is to these issues that I will turn in the next chapter. For now, I hope that this chapter has exemplified how a neurocritical dementia studies can make use of insights from critical psychiatry and critical gerontology. As I have attempted herein, such engagement can be bolstered by attending to cognitive neuroscience and clinical medicine in combination with critical social theory. This is important because the resulting insights can reveal marked resonances, e.g. molecular and clinical evidence regarding senescence and critical gerontological theorisation of aged heterogeneity. Collectively, such observations provide a rich toolkit with which a neurocritical dementia studies can address the neuropsychiatric biopolitics of dementia.

Notes

1 I order them as such throughout because this is the order in which they are typically used by associated stakeholders and endeavours.
2 Given the above discussion of biogenic legitimacy, there are inevitably some people who pursue neural correlates for suicidal ideation, however tentatively[49, 50].
3 The existence of AD in mice is an intriguing issue in its own right and is returned to in the next chapter.

References

1. Daly, T. (2023). Don't call older adults' lifestyles "unfavourable." *BMJ 380*. doi: 10.1136/bmj-2022-072691.
2. Berrios, G.E., and Marková, I.S. (2002). The concept of neuropsychiatry: A historical overview. *Journal of Psychosomatic Research 53*, 629–638. doi: 10.1016/S0022-3999(02)00427-0.

3. Alzheimer's Society (2022). What is dementia? Alzheimer's Society. https://www.alzheimers.org.uk/about-dementia/types-dementia/what-is-dementia.

4. The Office of David Cameron, D. (2018). David Cameron addresses the World Dementia Council. The Office of David Cameron. https://www.davidcameronoffice.org/david-cameron-addresses-the-world-dementia-council/.

5. Morrison, R. (2021). AI can now predict who will develop DEMENTIA, study reveals. Mail Online. https://www.dailymail.co.uk/sciencetech/article-10317707/AI-accurately-predict-develop-dementia-two-years-study-suggests.html.

6. ARUK (2018). Bryan Cranston confronts misunderstanding of dementia … using an orange. Alzheimer's Research UK. https://www.alzheimersresearchuk.org/bryan-cranston-confronts-misunderstanding-dementiausing-orange/.

7. Ballenger, J.F. (2017). Framing confusion: Dementia, society, and history. *AMA Journal of Ethics 19*, 713–719. doi: 10.1001/journalofethics.2017.19.7.mhst1-1707.

8. Rosenberg, C.E. (2002). The Tyranny of diagnosis: Specific entities and individual experience. *The Milbank Quarterly 80*, 237–260. doi: 10.1111/1468-0009.t01-1-00003.

9. Bzdok, D., and Meyer-Lindenberg, A. (2018). Machine learning for precision psychiatry: Opportunities and challenges. *Biological Psychiatry: Cognitive Neuroscience and Neuroimaging 3*, 223–230. doi: 10.1016/j.bpsc.2017.11.007.

10. Gupta, A. (2006). *Empiricism and Experience*. Oxford University Press.

11. Goff, P. (2019). *Galileo's Error: Foundations for a New Science of Consciousness*. Rider.

12. Temkin, O. (1963). The scientific approach to disease: Specific entity and individual sickness. In: A. C. Crombie (ed.), *Scientific Change: Historical Studies in the Intellectual, Social and Technical Conditions for Scientific Discovery and Technical Invention, from Antiquity to the Present*. Heinemann, pp. 629–647.

13. Fletcher, J.R. (2020). Mythical dementia and Alzheimerised senility: Discrepant and intersecting representations of cognitive decline in later life. *Social Theory & Health 18*, 50–65. doi: 10.1057/s41285-019-00117-w.

14. NIMH (2022). The NIMH strategic plan for research: An overview. National Institute of Mental Health. https://www.nimh.nih.gov/health/publications/strategic-plan-for-research.

15. Gupta, M. (2019). Mental illness is not a myth: Epistemic favoritism in research funding. In: C. V. Haldipur, J. L. Knoll, and E. V. D. Luft (eds.), *Thomas Szasz: An Appraisal of His Legacy*. Oxford University Press.

16. Nettleton, S. (2006). 'I just want permission to be ill': Towards a sociology of medically unexplained symptoms. *Social Science & Medicine 62*, 1167–1178. doi: 10.1016/j.socscimed.2005.07.030.

17. Fox, P. (1989). From senility to Alzheimer's disease: The rise of the Alzheimer's disease movement. *The Milbank Quarterly 67*, 58–102. doi: 10.2307/3350070.

18. Critchley, M. (1929). Critical review. *Journal of Neurology and Psychopathology 10*, 124–139.

19. Sachdev, P.S., Blacker, D., Blazer, D.G., Ganguli, M., Jeste, D.V., Paulsen, J.S., and Petersen, R.C. (2014). Classifying neurocognitive disorders: The DSM-5 approach. *Nature Reviews Neurology 10*, 634–642. doi: 10.1038/nrneurol.2014.181.

20. Higgs, P., and Gilleard, C. (2016). Interrogating personhood and dementia. *Aging & Mental Health 20*, 773–780. doi: 10.1080/13607863.2015.1118012.
21. Brain Health Scotland. https://www.alzscot.org/brain-health-scotland.
22. Beard, R.L. (2016). *Living with Alzheimer's: Managing Memory Loss, Identity, and Illness.* New York University Press.
23. Milne, R., Diaz, A., Badger, S., Bunnik, E., Fauria, K., and Wells, K. (2018). At, with and beyond risk: Expectations of living with the possibility of future dementia. *Sociology of Health & Illness 40*, 969–987. doi: 10.1111/1467-9566.12731.
24. Swallow, J. (2017). Expectant futures and an early diagnosis of Alzheimer's disease: Knowing and its consequences. *Social Science & Medicine 184*, 57–64. doi: 10.1016/j.socscimed.2017.05.017.
25. McKhann, G.M., Knopman, D.S., Chertkow, H., Hyman, B.T., Jack Jr., C.R., Kawas, C.H., Klunk, W.E., Koroshetz, W.J., Manly, J.J., Mayeux, R., et al. (2011). The diagnosis of dementia due to Alzheimer's disease: Recommendations from the National Institute on Aging-Alzheimer's Association workgroups on diagnostic guidelines for Alzheimer's disease. *Alzheimer's & Dementia 7*, 263–269. doi: 10.1016/j.jalz.2011.03.005.
26. Kuehn, B.M. (2015). The brain fights back: New approaches to mitigating cognitive decline. *JAMA 314*, 2492–2494. doi: 10.1001/jama.2015.15390.
27. Richard, E., Schmand, B., Eikelenboom, P., Westendorp, R.G., and Van Gool, W.A. (2012). The Alzheimer myth and biomarker research in Dementia. *Journal of Alzheimer's Disease 31* Supplement 3, S203–S209. doi: 10.3233/JAD-2012-112216.
28. Richards, M., and Brayne, C. (2010). What do we mean by Alzheimer's disease? *BMJ 341*, c4670. doi: 10.1136/bmj.c4670.
29. Scheltens, P., and Rockwood, K. (2011). How golden is the gold standard of neuropathology in dementia? *Alzheimer's & Dementia 7*, 486–489. doi: 10.1016/j.jalz.2011.04.011.
30. Zhang, M., Ganz, A.B., Rohde, S., Rozemuller, A.J.M., Bank, N.B., Reinders, M.J.T., Scheltens, P., Hulsman, M., Hoozemans, J.J.M., and Holstege, H. (2022). Resilience and resistance to the accumulation of amyloid plaques and neurofibrillary tangles in centenarians: An age-continuous perspective. *Alzheimer's & Dementia.* doi: 10.1002/alz.12899.
31. Giannakopoulos, P., Herrmann, F.R., Bussière, T., Bouras, C., Kövari, E., Perl, D.P., Morrison, J.H., Gold, G., and Hof, P.R. (2003). Tangle and neuron numbers, but not amyloid load, predict cognitive status in Alzheimer's disease. *Neurology 60*, 1495–1500. doi: 10.1212/01.WNL.0000063311.58879.01.
32. Jung, Y., Whitwell, J.L., Duffy, J.R., Strand, E.A., Machulda, M.M., Senjem, M.L., Jack, C.R., Lowe, V.J., and Josephs, K.A. (2016). Regional β-amyloid burden does not correlate with cognitive or language deficits in Alzheimer's disease presenting as aphasia. *European Journal of Neurology 23*, 313–319. doi: 10.1111/ene.12761.
33. Aizenstein, H.J., Nebes, R.D., Saxton, J.A., Price, J.C., Mathis, C.A., Tsopelas, N.D., Ziolko, S.K., James, J.A., Snitz, B.E., Houck, P.R., et al. (2008). Frequent amyloid deposition without significant cognitive impairment among the elderly. *Archives of Neurology 65*, 1509–1517. doi: 10.1001/archneur.65.11.1509.
34. Bennett, D.A., Schneider, J.A., Arvanitakis, Z., Kelly, J.F., Aggarwal, N.T., Shah, R.C., and Wilson, R.S. (2006). Neuropathology of older persons without

cognitive impairment from two community-based studies. *Neurology 66*, 1837–1844. doi: 10.1212/01.wnl.0000219668.47116.e6.

35. Høilund-Carlsen, P.F., Barrio, J.R., Gjedde, A., Werner, T.J., and Alavi, A. (2018). Circular inference in Dementia diagnostics. *Journal of Alzheimer's Disease 63*, 69–73. doi: 10.3233/JAD-180050.

36. Bouwman, F.H., Schoonenboom, N.S.M., Verwey, N.A., van Elk, E.J., Kok, A., Blankenstein, M.A., Scheltens, P., and van der Flier, W.M. (2009). CSF biomarker levels in early and late onset Alzheimer's disease. *Neurobiology of Aging 30*, 1895–1901. doi: 10.1016/j.neurobiolaging.2008.02.007.

37. Price, J.L., McKeel, D.W., Buckles, V.D., Roe, C.M., Xiong, C., Grundman, M., Hansen, L.A., Petersen, R.C., Parisi, J.E., Dickson, D.W., et al. (2009). Neuropathology of nondemented aging: Presumptive evidence for preclinical Alzheimer disease. *Neurobiology of Aging 30*, 1026–1036. doi: 10.1016/j.neurobiolaging.2009.04.002.

38. Fletcher, J.R., and Birk, R.H. (2019). Circularity, psychiatry & biomarkers: The operationalisation of Alzheimer's & stress in research. *Social Science & Medicine 239*, 112553. doi: 10.1016/j.socscimed.2019.112553.

39. Hunter, S. (2018). What is Aβ? *Journal of Alzheimer's Disease*. https://www.j-alz.com/editors-blog/posts/what-abeta.

40. Childs, B.G., Durik, M., Baker, D.J., and van Deursen, J.M. (2015). Cellular senescence in aging and age-related disease: From mechanisms to therapy. *Nature Medicine 21*, 1424–1435. doi: 10.1038/nm.4000.

41. Nelson, P.T., Braak, H., and Markesbery, W.R. (2009). Neuropathology and cognitive impairment in Alzheimer disease: A complex but coherent relationship. *Journal of Neuropathology & Experimental Neurology 68*, 1–14. doi: 10.1097/NEN.0b013e3181919a48.

42. Oh, H., Madison, C., Villeneuve, S., Markley, C., and Jagust, W.J. (2014). Association of gray matter atrophy with age, β-Amyloid, and cognition in aging. *Cerebral Cortex 24*, 1609–1618. doi: 10.1093/cercor/bht017.

43. Taylor, K. (2016). *The Fragile Brain: The Strange, Hopeful Science of dementia*. Oxford University Press.

44. Braak, H., Thal, D.R., Ghebremedhin, E., and Del Tredici, K. (2011). Stages of the pathologic process in Alzheimer disease: Age categories from 1 to 100 years. *Journal of Neuropathology & Experimental Neurology 70*, 960–969. doi: 10.1097/NEN.0b013e318232a379.

45. Tomlinson, B.E., Blessed, G., and Roth, M. (1968). Observations on the brains of non-demented old people. *Journal of the Neurological Sciences 7*, 331–356. doi: 10.1016/0022-510X(68)90154-8.

46. Tomlinson, B.E., Blessed, G., and Roth, M. (1970). Observations on the brains of demented old people. *Journal of the Neurological Sciences 11*, 205–242. doi: 10.1016/0022-510X(70)90063-8.

47. Leibing, A. (2016). On short cuts: The complexity of studying the early diagnosis and prevention of Alzheimer's disease. In: M. Boenink, H. van Lente, and E. Moors (eds.), *Emerging Technologies for Diagnosing Alzheimer's Disease: Innovating with Care*. Palgrave Macmillan, pp. 41–61. doi: 10.1057/978-1-137-54097-3_3.

48. Szasz, T.S. (1972). *The Myth of Mental Illness*. HarperCollins.

49. Ballard, E.D., Lally, N., Nugent, A.C., Furey, M.L., Luckenbaugh, D.A., and Zarate, C.A., Jr (2015). Neural correlates of suicidal ideation and its reduction

in depression. *International Journal of Neuropsychopharmacology 18*, 1–6. doi: 10.1093/ijnp/pyu069.

50. Auerbach, R.P., Pagliaccio, D., Allison, G.O., Alqueza, K.L., and Alonso, M.F. (2021). Neural correlates associated with suicide and nonsuicidal self-injury in youth. *Biological Psychiatry 89*, 119–133. doi: 10.1016/j.biopsych.2020.06.002.

51. Alzheimer's Society (2022). Five things you should know about dementia. Alzheimer's Society. https://www.alzheimers.org.uk/about-dementia/five-things-you-should-know-about-dementia.

52. Russell, A. (2017). David Cameron: I saw a world of darkness getting bigger and bigger. *Financial Times*. https://www.ft.com/content/7e16fd9e-d673-11e7-8c9a-d9c0a5c8d5c9.

53. Cannon, D.E. (2020). Dementia ISN'T part of old age - Nearly HALF of cases can be avoided. Mail Online. https://www.dailymail.co.uk/health/article-8583387/DR-ELLIE-CANNON-Dementia-ISNT-just-old-age-nearly-HALF-cases-avoided.html.

54. ARUK (2018). Alzheimer's Research UK's #ShareTheOrange with Bryan Cranston. Alzheimer's Research UK. https://www.youtube.com/watch?v=HvCBSGLD1HA.

55. Alzheimer's Society (2022). Normal ageing vs dementia. Alzheimer's Society. https://www.alzheimers.org.uk/about-dementia/symptoms-and-diagnosis/how-dementia-progresses/normal-ageing-vs-dementia.

56. Guerreiro, R., and Bras, J. (2015). The age factor in Alzheimer's disease. *Genome Medicine 7*, 106. doi: 10.1186/s13073-015-0232-5.

57. Ganguli, M., and Rodriguez, E. (2011). Age, Alzheimer's disease, and the big picture. *International Psychogeriatrics 23*, 1531–1534. doi: 10.1017/S1041610211001906.

58. Hebert, L.E., Weuve, J., Scherr, P.A., and Evans, D.A. (2013). Alzheimer disease in the United States (2010–2050) estimated using the 2010 census. *Neurology 80*, 1778–1783. doi: 10.1212/WNL.0b013e31828726f5.

59. Comfort, A. (1920). *The Biology of Senescence*. Rinehart.

60. Kirkwood, T.B.L. (2005). Understanding the odd science of aging. *Cell 120*, 437–447. doi: 10.1016/j.cell.2005.01.027.

61. Tchkonia, T., and Kirkland, J.L. (2018). Aging, cell senescence, and chronic disease: Emerging therapeutic strategies. *JAMA 320*, 1319–1320. doi: 10.1001/jama.2018.12440.

62. Jin, K. (2010). Modern biological theories of aging. *Aging and Disease 1*, 72–74.

63. Gawande, A. (2015). *Being Mortal: Illness, Medicine and What Matters in the End*. Profile Books Ltd.

64. Chinta, S.J., Woods, G., Rane, A., Demaria, M., Campisi, J., and Andersen, J.K. (2015). Cellular senescence and the aging brain. *Experimental Gerontology 68*, 3–7. doi: 10.1016/j.exger.2014.09.018.

65. Salthouse, T.A. (2009). When does age-related cognitive decline begin? *Neurobiology of Aging 30*, 507–514. doi: 10.1016/j.neurobiolaging.2008.09.023.

66. Lees, H., Walters, H., and Cox, L.S. (2016). Animal and human models to understand ageing. *Maturitas 93*, 18–27. doi: 10.1016/j.maturitas.2016.06.008.

67. Abrahams, S., Haylett, W.L., Johnson, G., Carr, J.A., and Bardien, S. (2019). Antioxidant effects of curcumin in models of neurodegeneration, aging, oxidative and nitrosative stress: A review. *Neuroscience 406*, 1–21. doi: 10.1016/j.neuroscience.2019.02.020.

68. Castellani, R.J., Lee, H.-G., Zhu, X., Nunomura, A., Perry, G., and Smith, M.A. (2006). Neuropathology of Alzheimer disease: Pathognomonic but not pathogenic. *Acta Neuropathologica 111*, 503–509. doi: 10.1007/s00401-006-0071-y.

69. Castellani, R.J., Lee, H., Zhu, X., Perry, G., and Smith, M.A. (2008). Alzheimer disease pathology as a host response. *Journal of Neuropathology & Experimental Neurology 67*, 523–531. doi: 10.1097/NEN.0b013e318177eaf4.

70. Castellani, R.J., and Perry, G. (2014). The complexities of the pathology–pathogenesis relationship in Alzheimer disease. *Biochemical Pharmacology 88*, 671–676. doi: 10.1016/j.bcp.2014.01.009.

71. Herrup, K. (2021). *How Not to Study a Disease: The Story of Alzheimer's*. MIT Press.

72. Vernooij, M.W., and Barkhof, F. (2019). Neuroimaging in normal brain aging. In: F. Barkhof, H. R. Jäger, M. M. Thurnher, and À. Rovira (eds.), *Clinical Neuroradiology: The ESNR Textbook*. Springer International Publishing, pp. 1277–1293. doi: 10.1007/978-3-319-68536-6_63.

73. NGMRC (2001). Pathological correlates of late-onset dementia in a multicentre, community-based population in England and Wales. Neuropathology Group of the Medical Research Council Cognitive Function and Ageing Study (MRC CFAS). *Lancet 357*, 169–175. doi: 10.1016/s0140-6736(00)03589-3.

74. Selvackadunco, S., Langford, K., Shah, Z., Hurley, S., Bodi, I., King, A., Aarsland, D., Troakes, C., and Al-Sarraj, S. (2019). Comparison of clinical and neuropathological diagnoses of neurodegenerative diseases in two centres from the Brains for Dementia Research (BDR) cohort. *Journal of Neural Transmission 126*, 327–337. doi: 10.1007/s00702-018-01967-w.

75. Lock, M. (2013). *The Alzheimer Conundrum: Entanglements of Dementia and Aging*. Princeton University Press.

76. Jellinger, K.A. (2010). Con: Can neuropathology really confirm the exact diagnosis? *Alzheimer's Research & Therapy 2*, 11. doi: 10.1186/alzrt34.

77. Coulthard, E.J., and Love, S. (2018). A broader view of dementia: Multiple co-pathologies are the norm. *Brain 141*, 1894–1897. doi: 10.1093/brain/awy153.

78. Whitehouse, P.J., and George, D.R. (2008). *The Myth of Alzheimer's: What You Aren't Being Told About Today's Most Dreaded Diagnosis*. St. Martin's Griffin.

79. Ballenger, J. (2010). DSM-5: Continuing the confusion about aging, Alzheimer's and Dementia. *Psychiatric Times*. https://www.psychiatrictimes.com/view/dsm-5-continuing-confusion-about-aging-alzheimers-and-dementia.

80. Whalley, L.J. (2002). Brain ageing and dementia: What makes the difference? *The British Journal of Psychiatry 181*, 369–371. doi: 10.1192/bjp.181.5.369.

81. Nelson, P.T., Dickson, D.W., Trojanowski, J.Q., Jack, C.R., Boyle, P.A., Arfanakis, K., Rademakers, R., Alafuzoff, I., Attems, J., Brayne, C., et al. (2019). Limbic-predominant age-related TDP-43 encephalopathy (LATE): Consensus working group report. *Brain 142*, 1503–1527. doi: 10.1093/brain/awz099.

82. Lo, R.Y. (2017). The borderland between normal aging and dementia. *Tzu-Chi Medical Journal 29*, 65–71. doi: 10.4103/tcmj.tcmj_18_17.

83. Boller, F., and Forbes, M.M. (1998). History of dementia and dementia in history: An overview. *Journal of the Neurological Sciences 158*, 125–133. doi: 10.1016/S0022-510X(98)00128-2.

84. Albert, M.L., and Mildworf, B. (1989). The concept of dementia. *Journal of Neurolinguistics 4*, 301–308. doi: 10.1016/0911-6044(89)90022-5.

85. Fukui, T. (2015). Historical review of academic concepts of dementia in the world and Japan: With a short history of representative diseases. *Neurocase 21*, 369–376. doi: 10.1080/13554794.2014.894532.

86. Yang, H.D., Kim, D.H., Lee, S.B., and Young, L.D. (2016). History of Alzheimer's disease. *Dementia and Neurocognitive Disorders 15*, 115–121. doi: 10.12779/dnd.2016.15.4.115.

87. Barrett, A. (1913). A case of Alzheimer's disease with unusual neurological disturbances. *The Journal of Nervous and Mental Disease 40*, 361–374. doi: 10.1097/00005053-191306000-00001.

88. Fuller, S.C., and Klopp, H.I. (1912). Further observations on Alzheimer's disease. *American Journal of Insanity 69*, 17–29.

89. Katzman, R., and Karasu, T. (1975). Differential diagnosis of dementia. In: W. S. Fields (ed.), *Neurological and Sensory Disorders in the Elderly*. Stratton Intercontinental Medical Book Corp.

90. Leibing, A., and Cohen, L. (2006). *Thinking about Dementia: Culture, Loss, and the Anthropology of Senility*. Rutgers University Press.

91. Rachner, T.D., Khosla, S., and Hofbauer, L.C. (2011). Osteoporosis: Now and the future. *The Lancet 377*, 1276–1287. doi: 10.1016/S0140-6736(10) 62349-5.

92. Canguilhem, G., and Foucault, M. (1991). *The Normal and the Pathological*. Zone Books.

93. Wilson, D. (2014). Quantifying the quiet epidemic: Diagnosing dementia in late 20th-century Britain. *History of the Human Sciences 27*, 126–146. doi: 10.1177/0952695114536715.

94. Wilson, D. (2017). Calculable people? Standardising assessment guidelines for Alzheimer's disease in 1980s Britain. *Medical History 61*, 500–524. doi: 10.1017/mdh.2017.56.

95. Dannefer, D. (1987). Aging as intracohort differentiation: Accentuation, the Matthew effect, and the life course. *Sociological Forum 2*, 211–236. doi: 10.1007/BF01124164.

96. Stone, M.E., Lin, J., Dannefer, D., and Kelley-Moore, J.A. (2017). The continued eclipse of heterogeneity in gerontological research. *The Journals of Gerontology: Series B 72*, 162–167. doi: 10.1093/geronb/gbv068.

97. Ferraro, K.F., and Shippee, T.P. (2009). Aging and cumulative inequality: How does inequality get under the skin? *The Gerontologist 49*, 333–343. doi: 10.1093/geront/gnp034.

98. Grenier, A. (2022). *Late-Life Homelessness: Experiences of Disadvantage and Unequal Aging*. McGill-Queen's Press.

99. Gonyea, J.G., and Grenier, A. (2021). Precarity in later life: Understanding risk, vulnerability, and resilence. *Generations: Journal of the American Society on Aging 45*, 1–12.

100. Anderson, L.N., McCaul, K.D., and Langley, L.K. (2011). Common-sense beliefs about the prevention of Alzheimer's disease. *Aging & Mental Health 15*, 922–931. doi: 10.1080/13607863.2011.569478.

101. Blay, S.L., and Piza Peluso, É. de T. (2008). The public's ability to recognize Alzheimer disease and their beliefs about its causes. *Alzheimer Disease & Associated Disorders 22*, 79–85. doi: 10.1097/WAD.0b013e31815ccd47.

102. Connell, C.M., Scott Roberts, J., and McLaughlin, S.J. (2007). Public opinion about Alzheimer disease among blacks, hispanics, and whites: Results from a National survey. *Alzheimer Disease & Associated Disorders 21*, 232–240. doi: 10.1097/WAD.0b013e3181461740.

103. Werner, P. (2005). Lay perceptions about mental health: Where is age and where is Alzheimer's disease? *International Psychogeriatrics 17*, 371–382. doi: 10.1017/S1041610205002255.

104. Zeng, F., Xie, W.-T., Wang, Y.-J., Luo, H.-B., Shi, X.-Q., Zou, H.-Q., Zeng, Y.-Q., Li, Y.-F., Zhang, S.-R., and Lian, Y. (2015). General public perceptions and attitudes toward Alzheimer's disease from five cities in China. *Journal of Alzheimer's Disease 43*, 511–518. doi: 10.3233/JAD-141371.

105. Fox, P. (1989). From senility to Alzheimer's disease: The rise of the Alzheimer's disease movement. *The Milbank Quarterly*, 58–102.

106. Partridge, B., Lucke, J., Bartlett, H., and Hall, W. (2011). Public attitudes towards human life extension by intervening in ageing. *Journal of Aging Studies 25*, 73–83. doi: 10.1016/j.jaging.2010.08.012.

107. Newman, J.C., Milman, S., Hashmi, S.K., Austad, S.N., Kirkland, J.L., Halter, J.B., and Barzilai, N. (2016). Strategies and challenges in clinical trials targeting human aging. *The Journals of Gerontology: Series A 71*, 1424–1434. doi: 10.1093/gerona/glw149.

108. Stambler, I. (2017). Recognizing degenerative aging as a treatable medical condition: Methodology and policy. *Aging and Disease 8*, 583–589. doi: 10.14336/AD.2017.0130.

109. Alzheimer's Society (2022). Early career researchers: You are the future of dementia research. *Alzheimer's Society*. https://www.alzheimers.org.uk/for -researchers/early-career-researchers-future-dementia-research.

110. Agency, S. (2013). Dementia cure "within our grasp", says David Cameron. https://www.standard.co.uk/news/health/dementia-cure-within-our-grasp-says -david-cameron-8998487.html.

111. Willgress, L. (2016). Sir Tony Robinson tells of anguish of losing parents to dementia. Mail Online. https://www.dailymail.co.uk/news/article-3391451 /Time-Team-star-Sir-Tony-Robinson-tells-anguish-losing-parents-dementia .html.

112. Brown, N., and Michael, M. (2003). A sociology of expectations: Retrospecting prospects and prospecting retrospects. *Technology Analysis & Strategic Management 15*, 3–18. doi: 10.1080/0953732032000046024.

113. Brown, N. (2003). Hope against hype - Accountability in biopasts, presents and futures. *Science & Technology Studies 16*, 3–21. doi: 10.23987/sts.55152.

114. Williams, S.J., Martin, P., and Gabe, J. (2011). The pharmaceuticalisation of society? A framework for analysis. *Sociology of Health & Illness 33*, 710–725. doi: 10.1111/j.1467-9566.2011.01320.x.

115. Pellizzoni, L. (2017). Intensifying embroilments: Technosciences, imaginaries and publics. *Public Understanding of Science 26*, 212–219. doi: 10.1177/0963662516663563.

116. Igini, M. (2022). Environmental pros and cons of self-driving cars. *Earth.Org*. https://earth.org/pros-and-cons-of-self-driving-cars/.

117. AutoTechInsight (2015). Auto Tech Report - Autonomous Driving: Question is when, not if. *AutoTechInsight*. https://autotechinsight.ihsmarkit.com/shop/ product/606/auto-tech-report-autonomous-driving-question-is-when-not-if.

118. Meyerson, B. (2016). Face it: You're a worse driver than an autonomous car. *World Economic Forum*. https://www.weforum.org/agenda/2016/06/autonomous-vehicles/.
119. Holley, P. (2018). Here's what happens when police pull over a driverless car. *Washington Post*. https://www.washingtonpost.com/technology/2018/10/24/heres-what-happens-when-police-pull-over-driverless-car/.
120. Schneider-Mayerson, M., and Leong, K.L. (2020). Eco-reproductive concerns in the age of climate change. *Climatic Change 163*, 1007–1023. doi: 10.1007/s10584-020-02923-y.
121. Swaffer, K. (2015). Dementia and prescribed dis-engagement. *Dementia 14*, 3–6. doi: 10.1177/1471301214548136.
122. Lyman, K.A. (1989). Bringing the social back. In: *A Critique of the Biomedicalization of Dementia. The Gerontologist 29*, 597–605. doi: 10.1093/geront/29.5.597.
123. Wong, G., and Knapp, M. (2020). Should we move dementia research funding from a cure to its care? *Expert Review of Neurotherapeutics 20*, 303–305. doi: 10.1080/14737175.2020.1735364.
124. Caspi, E. (2019). Trust at stake: Is the "dual mission" of the U.S. Alzheimer's Association out of balance? *Dementia 18*, 1629–1650. doi: 10.1177/1471301217719789.
125. BBC (2021). New Alzheimer's treatment hailed by researchers. BBC News. https://www.bbc.com/news/uk-england-leicestershire-59338044.
126. Li, X., Ng, K.P., Ba, M., Rosa-Neto, P., and Gauthier, S. (2017). Dementia and bioethics. In: H. Chiu and K. Shulman (eds.), *Mental Health and Illness of the Elderly Mental health and illness worldwide*. Springer, pp. 141–153. doi: 10.1007/978-981-10-2414-6_6.
127. Vanderschaeghe, G., Dierickx, K., and Vandenberghe, R. (2018). Review of the ethical issues of a biomarker-based diagnoses in the early stage of Alzheimer's disease. *Bioethical Inquiry 15*, 219–230. doi: 10.1007/s11673-018-9844-y.
128. Mastroleo, I., and Daly, T. (2021). Avoiding exceptionalism and silver bullets: Lessons from public health ethics and Alzheimer's disease. *The American Journal of Bioethics 21*, 25–28. doi: 10.1080/15265161.2021.1991049.
129. Liu, K.Y., Thambisetty, M., and Howard, R. (2022). How can secondary dementia prevention trials of Alzheimer's disease be clinically meaningful? *Alzheimer's & Dementia n/a*. doi: 10.1002/alz.12788.
130. WHO (2021). Towards a dementia inclusive society. *World Health Organisation*. https://www.who.int/publications-detail-redirect/9789240031531.
131. ARUK (2019). Dementia uncovered. Alzheimer's Research UK. https://www.alzheimersresearchuk.org/dementiauncovered/.
132. Fletcher, J.R. (2021). Destigmatising dementia: The dangers of felt stigma and benevolent othering. *Dementia 20*, 417–426. doi: 10.1177/1471301219884821.
133. Cooper, R. (2002). Disease. *Studies in History and Philosophy of Science Part C: Studies in History and Philosophy of Biological and Biomedical Sciences 33*, 263–282. doi: 10.1016/S0039-3681(02)00018-3.

5 Making Dementia Curable

Circling Cognition, Biomarkers and Meaningfulness

This chapter begins where the previous one ended, with the promise of future pharmaceutical cures for the dementias. So far, we have taken "cure" as a rather self-explanatory concept, denoting the overcoming of the affliction in question. Here, I want to make "cure" far more malleable. To do so, I consider two key issues: the nature of the problem that we seek to solve and the nature of what it would mean for that problem to be solved. Ultimately, these are questions of what matters, to whom and why. Too often, biopolitics can make dementia meaningful to corporate stakeholders and thereby serve their concerns first and foremost. At worst, this can be at odds with, and potentially detrimental to, the interests of people affected by dementia. In response, I argue that a neurocritical dementia studies should attempt to reimpose those interests on dementia and dementia research. I hence advocate a reappropriation of dementia.

In the first section, I provide an overview of the contemporary push for a cure by 2025 and the initiatives that have grown around that ambition. These initiatives have contributed to a high-stakes research field, characterised by an intimidating failure rate but promising rich rewards for the first companies to develop successful treatments. The field has recently been ignited by the FDA approval of aducanumab, the first disease-modifying treatment for AD, and the controversies that have emerged around it. I argue that aducanumab represents a triumph of neuropsychiatric biopolitics over traditional scientific and clinical considerations and that this story exemplifies the capacity – and indeed necessity – for dementia studies to respond to the issues raised (e.g. corporate collusion, lobbying and data misrepresentation) if only it can abandon its neuro-agnosticism.

In the second section, I explore how the repeated failure of clinical trials has led to the reconfiguration of dementia in relation to both biomarkers and the lifecourse. Dementia drug discovery is characterised by growing interest in presymptomatic neuropathology and the development of molecular landmarks to circumvent the unreliability of cognition as a basis for operationalising dementia. I suggest that

DOI: 10.4324/9781003398523-5

the move away from cognition and toward biomarkers represents a marked transformation of dementia as a technoscientific problem. The result is a new molecular imagining of dementia that is freed from the messiness of cognition and ageing and is therefore more amenable to traditional drug discovery research and the development of pharmaceutical products. Rather than finding a treatment that addresses dementia, dementia is made to fit the treatment.

Drawing on critical psychiatry, I argue that, in decoupling dementia from cognition, contemporary biomarker and drug discovery initiatives risk diagnosing and curing dementias, without having any meaningful impact on cognitive decline. In this context, it is increasingly difficult for trials to fail because the meanings of "failure" and "success" are themselves being reconfigured. In response to classic arguments that the amyloid hypothesis has become "too big to fail", I instead argue that neuropsychiatric biopolitics is transforming dementia into a new type of problem that is, to some extent, too small to fail. That is, dementia is increasingly defined in such an abstract and limited manner as to be easily remediable. The danger here is that such remedies will offer little to people affected by what we would traditionally consider to be dementia. Finally, I consider the recent case of the drug lecanemab, which further complicates the question of how we understand success as our outcomes are made smaller.

5.1 Drug Discovery, or Aducanumab

As dementia has grown in notoriety over recent decades, the prospect of a cure has become a holy grail in the pharmaceutical industry. The growth of dementia diagnoses across wealthy and ageing welfare states means that the first company to develop an effective treatment will reap vast financial returns. In December 2013, a dedicated G8 summit in London committed to a programme of increased dementia research funding with the goal of developing a cure or disease-modifying treatment by 2025.[1] This led to the creation of the Dementia Discovery Fund, a specialist investment fund that backs dementia-related therapeutic ventures and is currently worth £250 million.[2] In addition to fostering international corporate efforts, G8 states launched their own drug discovery initiatives. The British government established the UK Dementia Research Institute, providing £290 million of public and third-sector funding to therapeutic research.[3].

While a great deal of public and charitable funding is available, dementia drug discovery remains a high-stakes field for the pharmaceutical industry. Much of the Dementia Discovery Fund comes directly from these companies. The rewards for success will undoubtedly be huge, but success seems unlikely in the immediate future, and the costs of sustaining research programmes are substantial. AD ranks among the areas of drug discovery most blighted by failures, having a 99.6% failure rate among phase-III trials.[4] Each of these failed late-stage trials represents a substantial investment of capital, both financial and human, and generates a sense of foreboding regarding our prospects in the immediate future. In 2018, Pfizer, the second biggest pharmaceutical company in the world, opted to end its work in dementia drug discovery following a comprehensive review.[5] Though by no means signalling the death of dementia drug discovery, Pfizer's decision is indicative of the daunting scale of the task and the very real possibility that vast investments may never see a return. If an investor's aim is to back a successful treatment, then AD drug development offers relatively poor prospects.

This is terrible news for both drug companies and people affected by dementia. In Europe, only four treatments are typically used. These are all short-term symptom-modifying medications with substantial side effect profiles, the last of which was approved in 2003.[6–10] All but one of these are the acetylcholinesterase inhibitors discussed in Chapter 2. As noted, it was initially hoped, based on a collection of post-mortem and animal model evidence, that these treatments would prove to be disease-modifying and offer substantial results. However, those early hopes have failed to materialise, and the efficacy of acetylcholinesterase inhibitors is increasingly questioned. Indeed, France discontinued funding for them in 2018. Overall, there is a broad consensus that these drugs offer a statistically significant and clinically meaningful improvement in symptoms for a few months. It is then up to national authorities whether they deem the improvements substantial and/or reliable enough to warrant associated side effects and costs.[11]

Having mentioned it a couple of times so far, it is time to address the drug discovery elephant in the room: aducanumab. As discussed in Chapter 2, the amyloid hypothesis has dominated aetiological work for decades. This theory suggests that a toxic protein fragment called beta-amyloid builds up in the brain, causing neuron death and, by extension, progressive cognitive impairment. Aβ, often referred to as plaques, has been at the forefront of drug discovery attempts for several years. Much work has been dedicated to developing compounds which either remove Aβ aggregates or prevent aggregation in the first place. The theory goes that if we can prevent or remove Aβ, then we might prevent or remove its resulting cognitive effects. However, in practice, the amyloid hypothesis has been found wanting. So far, 23 separate agents have successfully targeted Aβ, yet none have produced obviously satisfactory results in terms of cognitive outcomes (at least until lecanemab, which I will discuss below)[12, 13]. Hence, molecular developments have far outpaced clinical progress.

It is against this backdrop that the FDA approval of aducanumab came as something of a surprise in June 2021. Aducanumab, marketed as Aduhelm, is another anti-Aβ monoclonal antibody, developed by the pharmaceutical company Biogen, that has consistently cleared Aβ in animal and human testing. After several years of development, aducanumab was subject to two randomised, double-blind, placebo-controlled phase-III trials, entitled ENGAGE and EMERGE, beginning in 2015. In 2019, these trials were ended following "futility analyses", early tests that convinced Biogen that aducanumab was not working and therefore did not justify further investment. However, a subsequent reanalysis of data collected immediately before termination showed a slight uptick in results. In particular, Biogen found that the higher-dose EMERGE trial revealed some statistically significant improvements across various cognitive outcomes.

Critics have noted that, in between the futility analysis and the in-house reanalysis, Biogen underwent significant management, consultant and statistics department reorganisations, with an eye to securing share prices that had become increasingly reliant on the fate of aducanumab.[14] Of note was the replacement of R&D chief Michael Ehlers, who had reportedly been uncomfortable with Biogen's approach. Following these changes, some investment analysts explicitly advised that, while the drug did not work, the personnel changes, statistical reanalyses and close FDA relationship made it likely that aducanumab would be approved nonetheless, rendering it an excellent investment opportunity.[15] The analysts were proven correct. The FDA and Biogen collaborated to reanalyse the data, concluding that EMERGE alone showed a positive result for high-dose treatment in participants with slow-progressing disease. The FDA, therefore, recommended that Biogen could reasonably apply for approval[16].

Aducanumab did not have an easy ride following Biogen's application to the FDA, facing external criticism and problems within the review process itself. The FDA's biostatistical review of ENGAGE and EMERGE found no correlation between Aβ removal and cognitive function. The FDA's Peripheral and Central Nervous System Drugs Advisory Committee unanimously voted that there was insufficient evidence for approval, with ten votes against and one uncertain.[17] The FDA typically respects its expert panel decisions, so at this point, the outlook for aducanumab seemed bleak. It was, therefore, something of a plot twist when the FDA granted aducanumab an accelerated approval based on Aβ as a surrogate endpoint, noting that there was reason to believe that Aβ removal would lead to clinical benefits.[18] This was particularly surprising because up until that point, the FDA had been coy about the prospects of treating Aβ as a surrogate.[17] Ultimately, a useful surrogate endpoint must be highly predictive of clinical benefit. Aβ is evidently not in such a position, at least yet.

The decision triggered substantial controversy. There were resignations from three members of the FDA's expert committee that had advised against approval,[16] and even denouncements from scientists who had worked on the development of aducanumab itself.[19] Several investigations were quickly launched into the approval, including by the US Department of Health and Human Services and the US House of Representatives. Of particular concern was the unusually close working relationship between the FDA and Biogen. Various sources have reported off-the-record collaborations between senior figures at the FDA and Biogen – collaborations that were not disclosed to the evaluating committee.[20]

Relatedly, the close involvement of the Alzheimer's Association in lobbying for approval has also provoked criticism. Following the initial negative decision by the FDA's expert panel, the Alzheimer's Association organised a listening event with FDA figures in which patients forwarded emotionally loaded personal appeals for approval.[21] When the FDA extended the review period for aducanumab in early 2021, the Alzheimer's Association issued an open letter in support of approval.[22] As condemnation grew following approval, the Alzheimer's Association CEO accused critics of not being "pro-patient".[23] In this manner, the Alzheimer's Association has consistently championed patient hopes as a legitimate basis for approval in spite of efficacy data. It has not gone unnoticed that Biogen's funding for the Alzheimer's Association increased from $275,000 in 2020 to $488,000 in 2021.[24]

The FDA provoked further criticism due to its initially lax stance toward defining the target population for Aduhelm when deciding on medication labelling. While aducanumab's approval, based on EMERGE, was predicated on an argument that the treatment was effective in a particular patient subset (very early and slow progressing with a substantial Aβ load), the approval was granted for AD generally. As we have seen, this is a vast prospective consumer base. Following further outcry, the FDA narrowed the approval to cover mild cognitive impairment and mild dementia due to AD. Nonetheless, this updated label still omitted any criteria based on the presence of Aβ, which was a critical component of the patient population defined during the trial and is key to aducanumab's proposed mechanism of action.[16]

The FDA's decision to exclude Aβ as a requirement for the prescription of aducanumab exemplifies another key tension in the development of anti-Aβ therapies. Aβ is becoming increasingly important in selecting trial populations and justifying the effectiveness of related drugs. However, after approval, it would require a major rollout of infrastructure to assess Aβ in prospective patients as a precondition for a prescription. Such a rollout would be a major undertaking and seems highly infeasible in the immediate future. Hence, Aβ is a risky play for stakeholders. It can offer an expedient means for gaining approval, but after approval, it can become a potential impediment to real-world uptake. With aducanumab, this pitfall was avoided by abandoning the Aβ focus once it had served its purpose of justifying accelerated approval.

In another highly unusual move, it took Biogen more than 2 years to publish its data in a peer-reviewed journal. Instead, the limited data shared with scientists over the entire consultation period largely came via Biogen presentations, often with pre-screened audience questions. During this time, Biogen did actually submit a paper to the *Journal of the American Medical Association* but then chose to withdraw the paper when the peer reviewers requested changes before publication.[25] It may also have done the same thing with the *New England Journal of Medicine*. The lack of publicly or even professionally available data on aducanumab left both critics and advocates in an uncertain position. Biogen finally published its work in March 2022 in *The Journal of Prevention of Alzheimer's Disease* (JPAD).[26] Having been subject to critical peer review elsewhere, JPAD finally presented an opportunity for Biogen to put forward its preferred argument – that aducanumab removed Aβ and therefore treated AD. Nonetheless, the paper seemed to confirm critics' fears, presenting a selective analysis of a biased dataset that still produced underwhelming results.[27]

Moreover, even if we accept the published results at face value, the meaningfulness of the effect size is debatable. While we often speak of "significance", a trial result can be statistically significant but clinically meaningless if the associated change is very small. For instance, if an intervention increases every recipient's cognitive ability by 1 point on a 1000-point scale, then the intervention's effect size is almost imperceptibly small but is nonetheless statistically significant because that tiny change has reliably happened in a lot of different individuals. Hence, we need full data availability to assess not only the significance of the results but also the extent to which they translate into desirable real-world outcomes. From what has now been made available, some critics have contended that the effect size is not clinically meaningful, being less than that typically produced by acetylcholinesterase inhibitors. The effect is even within the range of natural variability for AD symptom progression.[16]

Another issue for which good data are now available is side effects. Amyloid-related imaging abnormalities (ARIA) are a common side effect of anti-Aβ therapies, leading to brain bleeds and swelling. It is hypothesised that the removal of Aβ deposits can weaken the structural integrity of blood vessels and lead to an increased likelihood of haemorrhage. To understand this, we can imagine the brain as an old stone cottage and Aβ as ivy growing into the mortar. The ivy might be doing some damage, but it also becomes part of the building's fabric, so suddenly removing decades of growth will likely compromise the structural integrity. In December 2021, Biogen published the ARIA data from EMERGE and ENGAGE. The data showed that 41% of recipients experienced brain bleeds or swelling, though the majority were asymptomatic.[28] Most concerningly, while Aduhelm has hardly been prescribed to anybody amidst the ongoing controversy, it has already been linked to one death. While participating in a clinical trial, the victim was hospitalised with seizures and subsequently found to have brain swelling that is likely attributable to Aduhelm.[29]

Further fuel was added to the controversy when Biogen announced its pricing strategy. Analysts had anticipated a price of between $10,000 and $25,000. Aduhelm was instead offered at $56,000 per year. Executives justified the cost as proportionate to the economic impact of dementia on the US.[30] Several insurers and medical providers in the US were quick to announce that they would not be funding or administering Aduhelm in lieu of convincing data on clinical efficacy. In December 2021, facing sustained backlash, low uptake and the prospect of other anti-Aβ rivals gaining approval in the near future, Biogen cut the price of Aduhelm from $56,000 to $28,000.[31] The same month, the European Medicines Agency (EMA) refused a marketing licence for Aduhelm, citing a lack of evidence for both efficacy and safety.[32] Things got worse for Biogen when, in January 2022, the Centers for Medicare & Medicaid Services (CMS) proposed that Aduhelm would only be eligible for Medicare coverage if it was taken as part of a clinical trial.[33, 34] This was a major restriction to the rollout of Aduhelm, with relatively few patients becoming involved in clinical trials. The Alzheimer's Association responded angrily, describing the CMS decision as "shocking discrimination against everyone with Alzheimer's disease".[35] Ultimately, this final line of defence – physicians and funders simply refusing to use it – seems to have effectively ended the aducanumab saga. Nonetheless, we came surprisingly close to the mass-market availability of a lethal[1] anti-Aβ dementia treatment without clinical effectiveness. This should be a warning to us all.

As discussed, aducanumab is the latest addition to a collection of molecularly effective anti-Aβ therapies that have produced underwhelming clinical outcomes. Companies that have invested large sums in those failed treatments were watching the aducanumab saga with interest. It only took a few weeks for two other anti-Aβ monoclonal antibodies – donanemab, from Eli Lilly, and lecanemab, a joint Biogen and Eisai venture – to announce plans to seek similar approvals. Interestingly, Eli Lilly decided to trial donanemab against aducanumab.[38] By repositioning Aβ as a surrogate endpoint, the FDA reignited the hopes of several anti-Aβ projects that had previously been thwarted by clinical inefficacy. The wider effect on the drug development pipeline remains to be seen, but it may be difficult for the FDA to justify approvals for one treatment and not for similar compounds, as we have subsequently witnessed with lecanemab (which I will return to shortly). On top of existing, previously "failed" treatments, Aβ-targeting options also continue to comprise the largest proportion of candidates currently at the pre-clinical trial stage.[39]

The aducanumab saga is engrossing, but one might reasonably ask what it has to do with the neuro-agnosticism of dementia studies and the neuropsychiatric biopolitics of dementia. I would argue that the events have been partly enabled by neuro-agnosticism in dementia studies and that the relative silence of dementia studies in response has been telling. Critique has largely come from neuroscientists, psychiatrists and other physicians, who are incensed by technical shortcomings. However, much of this critique perpetuates a misconception that dementia drug discovery is simply a scientific matter, ignoring the more influential biopolitics that has led us to this point (as described in Chapters 3 and 4). Aducanumab's existence is decidedly biopolitical, regardless of, and perhaps in spite of, a range of traditional scientific and clinical considerations. It might seem bizarre, based on the science alone, that aducanumab remains on the market. However, under promissory biopolitics, we can understand aducanumab in the words of political scientist Luigi Pellizzoni as "an anticipated future retroacting on the present in the form of knowledge provisionally imperfect, hence justifying accidents and 'side effects'".[40] Debatable efficacy, brain bleeds and the undermining of the regulatory system all become regrettable but unavoidable steps on the road to progress. Scientific and clinical actors have obvious stakes in dementia drug discovery, but we cannot fairly expect them to be as well placed as social scientists when it comes to developing broader sociopolitical analyses and engagements with the public and legislative ecosystems of dementia. Aducanumab has posed a challenge to dementia studies, and dementia studies has largely looked the other way as our clinical and natural scientific peers have floundered, offering arguments predicated on a somewhat naïve faith in pure science.

As discussed, dementia studies is (or at least should be) comparatively well-equipped to critique normative neuropsychiatric commitments and develop transformative sociopolitical projects. Aducanumab provides a stark example of the real-world implications of adopting a largely agnostic stance toward neuropsychiatric biopolitics. In failing to engage robustly with that biopolitics by deconstructing and challenging its normative commitments, dementia studies partly facilitates the system that has allowed Aduhelm to come into existence. More than this, it actively participates to some extent. For instance, third-sector lobbying regarding the gravity of dementia as a problem likely informed FDA decision-making. Similarly, the argument that dementia is a huge economic burden was used by Biogen executives to justify Aduhelm's unexpectedly high initial pricing. These are ideas that are too often perpetuated in dementia studies, and their involvement in the aducanumab saga should give us pause to reflect on their potential consequences.

5.2 Biomarker Circularity

For all the problems bound up with aducanumab, it is at least useful in providing a stark example of how biopolitics, above and beyond simple science and (bio)medicine, can be crucial in shaping responses to dementia. Indeed, it is a useful example of how biopolitics, while never absolutely distinct, is often in tension with traditional ideals of science and clinical practice. In this section, I want to move on from the specificities of aducanumab to explore, in a broader manner, how the same neuropsychiatric biopolitics is fundamentally transforming dementia as an entity. This transformation is ultimately a process of making dementia more amenable to certain ends, specifically to sellable mass-market cures. As such, the recent machinations of aducanumab are indicative of a larger biopolitical trajectory that warrants serious critical attention in dementia studies. In particular, I want to consider the potential for a type of circular logic in these transformations of dementia, and what that means for people affected by dementia and our endeavours to address cognitive decline in later life as a specific type of problem. I argue that this circularity is a key symbolic machinery of neuropsychiatric biopolitics.

In a general sense, the term "circularity" denotes a type of conceptual feedback loop, wherein the conclusions that we make about a problem come to manifest the initial presumptions that we make about that problem.[41–43]

For example, if we define A as B, then addressing B is addressing A, and if we find that B is addressed, then we can assume that A is also addressed. The free interchange of A and B here is a sort of conceptual synonymisation. Two distinct things are treated as if they are the same thing. There are often good methodological reasons for doing this because if the synonym is a close match, then a very easy-to-measure thing may help us to work on an otherwise very difficult-to-measure thing. The downside to this approach is that we can lose important specificities. If I am interested in analysing letters, then B is a reasonable substitute for A. If I am interested in vowels, then B is a terrible proxy. Hence, the value of a conceptual synonym is dependent on which specificities of the original phenomenon we are interested in and which specificities are incidental or perhaps even unhelpful. Biomarkers for behavioural phenomena operate similarly, opening up questions about the value of our synonyms. Critically, that value is often conceived in terms of scientific accuracy, but it can also, somewhat cynically, be conceived in terms of stakeholder interest and hence its conductivity to biopolitical projects.

As discussed, Aβ has become a massively influential biomarker for AD over recent years. When Emil Kraepelin was popularising "plaques" at the beginning of the 20th century, the only way to assess a patient's neuropathological status was a post-mortem autopsy. In 1984, the National Institute on Neurological and Communicative Disorder and Stroke and the Alzheimer's Disease and Related Disorders Association published diagnostic criteria for AD. These guidelines made Aβ a precondition of a definitive diagnosis, an important development in the genesis of our contemporary biopolitics. This instituted the diagnostic approach that largely remains today, whereby a diagnosis of AD can only be "probable" until it is confirmed by observation of the presence of Aβ.[44] In practice, a great number of people are diagnosed with AD without recourse to biomarker assessments, but strictly speaking, Aβ is a requirement of diagnostic validity by-the-book, and the book has been actively enforced. In 1986, the NIA established the Consortium to Establish a Registry for Alzheimer's Disease, a yearly meeting of pathologists to police diagnoses and uphold gold-standard pathology. This was, and is, quite unusual because most psychiatric disorders do not require neuropathological evidence for diagnosis, based on an acceptance that overt signs of distress alone are sufficient to warrant treatment.[45] For instance, few clinicians would refuse to identify and assist a person with depression on the grounds that the person did not provide physical evidence of the condition.

Of course, if you were to ask most people what phenomena characterised AD, they would likely point to forgetfulness, confusion and other cognitive symptoms rather than Aβ. This highlights the observation that AD as a concept encompasses several facets, some neuropathological, some cognitive and that the relationship between the disease itself and what it is that makes up that disease varies according to who we ask. Different specificities matter to different people to different extents. Adopting a more explicitly biopolitical sensibility, we might say that the nature of the entity is amenable to stakeholder value commitments. If one specific facet of AD resonates with my own interests, then I might lean into that facet and emphasise how integral it is to the overarching phenomenon. This amenability is important because, while the cognitive characteristics of dementia may be the most noteworthy specificity for some, for others, cognition is a confounding factor that should be stripped away from dementia. Hence, many neuropsychiatric stakeholders view biomarkers as preferable to cognition as indicators of dementias, and an entire biomarker industry exists to service this preference.

Many stakeholders anticipate that the greater use of biomarkers will lead to more precisely differentiated dementia diagnoses, freed from the vagaries of cognitive symptoms.[44, 46] Readers will notice here the parallels with defining concepts of disease in relation to psychiatric disorder. As discussed in the previous chapter, pathophysiology offers a means of legitimising the existence of conditions by removing reliance on human interpretation of various signs and symptoms.[47] Joanna Latimer and Alex Hillman have characterised the pursuit of dementia biomarkers as an attempt to stabilise dementia as a solid and legitimate entity.[48] This has been particularly desirable in relation to psychiatric disorder because personal emotional and behavioural phenomena have traditionally played an important role in diagnosis.[49] Hence, the turn to biomarkers as the most apt specificity in dementia manifests the neuropsychiatric claim that dementias are caused by brain diseases, which itself overlaps concerns regarding the parameters of normality and pathology (as discussed in Chapter 4). Here we find one budding form of circularity that centres on and reinforces a core biopolitical commitment. Dementia is caused by brain diseases, so we must find the brain diseases that cause dementia.

Defining a disease entity in reference to cognition is difficult because the very nature of "cognition" is itself uncertain. Since the mid-20th century, much cognitive science has drawn inspiration from computer science to conceptualise cognition as an individual's intrinsic information-processing ability. This processing is typically depicted as occurring in the mind and/or brain, two mediums often used interchangeably to denote something happening inside the skull.[50] However, what cognition is, where it is, how it works and how we can measure it are all contested, and there are wildly different answers to these questions depending on who you ask.[51] Such questions are increasingly catalysed by the integration of digital technologies into our lives. Where once we might have placed things like mental arithmetic, memory or wayfinding within our skulls, now significant proportions of those functions occur in the smartphones in our hands. Practically speaking, even if we accept an old-school skull-contained view of cognition, it is difficult to use it to operationalise illness because the assessment of cognition is heavily socially mediated. For example, one study of a popular cognitive assessment tool (the mini-mental state examination) found that it had a false positive rate of 6% for white people compared with 42% for black people.[52] In response to such issues, it is easy to see why biomarkers are an appealing means of reimagining dementia, just as they are across much neuropsychiatric research more broadly.[53]

As well as manifesting longstanding desires to replace emotional and behavioural signs with physiological signs in psychiatric disorder, the increasing centrality of Aβ to AD is also bound up with reconceptualisations of dementia in relation to the lifecourse. As discussed, the failure of dominant hypotheses in drug trials, most notably anti-Aβ, but also anti-tau, has led some to reassess supposed aetiological timescales. In the lifecourse or presymptomatic reiteration of the amyloid hypothesis, the neuropathological process is slow and long. It begins decades before symptoms are first evident. Proponents theorise that, by the time the person begins to experience cognitive impairment, the physiological damage is already too advanced to be remedied. In this hypothesis, drug trials are failing because, while the targets are correct, the interventions are too late in the process.[54]

Following the longitudinal logic of dementia as a largely unnoticed lifelong process, the solution is to develop interventions similar to those currently failing trials but administering them earlier in the disease trajectory.[55–57] Naturally, to be able to intervene before the onset of cognitive symptoms requires a means of identifying the disease without recourse to cognition. Hence, a convergence of pathophysiological legitimacy and presymptomatic expansion has fuelled recent momentum toward generating new biomarker-based definitions, with a particular focus, as ever, on Aβ.[58–61] This approach was formally institutionalised in 2011 with the publication of a paper by the joint NIA and Alzheimer's Association workgroup regarding the definition of preclinical AD. This paper advocated for a lifecourse model of dementia, whereby neuropathologies (with an emphasis on Aβ) progress gradually for decades before the onset of cognitive symptoms.[62] From this perspective, it makes more sense to define AD in terms of Aβ than cognitive impairment. Doubling down on this position, the workgroup published a paper in 2018 stating that an AD diagnosis is based on pathophysiology and "is not based on the clinical consequences of the disease.[63]" In this context, AD has gradually been replaced by Aβ in much research and associated media output. It is now relatively conventional to claim that Aβ *is* AD, and vice versa, in a circular manner.[64] The result is a selection of specificities that align with neuropsychiatric biopolitics, centring brain disease and abnormality at the expense of cognition. This alignment of interests has guided research in a concordant manner so that circularity has alighted on and emphasised Aβ as the specificity most conducive to those interests.

An intriguing example of this circular use of Aβ can be found in animal research. It is not uncommon for initiatives that self-identify as (and are resultantly reported as) studying AD to be working with mice or worms. Dementia is not an easy thing to operationalise in animals. What does it mean for a tiny worm to experience cognitive decline? Does the worm have a mind that can become impaired? Does the worm forget? In practice, special worms are bred to produce Aβ. However, in the worms, Aβ leads to paralysis rather than lower mini-mental state scores. In the lab, worm AD is evidenced by the observation that the genetically altered worms, designed to express Aβ, do not thrash about as much as their natural counterparts.[48] Using this Aβ-based definition, it is common for animal studies, such as a study of immobile worms, to self-identify as AD research.[41] The development of Aβ-expressing animal models for studying AD is a hugely impressive technical achievement and offers great potential for scientific discovery. However, we must not make the mistake of anthropomorphising these animals. In practice, no non-human animal gets Aβ-dense dementia. Many animals have the appropriate proteins and proteases, age and experience functional degeneration, but only humans have been observed to develop AD.[45]

That biomarker-centred approach feeds through into media reports. It is common for headlines pertaining to breakthrough dementia cures to actually be referring to animal studies when one reads down into the article. Consider the following recent newspaper headlines: "Dementia breakthrough: new therapy 'could reduce the onset of Alzheimer's disease'"[65] and "Breakthrough on Alzheimer's cure as jab found to restore memory – for just £15 a dose".[66] Eye-catching claims, but read down in to the pieces and you will discover that the two studies in question used different methods to remove Aβ from mouse brains. The preponderance of this circularity in media accounts is unsurprising. The headline "jab cures dementia" is far more likely to sell newspapers than "jab removes protein from mouse". However, sensationalising journalists are only partly to blame here because a similar circularity afflicts the dementia research economy more broadly. Understandably so. In a competitive grant environment, a research proposal seeking a cure for dementia might seem more worthy of funding than the same proposal manipulating a molecule in a worm. For researchers and journalists alike, circularity is something of a survival strategy. It is not only methodologically useful but biopolitically useful as well.

Animal-based dementia research offers stark examples of circularity because, in lieu of cognition, it is often forced to be explicit. For example, a well-cited paper entitled "scanning ultrasound removes amyloid-β and restores memory in an Alzheimer's disease model mouse" includes the following observation: "Transgenic mice with increased amyloid-β (Aβ) production show several aspects of Alzheimer's disease, including Aβ deposition".[67] Here, we can see biomarker circularity at its most straightforward. Mice with Aβ have AD because they have Aβ. This circularity then feeds into the findings of animal model research. We can cure their AD because we can remove their Aβ, and we know that we have cured their AD because their Aβ is gone. Following this approach, research has been remarkably successful at curing AD in animals over recent years. Unfortunately, the continued failure of promising animal models to translate into comparable human interventions is a major source of frustration.[68] Nonetheless, some stakeholders view the stripping away of cognition as a major aid to dementia research. For instance, McColl and colleagues have championed worm models because they lack the behavioural complicatedness of rodent models.[69] Hence, circularity can become an aspiration.

The example of animal-based dementia research is also useful in highlighting the vast ontological distances that circularity can overcome. At a basic level, any person with experience of dementia will likely struggle to see meaningful parallels with a paralysed worm. Worm paralysis and human forgetfulness intuitively seem to be very different things. However, this is not necessarily as farcical as it may initially appear. Many proxies make substantial leaps to achieve instructive ends. Many conditions are characterised by heterogeneous individual indications that conceal the shared physiologies underpinning them. An interesting example of this is pregnancy. It stems from a relatively universal physiological process but is manifest in a variety of different experiences, from strange sensations and cravings to swelling feet and stretch marks. Stripping away the diverse presentations can help to standardise the disease entity and make it more amenable to our understanding and intervention.[70, 71] Of course, there are some important differences between lethargic worms and pregnant women. My point here is that circularity can sometimes span substantial ontological differences in meaningful, uncontroversial and useful ways. Hence, the distance between worm lethargy and human forgetfulness is not by itself the issue. Rather, it is the specificities of the switching that matter.

In social science, we often analyse social class or ethnicity, which are complex concepts and very difficult to operationalise. We do so by grouping people via income, occupation, skin colour or regional ancestry. That can be a problem, but it can also be useful as long as we are alert to the specificities that we have forfeited and reflect on whether those specificities are relevant to our particular research. When we are mindful of what we have lost by switching out one entity (e.g. dementia or class) for another (e.g. Aβ or income), we can cautiously but pragmatically pursue what we hope will prove to be enlightening research. This is a type of reductionism wherein the problem is made smaller so that we can better get at it. Inevitably, such switching is influenced by the interests of those doing the switching. Even this does not mean that switching is necessarily "bad" or "problematic" per se, but it does render such switching a valuable biopolitical tool with which things, such as dementia and class, can be fundamentally reformulated to suit different interests.

Similarly, reductionism (the switching of a big complex thing with a smaller and more straightforward thing) is often criticised outright, but it is not inherently flawed. It can be done intelligently, with an alertness to its consequences for findings, and produce useful insights that would otherwise be impractical. The problem arises when the proxy entity is embedded in the operationalisation of the problem and the results. To define dementia as Aβ and then cure dementia by targeting Aβ is akin to defining class inequality as income inequality and then addressing class inequality by addressing income inequality. Some difference may be made, but everything within class that falls beyond the parameters of income (e.g. wealth (e.g. assets), social capital) is forfeit. However, because the problem is defined in terms of the proxy, dealing with the proxy makes it look like we have dealt with the problem. In the case of dementia research, the discrepancy is particularly stark because we know that neurophysiology and cognition are not neatly correlated. Nonetheless, biomarkers are playing an increasingly important role in shaping the drug discovery pipeline, which is, in turn, feeding into wider research and media representations.[72] Hence, aducanumab represents one feature of an intensifying biopolitical avalanche.

Circularity and switching comprise some of the key mechanics through which a neuropsychiatric biopolitics of dementia is able to exert its influence. They are symbolic processes that facilitate the making and remaking of dementia into more or less desirable forms from the perspectives of those doing the making and those influenced by that making. If I sell drugs or study worms, then Aβ aggregation is far more conducive to my existential interests than cognitive impairment is (besides the latter's emotive usefulness as fodder for hard-hitting advertising campaigns). When circularity occurs in the context of biopolitical interests, it is unsurprising that it can often come to reflect those interests accordingly. The more it happens, the more ossified it can become, with little chance of natural change as long as it continues to serve substantive interests. To this end, commentators have long noted the stubbornness with which Aβ has become embedded in the dementia research economy and bemoaned the inability of science to dislodge it.

5.3 Too Small to Fail

For some time, critics of the amyloid hypothesis have claimed that it is too big to fail.[73, 74] In 2011, pathologists Rudy Castellani and Mark Smith published a blistering critique to this effect.[73] Their paper was instrumental in my personal development as a young dementia researcher because it was my first encounter with the problems of biomarker-led operationalisations of dementia. The authors lamented that each failed anti-Aβ trial seemed to be preceded by largely identical trials. They pointed to familiar issues: the lack of a clear relationship between pathophysiology and symptoms, the differences between rare familial AD and common sporadic dementia in later life, uncertainties regarding whether associated pathophysiologies preceded or followed disease onset, the variability of Aβ itself and its uses in the lab and the growing popularity of the presymptomatic lifecourse hypotheses that would be difficult to test robustly.[2] In a passage that seems prescient in light of aducanumab, they asked:

> Does expansion of trials run the risk of obtaining a kernel of positive data, purely out of randomness and the expanding denominator, thus perpetuating a fundamentally flawed paradigm and diverting attention from biological processes more worthy of targeting?

Castellani and Smith's conclusion that the amyloid hypothesis had become too big to fail remains a common criticism of AD drug development and associated enterprises. While there are merits to this argument, I would suggest that the "too big to fail" critique is only half the problem. The other is a sense in which things can be made too small to fail. Here, the very notion of "failure" can be reimagined within neuropsychiatric biopolitics.

Before delving into this issue, it is important to note that stakeholders have offered several perfectly sensible arguments against rejecting the amyloid hypothesis and related drug discovery efforts outright. Common arguments include (1) trials have started too late in the disease process, at a point when cognition could not be salvaged, (2) study samples are too heterogeneous and need to be more rigidly defined in terms of neuropathology and (3) assessments of cognitive outcomes are too unreliable[13, 75]. There is also an argument to be made that, while the involvement of public and government donations is ethically questionable, if private enterprises choose to invest in such drug trials, then that is their own prerogative. Moreover, these trials always have a chance, however tiny, of contributing to some important understanding, or maybe even stumbling across a miracle treatment. If nothing else, they create employment opportunities for researchers who may one day contribute to important developments in other areas. Of course, as aducanumab has shown, the ethics and usefulness of such enterprises do rely on the enforcement of robust scientific regulation, which is not always guaranteed. Hence, we must be wary of capital guiding research rather than research guiding capital, but that is not a good reason to curtail capital investment outright.

To unpack what I mean by "too small to fail", we must first attend more abstractly to what is being switched in biomarker-dementia circularity. Ultimately, this is an interchanging of two different conceptualisations of dysfunction, which in medical sociology we often refer to as "illness" and "disease". Illness here refers to a person's experience of dysfunction and the various perceived phenomena that come with it. This may contain pathophysiological components, e.g. a bruise is a very experiential physiologic entity but is often a collection of sensations, e.g. the pain of the bruise. Disease renders the same dysfunction in relation to different, but sometimes overlapping, phenomena. Here, experience is replaced by molecular considerations. The painfulness of the bruise is of less concern than the ruptured blood vessels.[70, 76] As discussed in Chapter 4, the basic concept of disease became popular during the nosological turn of the 19th century as a means of standardising and legitimising medical practice by moving away from the vagaries of illness and interpretation.[77] Hence, the contemporary neuropsychiatric biopolitics of dementia both relies on and propagates a longstanding concept of disease.

If we think of circularity as beginning with the replacement of illness (dementia) with disease (biomarker), then we get a sense of what is broadly being exchanged.[3] Experiences, sensations, behaviours, intuitions, cognition, etc. are taken out. Morphology, molecules, biochemical processes, etc. are brought in. The process is taken further in much dementia research because a great deal of the characteristic physiological messiness, as described in Chapter 3, is also replaced with a limited number of biomarkers, in many cases even one. An oft-repeated Kitwood quote cautions: "When you've met one person with dementia, you've met one person with dementia".[78] Indeed, one of the major impediments to clinical utility in dementia is the extreme variability of prognosis. In my research, I have worked with people who have experienced rapid decline over several months and people who retain some degree of independence after a decade. One person may remember my name after a 6-month interval, but be unable to articulate their thoughts in an interview, while another may forget who I am in an instant but be able to deftly talk their way around their impairments. The notion of aged heterogeneity,[4] discussed in Chapters 3 and 4, is echoed in a sort of dementia heterogeneity. Ultimately, by removing the highly variable subjective aspects of illness, the disease offers a more standardised and reliable entity to work with, and also typically a more concise and simplified one. As noted, this can be useful in research contexts. However, the approach becomes circular, and potentially problematic, when the synonymous entity becomes embedded within the conclusions or, indeed, becomes the conclusions.

The profound heterogeneity of personal manifestations of dementia poses a problem for research that seeks to understand and intervene in dementia at a level above the individual, especially when it comes to a population level. The swapping of illness for disease offers the most expedient means of approaching dementia in a way that has some applicability to a large number of people. However, by attending to the circumstances of more and more people, this process of abstraction risks attending to nobody's circumstances at all. By amalgamating numerous cases, a textbook definition of AD is unlikely to accurately apply to any specific individual. As an example of this discordance between average and individual characteristics, the average British family has 1.7 children and 0.5 dogs, but very few (if any) families will have 1.7 children and 0.5 dogs. Hence, in losing illness specificities, disease can come to represent a lot of people poorly but nobody well. This tendency is manifest in the use of words like "pseudo" and "atypical" in relation to health conditions.[47]

Circularity often begins with a swapping out of the problem to make it more easily interrogatable for pragmatic purposes. While very few people have 1.7 children, it is useful to know that the average person does if we are to plan family housing developments and the future provision of education. This useful reductionism becomes circular when it slips into swapping the problem outright and hence making it easier to solve. As a simplistic analogy, imagine that you are failing to solve a 10,000-piece jigsaw puzzle, so you replace it with a 1,000-piece jigsaw, which you then successfully solve. Even if you define it as the same jigsaw, the original 10,000-piece puzzle remains in its box unsolved. Framed as a puzzle to be solved, dementia is a huge challenge in several respects. We do not agree about what cognition is, let alone how to measure it.[79] Ageing is messy, massively heterogeneous and, for many people, something that they try not to think about. The brain is renowned for being enigmatic. Psychiatric disorder likewise, albeit with the added complication of widespread taboo and public fear. When faced with this collection of problems, biomarkers look appealingly simple, safe and comprehendible. A biomarker is an easier puzzle to tackle, but dementia remains unsolved.

The circularity of swapping a 10,000-piece puzzle for one with 1,000 pieces is precisely how a problem, in this case, dementia, is made smaller – potentially too small to fail. If you reduce the number of pieces far enough, right down to one piece, then the puzzle is effectively solved. Following this same logic, dementia has proved to be an incredibly difficult problem to solve, whereas Aβ, tau, etc. are far easier by comparison. They are easy enough that we can already solve them. As discussed, we have 23 successful Aβ-busting therapies, with the first successful anti-tau candidates now coming through.[80] Many people would be surprised to learn that we can cure dementia and have been able to do so for several years. The caveat, of course, is that this ability to cure depends on how we define dementia. The nature of the task has changed, and by extension, the nature of what it means to fail or succeed has changed accordingly. Those people would probably be equally surprised to learn that they have AD, given the ubiquity of Aβ. We were once healthy people with Aβ, but now we are diseased people without symptoms. Here, again, we find an example of dementia being conceptually amenable to particular normative commitments. Through the machinations of circularity, the biopolitics of "dementia is caused by diseases of the brain" leads to the removal of cognition from the entity that it was once an integral characteristic of. Historically, AD-Aβ circularity has not been solely driven by neuropsychiatric biopolitics, but it has come to resonate with that biopolitics and the interests it contains so that its straightforward practicality is no longer the only consideration governing its sustained existence.

One could reasonably argue that this approach is unsustainable. For those affected by dementia, it is obvious that we have not succeeded. That cold hard reality is surely unavoidable? This is an understandable position, but aducanumab stands as a cautionary tale of the extreme lengths that circularity can carry a clinically ineffective *success*, let alone one that is potentially deadly. The promissory capacities of neuropsychiatric biopolitics can insulate drug discovery efforts from the shortcomings of circularity and even turn them into evidence of progress. As noted above, current failings are recast as necessary incidents on the inevitable road to future utopias. This aligns with a view of science as trying, failing and trying again. Failure is positioned as a means of learning, but that only works if the failure leads to corresponding adjustments. The importance of failure as a learning aid is partly replaced by appeals to contemporary problems as merely indicative of science at work, irrespective of what is done in response to those problems.[40] Hence, under the influence of the biopolitics of "research will discover a cure", aducanumab remains a successful step along the road to progress, with any shortcomings only emphasising its contribution to the future. It is naïve to assume that some idealised version of *good science* will triumph by virtue of its own merits and that circularity cannot be sustained within neuropsychiatric biopolitics.

For evidence of this durability, we need only remember that this has been happening for a long time. In 2015, I gave an interview discussing some controversies regarding anti-Aβ drug development. My observations largely echoed those put forward in the aforementioned "too big to fail" paper published four years earlier. The interviewer was a little incredulous. He asked me why the pharmaceutical industry would continue to spend so much money doing the same studies despite continued failures. Admittedly, it is intuitively nonsensical that major companies with sincere profit motives would pursue costly projects that seem bound for failure. It is estimated that bringing a dementia drug to market now costs $5.7 billion.[81] Perhaps the interviewer's mistake here was to assume the fixed meaning of "failure" and "success" in drug discovery. In practice, both of these concepts are negotiable. Following FDA approval of aducanumab, Biogen's stock jumped 42%.[82] This was only a short-term gain, as mounting controversy eroded investor confidence, but it was a major financial boost, nonetheless. Ultimately, even if the drug is rapidly consigned to history, it will have been a momentous "success" for some stakeholders. Reflecting on the seemingly nonsensical reluctance of pharmaceutical companies to let go of the amyloid hypothesis, neurobiologist Karl Herrup has concluded that short-term stock market gains can provide sufficient motivation for continuing trials and emphasising positive results[45].

A major issue with redefining dementia, and by extension success, is that the successes of researchers, charities, journalists, pharmaceutical companies and shareholders are unlikely to feel like successes for people affected by dementia. Their interests are prised apart. In my work with people affected by dementia, I hear a lot about the cognitive problems that they experience and far less about the molecular problems they face. Of course, if switched-out successes, alienated from real-world experiences of cognitive impairment, are necessary steps toward real therapeutic successes, then they do warrant praise. However, too often, the apparent successes are merely variations on well-trodden themes that have long been found wanting when it comes to cognitive impairment. The ultimate risk that this circularity presents us with is that it leaves those affected by dementia behind, alienating them entirely. Few people run marathons in memory of loved ones with the intention of funding endless cycles of mouse protein removal. There is a difference between putting personal illness experiences to one side as a means of tackling those experiences, and simply discarding them outright in favour of something more conducive to biopolitical commitments.

This remaking of the parameters of dementia has latterly been exacerbated by the announcement of trial results for lecanemab and its subsequent accelerated FDA approval. Lecanemab is another anti-Aβ compound co-developed by Eisai and Biogen, the company behind aducanumab. In November 2022, Eisai presented results at the Clinical Trials on Alzheimer's Disease conference. Echoing aducanumab, the results indicated that lecanemab cleared Aβ and reduced cognitive decline, and the drug was subsequently hailed as a breakthrough treatment. The results were reminiscent of aducanumab in as much as Aβ was robustly cleared, and the cognitive effects of that clearing were statistically significant but had questionable real-world meaning. Rates of brain damage with lecanemab were high (21%), though lower than aducanumab, and three deaths have been associated.[83, 84] Media pieces on the new AD cure abounded, Biogen's share price increased by 40%,[85] and within hours, the lecanemab story had been appended to the bottom of the Alzheimer's Society's donations page.[86]

It is important to clarify that, procedurally, at least, lecanemab is not a repeat of the aducanumab debacle. The trial ran as planned, and we were promptly presented with the data and a range of reasonable analyses at a conference and via peer-review publication.[87] Eisai have been consistently cautious in their own claims and deserve considerable credit, especially when compared with Biogen. In January 2023, the FDA granted lecanemab, brand name Leqembi, accelerated approval. This is the same type of approval previously granted to aducanumab, but it seems that some lessons were learned from the aducanumab debacle. This time, lecanemab was licensed specifically for people with confirmed Aβ neuropathology, mirroring the study population, and the initial price was set at $26,500, even lower than aducanumab's cut price of $28,200.[88] At the time of writing (May 2023), a third anti-Aβ, donanemab, is being reviewed by the FDA. Again, Eli Lilly has released headline results to media and stakeholder fanfare without a full data release. Again, the cognitive testing results have been presented in strange ways that seemingly exaggerate what is a clinically meaningless effect size. Again, brain damage and deaths have been reported.[89, 90]

As with aducanumab, there are many scientific criticisms of lecanemab,[88, 91] and the "breakthrough" media and charity hype surrounding it is unjustified and irresponsible.[92] At worst, there is a risk that Castellani and Smith's "too big to fail" warning – that anti-Aβ therapies would eventually be minimally substantiated by virtue of expanding denominators and methodological artefacts – has now come to pass.[93] For brevity, I will focus on one issue here: the boundaries of meaningfulness. Lecanemab stirs most controversy by reigniting the question of what counts as clinical meaningfulness. To recap, trial results can be statistically significant but clinically meaningless if the associated change is reliable but very small. A drug that can consistently improve cognition by 1 point on a 1000-point scale is effectively useless. Lecanemab did much better than this. Specifically, the treatment group declined by 0.45 points less than the placebo group on an 18-point scale over an 18-month period. The treatment group declined by 1.21 points, and the control group declined by 1.66.[94] But what does this mean in practice? What amount of slowing is sufficient to be realistically appreciated by people affected by dementia? There are many attempts to define this,[83, 95] but despite a vague consensus of between 1 and 2 points (much more than is offered by aducanumab or lecanemab), no specific approach has been institutionalised in drug regulation.

Rather than the specifics of different operationalisations of meaningfulness, it is the ambiguity that is most important here. It offers conceptual wiggle room for stakeholders. In a post-aducanumab research economy, lecanemab gestures toward another viable means of "success". The recasting of AD as Aβ could be echoed in the recasting of meaningfulness as ever-smaller increments on an expanding roster of cognitive scales. To this end, the Alzheimer's Association convened an expert working group to better define clinical meaningfulness for future trials. Perhaps unsurprisingly, the resulting paper seeks to lower the bar of meaningfulness, emphasising the importance of biomarkers and appealing to preclinical treatment. It also argues for a greater attentiveness to patient advocacy when interpreting clinical meaningfulness, in line with the Alzheimer's Association's lobbying strategy regarding aducanumab, and stresses that minimal effect sizes today are baby steps on the long road to a more therapeutically substantial future.[96] Present expectations are lowered; future expectations are raised. The combined effect of this argument is to strengthen the case for current drug approvals and further research in the same vein.

As this chapter has shown in several instances, the nature of the problem is always up for grabs in dementia research. This means that the problem can be bent to suit the proposed solution. One attempt to manipulate dementia to fit biotech offerings is evident in the circular redefinition of dementia via Aβ. This circularity came to full fruition in the case of aducanumab, while lecanemab offers a glimpse into a concurrent strategy – the complexification of meaningfulness. Here, stakeholders do not even need to entirely decouple dementia from cognition. Rather, they just need to cultivate enough ambiguity to be able to make a seemingly reasonable claim about the success of an intervention. Again, decelerating decline by less than half a point is likely at odds with what most people affected by dementia would consider a successful response. Again, dementia moves from something that is known by those affected to something that is known numerically by those with access to that numerical language. Again, what are such questions of cognitive meaning and the experiential and ontological transformation of dementia, if not core concerns for dementia studies? No other field is so well placed to navigate these biopolitical frontiers.

* * *

The various successes in the dementia drug discovery pipeline are a cautionary tale regarding the neuropsychiatric biopolitics of dementia and the need for a critically engaged dementia studies to attend to neuropsychiatric matters. Too often, our mistake in dementia studies is to think that we are dealing with a scientific problem that is being shaped by science (that is, an idealised notion thereof) and is somewhat beyond our remit, rather than a biopolitical problem that is being shaped by biopolitics, the governance of personal experience and conduct through symbolically biologised and power-driven public normativities, and is hence at the heart of our expertise. While the previous chapter revealed the biopolitical determination of purportedly scientific issues at a conceptual level, this chapter has shown an equivalent process at the scale of practical interventions. Aducanumab is one of the most important developments in dementia research, certainly post-1970s and probably in history. While a coalition of physicians and medical scientists has offered some resistance to the potentially harmful ramifications of aducanumab, this has predictably been rather sociopolitically unsophisticated. Meanwhile, the relative silence of much dementia studies has been notable. The many panels that I have attended on aducanumab have never featured a dementia studies scholar, and I am yet to read a single critical dementia studies response. I would suggest that this silence is emblematic of neuro-agnosticism and a resulting hesitancy to attend to neuropsychiatric matters.

The post-1970s transformation of dementia into an entity that fits neuropsychiatric biopolitics should concern dementia studies scholars, especially given its intensification over recent years, but it should also give us a reason to be hopeful. It shows us the extent to which dementia is politically malleable. Neuropsychiatric biopolitics has been remarkably successful in generating an imaginary of dementia that has proved powerful enough to bend the world to suit it. In challenging the normative commitments of that biopolitics, dementia studies might also seek to nurture a counter-biopolitics (or a "sociopolitics", as I will argue in Chapters 8 and 9). Such a sociopolitics might embody the experiential and humanist ethics that dementia studies developed in opposition to the (bio)medical model. Hence, we might promote a sociopolitics of dementia that centres on the experiences, struggles and preferences of people affected by dementia. Methodologically, the history of much dementia studies is a story of significant efforts toward democratisation. With the aid of dementia studies, people with dementia have moved from subjects to participants, to co-researchers, to autonomous researchers in some instances. Dementia as an entity could feasibly undergo a similar process. I reflect on this potential more extensively in the concluding chapter.

It is important that we do not fall into the trap of saying what dementia is and is not. Dementia is not anything per se. All those who claim to know it definitively should inspire scepticism, especially when their definiteness comes at the expense of others. Assertive claims to the effect of "dementia is X" will not be properly challenged by similarly authoritative counterclaims to the effect of "dementia is *actually* X". A recognition that a biomarker, or a lethargic worm, or a 0.45-point differentiated decline rate is not the same thing as dementia does not require us to propose an opposing definition of what dementia is. The unknowns are not inherently problematic. Good science happily deals in uncertainties, qualifications and probabilities from a standpoint of curiosity. There is space for more pluralistic conceptualisations of dementia that also usefully strip out some specificities to help us work at a population level. Retreating into a heavily personalised and experiential approach to illness is unlikely to produce treatments that can systematically offer benefits to a large number of people, but we must nonetheless remain attentive to people affected by dementia and what matters to them. Importantly, this should be achieved through interpersonal relationships with a range of people affected by dementia rather than media campaigns featuring charity-approved advocates.

As the above Kitwood quote notes, in practice, no two dementias are alike. This is apt from a certain perspective. However, there is also value in the observation that millions of people around the world tend to experience loosely similar forms of mental dysfunction as they get older, with negative implications for their well-being. Hence, there is a case for grouping those millions of instances in reference to the things that are shared, and that will inherently require us to ignore some personal specificities. Some concept of dementia, senility, AD, or however it is articulated, is certainly worthwhile. In previous chapters, I have cautioned that the success of neuropsychiatric biopolitics in generating our contemporary dementia is not inherently bad. To a large extent, the growth of dementia studies and all that has come from it is greatly indebted to neuropsychiatric biopolitics. In attending critically to aspects of that biopolitics, such as circularity, there is little point in simply attempting to disprove it. Rather, there could be great utility in rearticulating it in a manner more expedient to the well-being of people affected by dementia. Circularity is one example of a feature of neuropsychiatric biopolitics that dementia studies could learn from and potentially even emulate, carefully selecting the specificities that befit our aims and, most importantly, the interests of those affected by dementia.

Notes

1 At the time of writing (May 2023), despite the small population of people who have been exposed to the drug, four deaths have been publicly linked with aducanumab.[36] Lecanemab and donanemab (discussed below) are currently linked with three deaths each.[37] One wonders how much greater the outrage might be if these deaths were not limited to older people with dementia.

2 Lifecourse hypotheses posit mechanisms over such large timescales that the proposed aetiologies become practically unfalsifiable. If I claim that giving 30-year-olds anti-Aβ medication will prevent the onset of dementia in their 80s, you will be hard-pressed to disprove my claim with an RCT.

3 I mean this in terms of the sociological concepts of course. Literally speaking, dementia is not an illness, but rather a syndrome, and biomarkers are not diseases, but rather indicators of diseases.

4 As discussed in Chapters 3 and 4, aged heterogeneity describes the tendency for inequality to increase over time with the result that older people are an especially diverse population across many different social, economic, physiological and psychological measures.

References

1. Pickett, J., Bird, C., Ballard, C., Banerjee, S., Brayne, C., Cowan, K., Clare, L., Comas-Herrera, A., Corner, L., Daley, S., et al. (2018). A roadmap to

advance dementia research in prevention, diagnosis, intervention, and care by 2025. *International Journal of Geriatric Psychiatry 33*, 900–906. doi: 10.1002/gps.4868.

2. Dementia Discovery Fund (2022). https://svhealthinvestors.com/funds/the-dementia-discovery-fund.

3. UK DRI (2021). About us. UK Dementia Research Institute. https://ukdri.ac.uk/about-us.

4. Cummings, J.L., Morstorf, T., and Zhong, K. (2014). Alzheimer's disease drug-development pipeline: Few candidates, frequent failures. *Alzheimer's Research & Therapy 6*, 37. doi: 10.1186/alzrt269.

5. Watts, G. (2018). Prospects for dementia research. *The Lancet 391*, 416. doi: 10.1016/S0140-6736(18)30190-9.

6. Herrmann, N., Chau, S.A., Kircanski, I., and Lanctôt, K.L. (2011). Current and emerging drug treatment options for Alzheimer's disease. *Drugs 71*, 2031–2065. doi: 10.2165/11595870-000000000-00000.

7. Salomone, S., Caraci, F., Leggio, G.M., Fedotova, J., and Drago, F. (2012). New pharmacological strategies for treatment of Alzheimer's disease: Focus on disease modifying drugs. *British Journal of Clinical Pharmacology 73*, 504–517. doi: 10.1111/j.1365-2125.2011.04134.x.

8. Schneider, L.S., Mangialasche, F., Andreasen, N., Feldman, H., Giacobini, E., Jones, R., Mantua, V., Mecocci, P., Pani, L., Winblad, B., et al. (2014). Clinical trials and late-stage drug development for Alzheimer's disease: An appraisal from 1984 to 2014. *Journal of Internal Medicine 275*, 251–283. doi: 10.1111/joim.12191.

9. Vaci, N., Koychev, I., Kim, C.-H., Kormilitzin, A., Liu, Q., Lucas, C., Dehghan, A., Nenadic, G., and Nevado-Holgado, A. (2021). Real-world effectiveness, its predictors and onset of action of cholinesterase inhibitors and memantine in dementia: Retrospective health record study. *The British Journal of Psychiatry 218*, 261–267. doi: 10.1192/bjp.2020.136.

10. Valenzuela, M., Sachdev, P., and Brodaty, H. (2021). Concerns about cholinesterase inhibitor recommendations. *Neurology*. https://n.neurology.org/content/concerns-about-cholinesterase-inhibitor-recommendations.

11. Walsh, S., King, E., and Brayne, C. (2019). France removes state funding for dementia drugs. *BMJ 367*, l6930. doi: 10.1136/bmj.l6930.

12. Mehta, D., Jackson, R., Paul, G., Shi, J., and Sabbagh, M. (2017). Why do trials for Alzheimer's disease drugs keep failing? A discontinued drug perspective for 2010–2015. *Expert Opinion on Investigational Drugs 26*, 735–739. doi: 10.1080/13543784.2017.1323868.

13. Rubin, R. (2021). Recently approved Alzheimer drug raises questions that might never be answered. *JAMA 326*, 469–472. doi: 10.1001/jama.2021.11558.

14. George, D.R., and Whitehouse, P.J. (2021). *American Dementia: Brain Health in an Unhealthy Society*. Johns Hopkins University Press.

15. Erickson, T. (2020). Biogen's statistical gymnastics and PR maneuvering will likely turn Aducanumab straw into mega blockbuster gold. *Seeking Alpha*. https://seekingalpha.com/article/4355504-biogens-statistical-gymnastics-and-pr-maneuvering-will-likely-turn-aducanumab-straw-mega, https://seekingalpha.com/article/4355504-biogens-statistical-gymnastics-and-pr-maneuvering-will-likely-turn-aducanumab-straw-mega.

16. Liu, K.Y., and Howard, R. (2021). Can we learn lessons from the FDA's approval of aducanumab? *Nature Reviews Neurology 17*, 715–722. doi: 10.1038/s41582-021-00557-x.

17. Alexander, G.C., Knopman, D.S., Emerson, S.S., Ovbiagele, B., Kryscio, R.J., Perlmutter, J.S., and Kesselheim, A.S. (2021). Revisiting FDA approval of Aducanumab. *New England Journal of Medicine 385*, 769–771. doi: 10.1056/NEJMp2110468.

18. Cavazzoni, P. (2021). FDA's decision to approve new treatment for Alzheimer's disease. U.S. Food and Drug Administration. https://www.fda.gov/drugs/news-events-human-drugs/fdas-decision-approve-new-treatment-alzheimers-disease.

19. Belluck, P., Kaplan, S., and Robbins, R. (2021). How an unproven Alzheimer's drug got approved. *The New York Times*. https://www.nytimes.com/2021/07/19/health/alzheimers-drug-aduhelm-fda.html.

20. Rogers, M.B. (2021). Flurry of investigations besets Aducanumab. *ALZFORUM*. https://www.alzforum.org/news/conference-coverage/flurry-investigations-besets-aducanumab.

21. Gingery, D. (2021). Patient support may have helped push Aduhelm toward approval. *Pink Sheet*. https://pink.pharmaintelligence.informa.com/PS144438/Patient-Support-May-Have-Helped-Push-Aduhelm-Toward-Approval.

22. Norins, L. (2021). Alzheimer's Association again endorses Biogen drug despite mystery data analysis and financial conflict of interest. *AP NEWS*. https://apnews.com/press-release/pr-newswire/technology-seniors-health-special-interest-groups-data-management-neurological-disorders-3bdacd1821ed405570aded6244b7c9de.

23. Sinha, M.S., and Latham, S. (2021). Patient advocacy organizations and FDA drug approval: Lessons from Aduhelm. *STAT*. https://www.statnews.com/2021/07/23/patient-advocacy-organizations-lessons-from-aducanumab/.

24. Alzheimer's Association (2022). Our commitment to transparency. Alzheimer's Association. https://alz.org/about/transparency.

25. Herman, B. (2021). Biogen pulled Aduhelm paper after JAMA demanded edits. *Axios*. https://www.axios.com/biogen-jama-aduhelm-clinical-trial-results-publish-fc7c2876-a684-4bfc-8462-4165f57d735a.html.

26. Budd Haeberlein, S., Aisen, P.S., Barkhof, F., Chalkias, S., Chen, T., Cohen, S., Dent, G., Hansson, O., Harrison, K., von Hehn, C., et al. (2022). Two randomized phase 3 studies of Aducanumab in early Alzheimer's disease. *The Journal of Prevention of Alzheimer's Disease*. doi: 10.14283/jpad.2022.30.

27. Schneider, L.S. (2022). Aducanumab trials emerge but don't engage. *The Journal of Prevention of Alzheimer's Disease*. doi: 10.14283/jpad.2022.37.

28. Salloway, S., Chalkias, S., Barkhof, F., Burkett, P., Barakos, J., Purcell, D., Suhy, J., Forrestal, F., Tian, Y., Umans, K., et al. (2022). Amyloid-related imaging abnormalities in 2 phase 3 studies evaluating Aducanumab in patients with early Alzheimer disease. *JAMA Neurology 79*, 13–21. doi: 10.1001/jamaneurol.2021.4161.

29. Belluck, P. (2021). Concerns grow over safety of Aduhelm after death of patient who got the drug. *The New York Times*. https://www.nytimes.com/2021/11/22/health/aduhelm-death-safety.html.

30. Lovelace, B. (2021). Biogen faces tough questions over $56K-a-year price of newly approved Alzheimer's drug. CNBC. https://www.cnbc.com/2021/06

/08/biogen-faces-tough-questions-over-56k-a-year-price-of-newly-approved -alzheimers-drug.html.

31. Gleckman, H. (2021). What's behind Biogen's move to cut prices on its controversial Alzheimer's drug Aduhelm? Forbes. https://www.forbes.com/sites /howardgleckman/2021/12/23/whats-behind-biogens-move-to-cut-prices-on-its -controversial-alzheimers-drug-aduhelm/.

32. EMA (2021). Aduhelm: Pending EC decision. European Medicines Agency. https://www.ema.europa.eu/en/medicines/human/summaries-opinion/aduhelm.

33. CMS (2022). CMS proposes Medicare coverage policy for monoclonal antibodies directed against amyloid for the treatment of Alzheimer's disease. *CMS.gov.* https://www.cms.gov/newsroom/press-releases/cms-proposes -medicare-coverage-policy-monoclonal-antibodies-directed-against-amyloid -treatment.

34. CMS (2022). Monoclonal antibodies directed against amyloid for the treatment of Alzheimer's disease. *CMS.gov.* https://www.cms.gov/medicare-coverage -database/view/ncacal-decision-memo.aspx?proposed=Y&NCAId=305.

35. Alzheimer's Association (2022). Alzheimer's Association statement on CMS draft decision. *Alzheimer's Disease and Dementia.* https://alz.org/news/2022/ alzheimers-association-statement-on-cms-draft-deci.

36. Dunleavy, K., and 2022 06:35pm (2022). 3 more deaths among patients on Biogen's Aduhelm fuel safety concerns, though no link established. Fierce Pharma. https://www.fiercepharma.com/pharma/death-3-more-patients-biogen -s-aduhelm-fuel-more-concern-about-drug-s-safety-though-no-link.

37. Simonian, L. (2023). Eli Lilly's Donanemab: The Anti-Amyloid Saga Continues. https://seekingalpha.com/article/4600816-eli-lillys-donanemab-the-anti -amyloid-saga-continues, https://seekingalpha.com/article/4600816-eli-lillys -donanemab-the-anti-amyloid-saga-continues.

38. Mullard, A. (2021). More Alzheimer's drugs head for FDA review: What scientists are watching. *Nature* 599, 544–545. doi: 10.1038/d41586-021-03410-9.

39. van Bokhoven, P., de Wilde, A., Vermunt, L., Leferink, P.S., Heetveld, S., Cummings, J., Scheltens, P., and Vijverberg, E.G.B. (2021). The Alzheimer's disease drug development landscape. *Alzheimer's Research & Therapy* 13, 186. doi: 10.1186/s13195-021-00927-z.

40. Pellizzoni, L. (2017). Intensifying embroilments: Technosciences, imaginaries and publics. *Public Understanding of Science* 26, 212–219. doi: 10.1177/0963662516663563.

41. Fletcher, J.R., and Birk, R.H. (2019). Circularity, psychiatry & biomarkers: The operationalisation of Alzheimer's & stress in research. *Social Science & Medicine* 239, 112553. doi: 10.1016/j.socscimed.2019.112553.

42. Hahn, U. (2011). The problem of circularity in evidence, argument, and explanation. *Perspectives on Psychological Science* 6, 172–182. doi: 10.1177/1745691611400240.

43. Kriegeskorte, N., Simmons, W.K., Bellgowan, P.S.F., and Baker, C.I. (2009). Circular analysis in systems neuroscience: The dangers of double dipping. *Nature Neuroscience* 12, 535–540. doi: 10.1038/nn.2303.

44. Reitz, C., Brayne, C., and Mayeux, R. (2011). Epidemiology of Alzheimer disease. *Nature Reviews Neurology* 7, 137–152. doi: 10.1038/nrneurol.2011.2.

45. Herrup, K. (2021). *How Not to Study a Disease: The Story of Alzheimer's.* MIT Press.

46. Ahmed, T.F., Ahmed, A., and Imtiaz, F. (2021). History in perspective: How Alzheimer's Disease came to be where it is? *Brain Research 1758*, 147342. doi: 10.1016/j.brainres.2021.147342.

47. Rosenberg, C.E. (2002). The Tyranny of diagnosis: Specific entities and individual experience. *The Milbank Quarterly 80*, 237–260. doi: 10.1111/1468-0009.t01-1-00003.

48. Latimer, J., and Hillman, A. (2020). Biomarkers and brains: Situating dementia in the laboratory and in the memory clinic. *New Genetics and Society 39*, 80–100. doi: 10.1080/14636778.2019.1652804.

49. Bzdok, D., and Meyer-Lindenberg, A. (2018). Machine learning for precision psychiatry: Opportunities and challenges. *Biological Psychiatry: Cognitive Neuroscience and Neuroimaging 3*, 223–230. doi: 10.1016/j.bpsc.2017.11.007.

50. Teubert, W. (2010). *Meaning, Discourse and Society*. Cambridge University Press.

51. Newen, A., Bruin, L.D., and Gallagher, S. eds. (2018). *The Oxford Handbook of 4E Cognition*. Oxford University Press.

52. Khan, F., and Tadros, G. (2014). Complexity in cognitive assessment of elderly British minority ethnic groups: Cultural perspective. *Dementia 13*, 467–482. doi: 10.1177/1471301213475539.

53. Singh, I., and Rose, N. (2009). Biomarkers in psychiatry. *Nature 460*, 202–207. doi: 10.1038/460202a.

54. Fahey, M., Tinker, A., and Fletcher, J.R. (2023). Dementia's preventative futures: Researcher perspectives on prospective developments in the UK. *Working with Older People*. doi: 10.1108/WWOP-10-2022-0049.

55. Lock, M. (2013). *The Alzheimer Conundrum: Entanglements of Dementia and Aging*. Princeton University Press.

56. Leibing, A., and Schicktanz, S. eds. (2020). *Preventing Dementia?: Critical Perspectives on a New Paradigm of Preparing for Old Age*. Berghahn Books.

57. Milne, R., Diaz, A., Badger, S., Bunnik, E., Fauria, K., and Wells, K. (2018). At, with and beyond risk: Expectations of living with the possibility of future dementia. *Sociology of Health & Illness 40*, 969–987. doi: 10.1111/1467-9566.12731.

58. Beard, R.L. (2016). *Living with Alzheimer's: Managing Memory Loss, Identity, and Illness*. New York University Press.

59. Beard, R.L., and Neary, T.M. (2013). Making sense of nonsense: Experiences of mild cognitive impairment. *Sociology of Health & Illness 35*, 130–146. doi: 10.1111/j.1467-9566.2012.01481.x.

60. Hampel, H., Prvulovic, D., Teipel, S., Jessen, F., Luckhaus, C., Frölich, L., Riepe, M.W., Dodel, R., Leyhe, T., Bertram, L., et al. (2011). The future of Alzheimer's disease: The next 10 years. *Progress in Neurobiology 95*, 718–728. doi: 10.1016/j.pneurobio.2011.11.008.

61. Leibing, A. (2014). The earlier the better: Alzheimer's prevention, early detection, and the quest for pharmacological interventions. *Culture, Medicine, and Psychiatry 38*, 217–236. doi: 10.1007/s11013-014-9370-2.

62. Sperling, R.A., Aisen, P.S., Beckett, L.A., Bennett, D.A., Craft, S., Fagan, A.M., Iwatsubo, T., Jack, C.R., Kaye, J., Montine, T.J., et al. (2011). Toward defining the preclinical stages of Alzheimer's disease: Recommendations from the National Institute on Aging-Alzheimer's Association workgroups on diagnostic

guidelines for Alzheimer's disease. *Alzheimer's & Dementia* 7, 280–292. doi: 10.1016/j.jalz.2011.03.003.

63. Jack, C.R., Bennett, D.A., Blennow, K., Carrillo, M.C., Dunn, B., Haeberlein, S.B., Holtzman, D.M., Jagust, W., Jessen, F., Karlawish, J., et al. (2018). NIA-AA Research Framework: Toward a biological definition of Alzheimer's disease. *Alzheimer's & Dementia* 14, 535–562. doi: 10.1016/j.jalz.2018.02.018.

64. Høilund-Carlsen, P.F., Barrio, J.R., Gjedde, A., Werner, T.J., and Alavi, A. (2018). Circular Inference in Dementia Diagnostics. *Journal of Alzheimer's Disease* 63, 69–73. doi: 10.3233/JAD-180050.

65. Buntajova, D. (2022). Dementia breakthrough: New therapy 'could reduce the onset of Alzheimer's disease".' *Express*. https://www.express.co.uk/life -style/health/1556456/dementia-breakthrough-ultrasound-stimulation-reduces -alzheimers-disease-onset.

66. Fricker, M. (2021). Breakthrough on Alzheimer's cure as jab found to restore memory – For just £15. *Mirror*. https://www.mirror.co.uk/news/uk-news/ breakthrough-alzheimers-cure-jab-found-25457407.

67. Leinenga, G., and Götz, J. (2015). Scanning ultrasound removes amyloid-β and restores memory in an Alzheimer's disease mouse model. *Science Translational Medicine* 7, 278ra33. doi: 10.1126/scitranslmed.aaa2512.

68. Milne, R. (2016). In search of lost time: Age and the promise of induced pluripotent stem cell models of the brain. *New Genetics and Society* 35, 393–408. doi: 10.1080/14636778.2016.1257934.

69. McColl, G., Roberts, B.R., Pukala, T.L., Kenche, V.B., Roberts, C.M., Link, C.D., Ryan, T.M., Masters, C.L., Barnham, K.J., Bush, A.I., et al. (2012). Utility of an improved model of amyloid-beta (Aβ1-42) toxicity in Caenorhabditis elegans for drug screening for Alzheimer's disease. *Molecular Neurodegeneration* 7, 57. doi: 10.1186/1750-1326-7-57.

70. Jutel, A. (2009). Sociology of diagnosis: A preliminary review. *Sociology of Health & Illness* 31, 278–299. doi: 10.1111/j.1467-9566.2008.01152.x.

71. Bell, V. (2017). Why we need to get better at critiquing psychiatric diagnosis. *Mind Hacks*. https://mindhacks.com/2017/09/19/why-we-need-to-get-better-at -critiquing-diagnosis/.

72. Cummings, J., Lee, G., Zhong, K., Fonseca, J., and Taghva, K. (2021). Alzheimer's disease drug development pipeline: 2021. *Alzheimer's & Dementia: Translational Research & Clinical Interventions* 7, e12179. doi: 10.1002/ trc2.12179.

73. Castellani, R.J., and Smith, M.A. (2011). Compounding artefacts with uncertainty, and an amyloid cascade hypothesis that is 'too big to fail.' *The Journal of Pathology* 224, 147–152. doi: 10.1002/path.2885.

74. Couteur, D.G.L., Hunter, S., and Brayne, C. (2016). Solanezumab and the amyloid hypothesis for Alzheimer's disease. *BMJ* 355, i6771. doi: 10.1136/bmj. i6771.

75. Tian Hui Kwan, A., Arfaie, S., Therriault, J., Rosa-Neto, P., and Gauthier, S. (2020). Lessons learnt from the second generation of anti-amyloid monoclonal antibodies clinical trials. *Dementia and Geriatric Cognitive Disorders* 49, 334–348. doi: 10.1159/000511506.

76. Kleinman, A., Eisenberg, L., and Good, B. (1978). Culture, illness, and care: Clinical lessons from anthropologic and cross-cultural research. *Annals of Internal Medicine* 88, 251–258. doi: 10.7326/0003-4819-88-2-251.

77. Lupton, D. (2012). *Medicine as Culture: Illness, Disease and the Body*. SAGE.

78. SCIE (2020). Understanding dementia. Social Care Institute for Excellence. https://www.scie.org.uk/dementia/after-diagnosis/communication/understanding-dementia.asp.

79. Bayne, T., Brainard, D., Byrne, R.W., Chittka, L., Clayton, N., Heyes, C., Mather, J., Ölveczky, B., Shadlen, M., Suddendorf, T., et al. (2019). What is cognition? *Current Biology 29*, R608–R615. doi: 10.1016/j.cub.2019.05.044.

80. Mullard, A. (2021). Failure of first anti-tau antibody in Alzheimer disease highlights risks of history repeating. *Nature Reviews Drug Discovery 20*, 3–5. doi: 10.1038/d41573-020-00217-7.

81. Daly, T., and Epelbaum, S. (2022). The accelerated approval of Aducanumab invites a rethink of the current model of drug development for Alzheimer's disease. *AJOB Neuroscience 0*, 1–4. doi: 10.1080/21507740.2022.2048721.

82. Lovelace, B. (2020). Biogen's stock jumps 42% after FDA staff says it has enough data to support approving Alzheimer's drug.*CNBC*. https://www.cnbc.com/2020/11/04/biogens-stock-jumps-30percent-after-fda-staff-says-it-has-enough-data-to-support-approving-alzheimers-drug-.html.

83. *The Lancet* (2022). Lecanemab for Alzheimer's disease: Tempering hype and hope. *The Lancet 400*, 1899. doi: 10.1016/S0140-6736(22)02480-1.

84. Piller, C. (2022). Scientists tie third clinical trial death to experimental Alzheimer's drug. *Science*. https://www.science.org/content/article/scientists-tie-third-clinical-trial-death-experimental-alzheimer-s-drug.

85. Philippidis, A. (2022). StockWatch: Biogen shares rebound as Alzheimer's drug aces phase III trial. *GEN Edge 4*, 728–732. doi: 10.1089/genedge.4.1.119.

86. Alzheimer's Society (2022). Help fund the next dementia breakthrough. Alzheimer's Society. https://secure.alzheimers.org.uk/breakthrough/.

87. van Dyck, C.H., Swanson, C.J., Aisen, P., Bateman, R.J., Chen, C., Gee, M., Kanekiyo, M., Li, D., Reyderman, L., Cohen, S., et al. (2022). Lecanemab in early Alzheimer's disease. *New England Journal of Medicine*. doi: 10.1056/NEJMoa2212948.

88. LaHucik, K. (2023). Breaking: FDA clears second Alzheimer's drug in "foundational spark" for field. Endpoints News. https://endpts.com/fda-approves-alzheimers-drug-lecanemab-from-eisai/.

89. Alzforum (2023). Donanemab. https://www.alzforum.org/therapeutics/donanemab.

90. Cross, R. (2023). Lilly's Alzheimer's drug donanemab slows cognitive decline by 35% in PhIII, setting up showdown with Eisai's Leqembi. *Endpoints News*. https://endpts.com/lillys-alzheimers-drug-donanemab-succeeds-in-phase-iii-trial/.

91. Lowe, D. (2022). Brain Shrinkage as a Side Effect. *Science*. https://www.science.org/content/blog-post/brain-shrinkage-side-effect.

92. Alzheimer's Society (2022). Alzheimer's Society comment on today's "breakthrough" Alzheimer's drug news. Alzheimer's Society. https://www.alzheimers.org.uk/news/2022-12-02/alzheimers-society-comment-todays-breakthrough-alzheimers-drug-news.

93. Thambisetty, M., and Howard, R. (2023). Lecanemab trial in AD brings hope but requires greater clarity. *Nature Reviews Neurology 19*, 132–133. doi: 10.1038/s41582-022-00768-w.

94. Mahase, E. (2022). Lecanemab trial finds slight slowing of cognitive decline, but clinical benefits are uncertain. *BMJ 379*, o2912. doi: 10.1136/bmj.o2912.

95. Lansdall, C.J., McDougall, F., Butler, L.M., Delmar, P., Pross, N., Qin, S., McLeod, L., Zhou, X., Kerchner, G.A., and Doody, R.S. (2022). Establishing clinically meaningful change on outcome assessments frequently used in trials of mild cognitive impairment due to Alzheimer's disease. *The Journal of Prevention of Alzheimer's Disease*. doi: 10.14283/jpad.2022.102.
96. Petersen, R.C., Aisen, P.S., Andrews, J.S., Atri, A., Matthews, B.R., Rentz, D.M., Siemers, E.R., Weber, C.J., and Carrillo, M.C. Expectations and clinical meaningfulness of randomized controlled trials. *Alzheimer's & Dementia*. doi: 10.1002/alz.12959.

6 Destigmatising Normality

How the Awareness Economy Misconstrues and Perpetuates Stigma

Having argued for a more neurocritical dementia studies and provided examples of some of the key areas where critical analyses are currently wanting, this chapter turns to more familiar territory for dementia studies. In it, I critically analyse dementia awareness and anti-stigma campaigns. I begin by charting the development of dementia awareness campaigns as a response to reports of the widespread stigmatisation of dementia. I contextualise this development within the broader trend toward mental health awareness raising as a means of combatting stigma. I argue that the evidence base regarding stigma and dementia has traditionally relied on questionable definitions and interpretations of stigma. I ask what stigma means, exploring several ways in which the concept has been operationalised in research. Drawing on my own research with people affected by dementia, I argue that we need a more conceptually robust approach to understanding people's experiences of derogatory attitudes and reactions as echoing wider contexts of stigma. This is especially true when it comes to recognising (1) the extent to which stigma is intuitively felt and applied to oneself irrespective of direct discrimination and (2) the biopolitical structuring of that stigma by awareness-raising initiatives that may serve to further the interests of select stakeholders. I argue that discussions of stigma too often individualise and psychologise structural forces that are extrinsic to individuals but that are nonetheless experienced personally and potently. Hence, we need to theorise stigma as something experientially poignant but generated by conditions beyond the personal and interpersonal.

Having unpacked notions of stigma in relation to dementia, I then critically evaluate some of the core tenets of dementia awareness raising as an anti-stigma strategy, arguing that these are predicated on a neuropsychiatric biopolitics that is often perpetuated by uncritical dementia studies. In particular, I focus on two of the claims discussed in Chapter 4: "dementia is not a normal part of ageing" and "dementia is caused by diseases of the brain". I question the idea that biogenic accounts of psychiatric disorder lead to reduced stigma. Taking a critical gerontological perspective on the separation of dementia from normal ageing, I explore the apparent contradiction of destigmatising a

DOI: 10.4324/9781003398523-6

phenomenon by denormalising it. I argue that these claims, and the roles that they play in the wider awareness economy, could risk exacerbating certain forms of stigma, particularly via unintentional othering that resonates with structural disadvantages faced by people affected by dementia. I conclude that awareness raising is another key area where critical dementia studies could engage with neuropsychiatric biopolitics and question the role of some dementia studies in furthering the stigmatisation of cognitive decline in later life.

6.1 Awareness as Biopolitics

During the latter half of the 20th century and the early 21st century, campaigns to convey health-related information to the general public have become increasingly central to public health strategy. It is now widely recognised by major public health institutions that a key function of their field is the advertising of health information. Indeed, many renowned organisations provide resources, offering guidance on how to maximise the effectiveness of public messaging, and the field of health communication has grown significantly, with departments being established in many educational and government institutions.[1, 2] This health communication field can point to a proud history of improving public health through awareness-raising initiatives. The promotion of vaccinations, smoking cessation and contraceptives are a few well-known examples of areas where dedicated public messaging has contributed to population health improvements.

The concept of "awareness"[1] plays an important role in neuropsychiatric biopolitics generally. An emphasis on awareness, both making claims about its current state and seeking to change it, has become a key feature of public health responses to mental illness. This is represented by the growing collection of high-profile celebrity disclosures of personal experiences of psychiatric disorder[3] Examples are commonplace. For instance, in 2019, the BBC produced an acclaimed documentary in which the popular singer Jesy Nelson disclosed her experiences with mental illness.[4] In 2020, Public Health England partnered with Prince William and various premier league football players to produce a film focusing on raising awareness about actions to support positive mental health.[5] In 2021, the popstar Demi Lovato starred in a YouTube original documentary series focusing on her history of mental disorder.[6] While each of these instances has its own specificities, they collectively exemplify a long and growing list of celebrity mental health awareness projects. Across such initiatives, the value of openness and understanding is repeatedly championed as a key rationale and basis for action. The openness of celebrity figureheads is supposed to encourage publics to emulate their conduct and become similarly open. These initiatives rarely acknowledge that the celebrities involved may have different circumstantial capacities for responding to mental illness than other members of the public. Prince William is unlikely to have to navigate the relevant bureaucracies and waiting lists for

NHS CBT, etc. As such, awareness is often decontextualised as somehow resource neutral or independent (an issue returned to in Chapter 8).

As with the broader post-1970s neuropsychiatric biopolitics, dementia resonates with the turn to awareness. Campaigns seeking to raise awareness now comprise a core function of public health and third-sector reactions to dementia. Indeed, improved awareness of dementia is enshrined in the National Dementia Strategies of England,[7] Scotland[8] and Wales.[9] The public is encouraged to develop their understanding of dementia, treat those affected kindly and perhaps donate to worthy associated causes. Those affected, or potentially affected, by dementia, are advised to be open about their problems and seek formal help, typically in terms of official diagnosis. As with the above examples, celebrity endorsement and glossy productions, decontextualised through vague psychological vocabularies of greater "understanding", "hope", "positivity", etc. are central to dementia awareness campaigning. For example, ARUK has partnered with several high-profile celebrities to produce powerful awareness-raising media content. Speaking about one of these initiatives, the charity's chief executive, Hilary Evans, stated:

> Samuel L. Jackson's role in our #ShareTheOrange campaign will put a global spotlight on the seriousness of dementia and the huge impact it has on society … We're calling on the public to #ShareTheOrange, turn fatalism into hope.[10]

In a similar manner, the Alzheimer's Society employs a range of celebrity "ambassadors" who use their profiles to raise public awareness about dementia. For example, famous actress and Alzheimer's Society ambassador Carey Mulligan states: "I want every person in every corner of the world to be dementia aware … we need to change the way people think, act and talk about the condition.[11]" Here, the biopolitical aim of transforming public thought and conduct is explicit. The material aims of resource distribution, service provision and effective evidence-based intervention are missing. Change is first and foremost demanded of the individual.

The aforementioned #ShareTheOrange initiative, developed by ARUK, is among the most well-known British dementia awareness campaigns.[12] The Bryan Cranston quotes at the beginning of each section in Chapter 4 are taken from this campaign. To recap:

> It all starts and ends with the brain … Dementia is caused by diseases, most commonly Alzheimer's. It physically destroys cells.
> Too many people still believe that dementia is just a natural part of ageing.
> Alzheimer's is a physical disease that we can fight. Research has already made great breakthroughs in other diseases, like cancer and AIDS, and with your support, Alzheimer's Research UK will breakthrough against dementia.[13]

They relay core neuropsychiatric claims and, as will become apparent in this chapter, are an important component of the translation of the biopolitics of dementia into awareness raising. The #ShareTheOrange initiative is an impressive high-production media campaign. Running since 2015, it has been fronted by Christopher Eccleston, Bryan Cranston and Samuel L Jackson. A key feature of the campaign is its conduciveness to social media, intentionally embedded in the title via the "#Share" component, and also manifest in its use of the orange emoji, which can easily be added to profile names and descriptions. By 2019, it had already been shared more than two million times.[14]

The Alzheimer's Society's Dementia Friends[15] programme is another awareness campaign of comparable scope to ARUK's #ShareTheOrange initiative. The core premise of Dementia Friends is that the well-being of people affected by dementia can be better supported if the public has greater awareness of dementia and associated issues (which in practice entails learning five core principles). Organisations and members of the public can sign up for 45-minute training sessions with an awareness facilitator. Alternatively, the Alzheimer's Society offers a short online awareness-raising video. After attending the session or watching the video, the newly aware participants can get a Dementia Friends badge. In 2019, the scheme announced its three millionth Friend, and comparable worldwide initiatives had reached 20 million people.[11, 16] As with the #ShareTheOrange initiative, Dementia Friends awareness raising is heavily indebted to neuropsychiatric biopolitics, with the claims discussed in Chapter 4 forming core components of its messaging. Indeed, two of the five core principles are "dementia is not a normal part of ageing" and "dementia is caused by diseases of the brain".

6.2 Awareness in Dementia Studies

As well as the high-production national and international initiatives of major institutions that reach millions of people, awareness campaigning is manifest on a smaller scale. Children and minoritised ethnic people are popular targets for such programmes, the latter of which I will explore in depth in Chapter 7. Examples include the "Kids4Dementia" scheme, which works across several Australian schools to raise dementia awareness in children.[17] In the UK, "Dementia Detectives" runs awareness sessions in secondary schools.[18] In the US, the "Psycho-educational Intervention for African American Caregivers" provides several awareness modules targeting African Americans,[19] while a series of fotonovelas have been designed to spread dementia awareness in Latino communities.[20] Again, these initiatives are heavily reliant on neuropsychiatric biopolitics, promoting biogenic disease-centred, anti-"normal ageing" conceptualisations and decontextualised pseudo-psychological solutions. They represent the explicit participation of dementia studies in neuropsychiatric biopolitics because many such initiatives are designed, run and assessed by social dementia scholars. This active involvement is a common feature of dementia awareness enterprises more broadly. All these examples manifest social scientific efforts to assess and intervene in awareness, with the aim of improving dementia-related outcomes, albeit heterogeneously defined.

As awareness campaigns have become an increasingly influential strand of neuropsychiatric biopolitics, a concomitant sub-genre of dementia studies has grown around it. The above examples of specific awareness interventions are outweighed by a far larger collection of assessments that seek to measure what a certain population knows about dementia and appraise the goodness/ badness of that knowing. Some research that I did in 2020 revealed the rapid proliferation of research publications attending to dementia "awareness", "literacy", "understanding" and "knowledge" from 1970 to 2020. Based on PubMed records, while dementia-related publications increased substantially but steadily as a proportion of overall research publications over this period, the proportion of awareness-focused dementia papers proliferated massively from the early 2000s onward.[21] As a result, there now exists a sizeable canon of literature offering assessments of the dementia awareness (again using various terms to indicate what people think about dementia) of many different populations, including people with dementia,[22, 23] family carers,[24-26] healthcare professionals[27-29] and the general public, both nationally[30-33] and internationally.[34, 35]

These efforts to appraise dementia awareness entail the creation of various tools to operationalise and measure a subject's knowledge about dementia.[36] The tools typically work by establishing a series of truths about dementia, asking the target population questions relating to those truths, and then comparing the (in)congruences between the truths and the participants' responses. Another common way of achieving this comparison is by presenting participants with a series of true and false statements about dementia and asking them whether they believe the statements to be true or false. The truths and falsehoods that are used in these tools typically manifest neuropsychiatric claims regarding dementia. For instance, the following is a collection of statements about dementia from various studies. In each instance, participants were asked to evaluate whether the statements were true or false:

Alzheimer's disease is a normal process of aging, like graying of hair or wrinkles. [37]
Significant loss of memory and mental ability, commonly known as senility, is a normal part of aging. [38]
All humans if they live long enough, will probably develop Alzheimer's disease. [39]

The correct[2] answer in all of these cases was "false". If participants deemed the statements to be true, then this was interpreted by the researchers as evidence of poor dementia awareness. The falseness of each of these statements largely relies on the claim that dementia is not a normal part of ageing. As discussed in Chapter 3, this differentiation of normal from abnormal and ageing from dementia is difficult to sustain from a molecular or clinical perspective. It contains within it a series of political considerations, ranging from the attempt to establish value-neutrality through quantified operationalisations of (ab)normality, to the regulation of clinical trials for age-related syndromes (i.e. "ageing" is not a sanctioned FDA indication). With this in mind, these awareness assessments can be understood as measuring the extent to which participants are aligned with neuropsychiatric biopolitics. A great deal of dementia studies scholarship appears relatively unalert to the relations between "awareness" and neuropsychiatric biopolitics, too often assuming that the implicated truths and falsehoods are somehow absolute. Again, an aura of scientism perhaps discourages our criticality.

Beyond the development of awareness questionnaires and the application of direct statements, a parallel body of dementia awareness evaluation scholarship achieves similar ends through qualitative means. In these instances, researchers typically conduct more discursive interviews with select populations. Evidence of (un)awareness is subsequently located within these discussions when researchers analyse them, looking for particular utterances that relate to neuropsychiatric claims. In a similar manner to the studies relying on statement-based assessment tools, such analyses position participant concordance with neuropsychiatric biopolitics as evidence of awareness and discordance as evidence of a lack of awareness. Hence, across the sub-field of dementia awareness scholarship, awareness is operationalised as an analogue for compliance with neuropsychiatric biopolitics and acceptance of its normative claims.

Neuro-agnosticism has contributed to the proliferation of biopolitical awareness in dementia studies because assessment methods are often based on previous assessment methods. Once established, such assessments furnish precedents for further assessments and so on. Much contemporary awareness work can trace its heritage back to the Alzheimer's Disease Knowledge Test,[40] published in 1988, which is the oldest and most widely used awareness assessment tool.[41] Developed during the NIA's early attempts to promote public awareness of Alzheimer's disease, the Knowledge Test was positioned as the first robust means of measuring existing public knowledge and appraising the efficacy of emerging awareness campaigns. With this in mind, the familiar approach of providing correct and incorrect statements was chosen because it was conducive to assessing participants' instruction-based knowledge, i.e. specific knowledge they had gained from dedicated instructional sources such as dedicated awareness-raising interventions. The original statements were based on advice from ten experts, including neurologists, psychologists and epidemiologists. The authors note that advisers disagreed on some statements, with the most common criticism being that statements lacked empirical evidence. In these instances, the authors followed the advice of the expert that they deemed most relevant to the statement in question. The result was a 20-item tool that laid the conceptual and methodological foundations for contemporary assessments of dementia truths and falsehoods.[40] Here, again, we can trace a contemporary strand of the neuropsychiatric biopolitics of dementia back to the development of the AD movement and its various initiatives in the late 20th century, working to solidify normative commitments in reference to numerical scales.

The growth of dementia studies projects that seek to measure the awareness of various populations is integral to the broader awareness economy of neuropsychiatric biopolitics because it produces an evidence base from which awareness initiatives can be developed. One of the most substantial exercises in assessing dementia awareness is the work undertaken for the Alzheimer's Disease International World Report.[42] This report presents the results of a huge survey of dementia awareness involving nearly 700,000 people from 155 countries. The official press release of this report opened with an appeal to the overall lack of dementia awareness that its results suggested:

> Results from the world's largest survey on attitudes to dementia reveals a startling lack of global knowledge around dementia, with two- thirds of people still thinking[3] the disease is a normal part of ageing rather than a neurodegenerative disorder [sic].[43]

This headline appeal to normal ageing, as with the report generally, manifests a particular form of awareness as beliefs aligned with neuropsychiatric biopolitical commitments. The sheer scale of the World Report positions it as a particularly potent piece of evidence regarding the state of public dementia awareness (or lack thereof) around the world. It quickly gained much attention, including across dementia studies, being shared via social and traditional media as evidence of the lack of and importance of awareness.[44, 45] As such, the report has become key source material for those who are critical of poor dementia awareness and advocate further campaigns to address knowledge deficits.

6.3 Anti-Stigma

As mentioned, the contemporary popularity of dementia awareness sits within a larger history of public health improvements led by educational campaigns. Smoking cessation and sexual health are examples of areas where targeted messaging has influenced public thought, inspired behaviour change, and thereby contributed to advances in population health outcomes. A rather intuitive example of an awareness-to-health pathway is making people aware of the adverse effects of smoking, with the aim of leading them to smoke less, leading to a lower incidence of smoking-related diseases. However, few would suggest that making people aware that dementia is not a normal part of ageing is going to lead to behavioural change that will, in turn, lead to reduced dementia incidence. This begs the question – what are we trying to achieve by raising public awareness of dementia? In essence, there are three answers here, each manifest in the WHO's *Global Action Plan* for addressing dementia.[46] The first is a relatively new and as yet underdeveloped prevention agenda, focusing on persuading people to adopt familiar health behaviours (less alcohol, more vegetables, less smoking, more exercise, etc.) in the hope that this will reduce future dementia incidence.[33, 47, 48] I reflect on the new problems that this tradition is generating in Chapter 9. The second is focused on encouraging people to seek a diagnosis for themselves and others, an issue that I unpack in Chapter 7. The third, and I would argue most substantive, answer is to change how people think about, and hence act toward, dementia and those affected by it in order to intervene in phenomena that are commonly defined as "stigma". It is this third rationale that I focus on here.

Cynically, one might argue that greater public adherence to the biopolitics espoused by charitable institutions may improve the financial fortunes of said institutions. However, putting such cynicism to one side, I think it is important to attend to the underlying rationale of the aforementioned Dementia Friends scheme run by the Alzheimer's Society. As noted, Dementia Friends is predicated on the notion that a more dementia-aware public will conduct themselves in ways that will improve the circumstances and experiences of people affected by dementia. Central to this argument is the idea that dementia is stigmatised. By this, proponents typically mean that dementia is viewed in a derogatory manner, meaning that those affected by it are similarly viewed in a negative light, and people act toward them in problematic ways, informed by the stigma. Much of this work falls back on a popular, albeit often implicit, conceptualisation of stigma as tripartite, being made up of ignorance, prejudice and discrimination, as popularised by the psychiatrist Graham Thornicroft.[49] We will return to this notion of stigma shortly because the field is afflicted by poor conceptualisations, but for now, suffice to say that a lot of work relies on a basic definition of stigma as ignorance, prejudice and discrimination blending into a sort of vague badness. Awareness is presented as a means of addressing stigma, purportedly making people think about and act differently (i.e. preferably) toward people affected by dementia.

Neuropsychiatric stakeholders are instrumental in linking awareness and stigma. As an example, the Alzheimer's Society ambassador Carey Mulligan has charted her own involvement in "promoting greater awareness and tackling stigma around dementia".[50] The 2012 edition of the annual World Alzheimer's Report produced by Alzheimer's Disease International was entitled *Overcoming the Stigma of Dementia* and opened with the claim: "It is very important that there is better public awareness and understanding to reduce the stigma associated with dementia".[51] Both the Alzheimer's Society and the Alzheimer's Association have produced separate resources listing reasons and methods to overcome stigma.[52, 53] Four of the five items on the Alzheimer's Association list centre on raising awareness and educating other people. For example, point five reads:

> Be a part of the solution. As an individual living with the disease, yours
> is the most powerful voice to help raise awareness, end stigma, and
> advocate for more Alzheimer's support and research.

Beyond third-sector organisations, stigma has also become a major issue in
dementia studies. According to PubMed, between 2000 and 2020, publications citing "dementia" increased by around 400%, whereas publications citing "dementia" and "stigma" increased by roughly 2500%. As a proportion
of all publications, "dementia" + "stigma" increased by 600% compared
with an increase of around 150% for "dementia" alone. Before the 21st century, stigma was rarely mentioned explicitly in the academic dementia literature, with only four registered publications in the 1990s and one publication
in the 1980s. These are crude metrics.[4] That said, the sheer scale suggests
that, within the general growth of dementia studies, stigma has recently and
rapidly become a big concern, aligning with the rise of awareness described
above. Within this contemporary tradition of stigma-focused dementia studies, a sizeable body of work now exists exploring the attitudes of various
populations toward dementia and finding that dementia is generally stigmatised across society.[55–59] Another notable strand of stigma-focused dementia
studies attends to media representations, documenting the ways in which
dementia and those affected by it are depicted in a negative manner.[60–63]
This literature largely paints a picture of dementia as heavily stigmatised in
a general sense.

It may have already struck you that the hypothesis that dementia is stigmatised could be difficult to evaluate. For instance, in a piece of media, it may
not be immediately clear what constitutes a negative depiction of dementia.
If a film depicts a person with dementia forgetting her child's name, is it
stigmatising dementia? What particular qualities of a depiction make it stigmatising? Is it simply a case of whether a depiction is broadly sad or happy?
There are related questions about whether the justification for viewing something negatively influences whether or not that negativity is stigmatising.
For instance, dementia is seen as a bad thing by a lot of people, and many
would argue that this assumed badness is apt. Indeed, much neuropsychiatric
biopolitics explicitly promises to abolish dementia because it is bad. I personally would not want anyone I know to go through it because I have plenty
of experience of dementia, and it can be deeply unpleasant. By thinking and
writing this, am I stigmatising dementia? If I am, does that mean that the
stigma is justified? There are blurred boundaries between stigma, pessimism
and realism here, a blurriness partly owing to that expansive definition of
"stigma" as ignorance, prejudice and discrimination. By effectively equating
stigma with badness generally, as opposed to some more particular problem,
the concept can be made applicable to a wide range of phenomena that are
deemed bad by those invoking it.

The simplistic conflation of stigma and badness has led to a research literature characterised by questionable arguments emphasising the widespread

stigmatisation of dementia. One straightforward example of this is the use of negative language about dementia as evidence of stigma. A classic example is the word "suffering", which has long been condemned across much dementia studies for inaccurately homogenising dementia as a bad experience. The "homogenising" qualification is key here. It is certainly inaccurate to say that people inherently and universally suffer with dementia. However, it is not inaccurate to say that some people suffer sometimes or even that a lot of people suffer a lot of the time. With this is mind, we understandably refrain from generalising people as "dementia sufferers" in dementia studies.[64] Unfortunately, the rationale behind this convention is too often overlooked in associated scholarship, so the use of the word "suffer" and similarly negative words in any instance is presented as stigma in and of itself. At worst, this leads to ill-tempered and inane debates over language.[14] Ultimately, individuals themselves are best placed to evaluate and articulate the extent to which they do or do not suffer, and experiences vary widely.

Besides conflations with negative language, there is also an unfortunate tendency to produce circular arguments whereby stigma is defined as incorrect beliefs about dementia. A lack of awareness is itself described as a form of stigma, meaning that raising awareness will, by definition, decrease stigma because they are defined as direct opposites. Critically, awareness here equates to complicity with neuropsychiatric biopolitics. The conflation of awareness and stigma, leaning into the "ignorance" qualification, is strange because most of us do not understand lots of different things, but we do not typically view our lack of knowledge as meaning that we are stigmatising those things. I do not know how aeroplanes work, but few would suggest that my ignorance is stigmatising aviation. Nonetheless, as with negative language, a lack of neuropsychiatric awareness is used as evidence of stigma regarding dementia. This issue is distinct from the "suffering" debate, which typically relies on the "badness" approach to stigma, but occasionally plays a role in arguments to the effect that a person does not properly understand the true nature of dementia, be that suffering or not suffering.

Echoing the aforementioned approaches to awareness, much of the stigma-as-ignorance evidence base is derived from a range of statement-based questionnaires that have been developed to measure stigma in relation to dementia. Again, we can find a range of interesting operationalisations within the various items employed in research, which participants are asked to express their relative dis/agreement with. For example, Cheng and colleagues' stigma questionnaire includes the statement, "Research on dementia is nothing but a good way for pharmaceutical companies to make profits".[65] Woo and Chung's questionnaire includes the statement, "This illness is different from other physical illnesses (e.g., high blood pressure)".[66] In the studies, agreeing with these statements is indicative of stigma. It is important to note that, while these are real examples, I am deliberately cherry-picking for dramatic (perhaps comic) effect. There are other statements that at least intuitively appear to be more relevant to stigma. For instance, one of Piver and colleagues' items asks: "Would this disease cause you shame or embarrassment?"[67] The point here is that between badness, ignorance and questionnaires, the evidence base regarding stigma in dementia studies is a mess. In a systematic review of AD stigma research, Perla Werner noted: "The term stigma is used in these studies in a conversational way, without any conceptual or operational definition".[68] This is not to refute the existence of stigma in some sense but rather to note that engagements with the topic in dementia studies are vulnerable to corruption in relation to neuropsychiatric biopolitics.

Nonetheless, stigma has become embedded in dementia studies as a frequent claim. This is evident in the common invocation of stigma as an opening gambit in various outputs. Consider the following examples from the introductions of various recent articles in the *Dementia* journal:

> Stigma negatively impacts quality of life of people with dementia and their family members.[69]
>
> Despite the high prevalence and incidence, dementia is still perceived as a highly stigmatised condition.[70]
>
> Low levels of public understanding can contribute to the fear, stigma and social exclusion associated with living with dementia.[71]

In this manner, stigma has become embedded in dementia studies literature. The existence of this stigma is used to develop and justify awareness raising. As we have seen, this awareness-raising typically entails promoting neuropsychiatric biopolitics. Again, we find a situation in which a body of neuro-agnostic dementia studies has become complicit in neuropsychiatric biopolitics. The growth of this anti-stigma awareness economy is also another example of how the interests of neuropsychiatric biopolitics and dementia studies are partially entwined in the problematisation of dementia-related phenomena. The existence of stigma as a problem warrants a corresponding assemblage of stakeholders, resources and initiatives to interrogate and address the problem. None of this is to say that stigma, or something approaching it, is not pertinent to dementia and the experiences of those affected by it. Rather, I would suggest that we need to reflect more critically on the manner in which, over a relatively brief period of time, simplistic conceptions and lax definitions of stigma have flourished within dementia studies that are remarkably concordant with certain biopolitical interests.

6.4 Anti-What?

To challenge those interests, we might do well to consider more carefully the ways in which we are conceptualising stigma and how dementia studies relates to it. Stigma has long been a substantive topic of interest in medical sociology. The touchstone for much work in this area is the seminal scholarship of Erving Goffman, one of the most influential sociologists of the 20th century. This is a useful foundation for us to begin to counter under-conceptualised appeals to stigma. However, as will become clear, by attending to interpersonal phenomena, such work does not go far enough in demarcating the structural conditions of stigma. I will expand on that point below, but first, I will better define stigma in relation to Goffman's highly influential writing. Goffman produced several ethnographic accounts of social phenomena surrounding psychiatric disorder, and one of his most renowned texts is actually entitled *Stigma*.[72] Goffman noted that, etymologically, stigma initially described signs or indicators of a badness in a person. For example, the Nazi regime infamously affixed badges to Jewish people to visibly demarcate their badness. Here, the badge is the stigma. However, the meaning of stigma has shifted over time so that it is now often applied to the badness itself. Goffman distinguished three forms of this stigma: (1) abominations of the body, (2) blemishes of individual character and (3) tribal stigma of race, nation or religion. Dementia fits most neatly into the second category, which Goffman contended is typically viewed as a matter of "Weak will, domineering or unnatural passions, treacherous beliefs, and dishonesty, these being inferred from a known record of, for example, mental disorder".

Another important means of differentiating types of stigma for Goffman was the notion of discreditation. A person with a stigma can be either discredited or discreditable. The former typically has some form of difference that is immediately tangible to others, such as a visible physical deformity. The latter has a difference that is not instantly obvious and can potentially be concealed from others so that the person might partly evade the stigma and its social implications. Like many other psychiatric disorders, dementia is often discreditable. It can be difficult to tell whether a person has dementia simply by looking at him or her. When encountering a person, we can see neither their cognition nor neurophysiology. It is usually only through the discovery of additional information, perhaps from the person's behaviour or the testimony of family members, that we come to suspect that something is amiss. In light of this, I have researched and written about the attempts of people with dementia to protect themselves from the discreditation of social stigma by concealing their impairments.[73–75] In the everyday lives of people with dementia, this means that personal experiences of stigma can be potential rather than automatically assured.

I have repeatedly found evidence of this potential stigma in my research. When I interview people affected by dementia, they typically speak of "stigma" when referring to their belief that people generally perceive dementia in a derogatory manner, a finding echoed in other studies.[76, 77] The conviction that other people view dementia, and therefore those affected by it, in this stigmatising way, feeds into fears about being perceived to be a person with dementia and treated differently, perhaps badly. I have found that this fear of the perceptions and responses of others can lead people with dementia to conceal their diagnoses where practicable. Likewise, carers have often told me of their concerns that their loved one will be viewed and treated badly by other people because of the dementia.[73, 74] Again, this finding is echoed in the wider literature, though it is important to note that some people find it helpful to openly engage with their diagnoses as a means of resisting the potentially stigmatising perceptions and actions of others.[78] There is, then, evidently a sense in which dementia is subject to stigma in the experiences of those affected.

When considering these conversations, I am struck by the way in which stigma is articulated as something that others *will have/do* if the presence of a dementia is made apparent. People with dementia do encounter palpable stigma in their interactions with others, but my interviewees mostly speak of stigma in more general terms rather than as something manifest in specific incidents. In these discussions, stigma is a potential evil to guard against rather than something that has happened or is happening. It might be tempting to deem this anticipation of stigma as somehow less bad than the more active stigma that is represented in much literature. However, the effects of anticipated stigma on those who anticipate it are not necessarily any less detrimental. In practice, the assumption that dementia is stigmatised by others can trigger experiences of anxiety and self-derision that dramatically worsen people's lives, irrespective of whether the assumption is correct. Hence, stigma can have a harmful potency simply by virtue of its possibility.

This observation of stigma – as something that is anticipated – resonates with the work of sociologist Graham Scambler on the distinctions between felt and enacted stigma. Writing on the experiences of people with epilepsy in the 1980s, Scambler contested the dominant sociological conceptualisation of stigma as mainly manifest in the discriminatory attitudes and behaviours of other people. Instead of this "enacted" stigma, Scambler argued that stigma was more typically rooted in the perceptions of people with the stigmatised condition. This "felt" stigma was no less problematic than enacted stigma. It was characterised by shame, fear and self-isolation as a means of guarding against the possible enacted stigma of others. Ultimately, the effects of felt and enacted stigma are similarly realised in as much as the person feels bad about themselves and is socially isolated, but the mechanisms differ. Hence, an expectation of stigma can be as painful as an outward experience of stigma.[79, 80]

My most affecting experience of felt stigma and the dramatic impact that it can have on somebody's life occurred during some interviews that I conducted with Brian,[5] who had been diagnosed with mixed dementia. His most pronounced symptom was aphasia, which significantly impaired his ability to speak. Aphasia is a clear example of a discreditable stigma. To observe Brian as a passer-by, you would see an ordinary man going about his business in an unremarkable fashion. However, if you were to engage him in conversation, his word-finding and pronunciation impairments would immediately reveal some form of cognitive dysfunction. Brian repeatedly lamented the risk that his dementia would be discovered if he spoke to people. He was convinced that any interlocutor would quickly recognise his dementia and judge him harshly because of it. His family members refuted his fears, claiming that this did not happen in practice, but Brian was adamant in his belief and reiterated it with considerable emotion several times. In consequence, Brian deliberately removed himself from interaction with others. He preferred the perceived safety of self-imposed isolation to the risk that people would view him detrimentally. Felt stigma caused him substantial unhappiness and loneliness, and hence qualitatively worsened his life irrespective of enacted stigma.

There are important points to clarify in relation to felt stigma: (1) it matters and can have profoundly negative effects, irrespective of any questions regarding the "validity" of the stigma, (2) it does not mean that enactive discrimination does not exist and (3) it is structurally constituted rather than representing some intrinsic psychic characteristic. This latter point is critical, and I will return to it shortly. It is important to state clearly here that Brian's story demonstrates the gravity of felt stigma. It does not refute the reality or severity of the ways in which people with dementia are viewed and treated by others. Many people with dementia are treated badly because of derogatory assumptions that others make about them based on their diagnoses. Several people have told me of various instances where others have treated them differently because of their dementias. One woman told me how her husband's friends steadily lost contact following his diagnosis. Another woman described overhearing a group of acquaintances talking disparagingly about her husband and his illness. One man with dementia lamented the way in which his doctor would talk to his wife on his behalf despite him being in the room. These instances of hurtful treatment by others, enacted under the influence of assumptions regarding dementia, evidence the manifest reality of something, faced by people affected by dementia at the hands of others, that we might understandably put into a category called "stigma". However, we would be remiss to think that stigma is solely enacted by others, thereby overlooking the substantial harm that is realised through the felt stigma of the discreditable.

Some contemporary dementia studies literature recognises the need to be attentive to felt stigma, or at least similar conceptualisations.[64, 81] That said, a large body of scholarship simply treats stigma as either derogatory or mistaken views about dementia held by other people and realised in the negative treatment of people with dementia. Again, this is the simplistic approach to a badness made up of ignorance, prejudice and discrimination. As noted, the *correct* views of dementia are aligned with neuropsychiatric biopolitics, so the anti-stigma awareness economy that has flourished around these ideas can be understood as another example of neuro-agnostic complicity. To clarify, this is not to say that no good has or can come of that economy, but its own explicit aims (i.e. stigma reduction) do not appear to have been satisfied.[82] A lack of critical attentiveness has led to a body of dementia studies inadvertently serving a particular biopolitics and its normative commitments. The problem here is not simply that these endeavours are conceptually and empirically flawed, nor that they are straightforwardly uncritical. As well as these concerns, there is also a risk that anti-stigma awareness biopolitics inadvertently exacerbates stigma and thereby worsens the circumstances of people affected by dementia. In this manner, as I will explicate in the next section, felt stigma is structurally determined by wider biopolitical machinations.

Ultimately, "stigma", in its contemporary messy form, can be an unhelpful concept in dementia studies. This is not only because of its conceptual impoverishment but also because it too often serves to individualise (either enacted by a perpetrator or felt by a victim) what is better conceptualised as biopolitical structural positioning. By this, I mean that the neuropsychiatric biopolitics of dementia generates the conditions within which felt stigma is not only possible but probable. It positions us as the enactors and feelers of stigma, as I will outline in the next section. With this in mind, I argue that stigma can be more astutely understood as the constitution of people in relation to ideas, particularly the othering of those that fall on the wrong side of governing definitions. Even a more conceptually robust appreciation of discreditation and felt stigma can easily be misconstrued as something that is either attributable to the personal or the interpersonal. Such a reading risks reiterating the shortcomings of early psychosocial dementia studies in a manner that has been roundly critiqued over recent years for its sociopolitical naivety and concurrent blaming of individuals. Here, Goffman's continued influence on stigma theorisation, while helpful in encouraging richer and more precise definitions of stigma as it is immediately manifest and experienced, can lead to misleadingly astructural analyses that obscure the wider determinants of those experiences. The challenge, then, is to take intellectually robust and experientially meaningful theorisations of stigma and to develop more critical social scientific sensitivities toward the structural determination of that stigma.

Advocating for a more structural interrogation of stigma, Heather Stuart and Norman Sartorius have argued that awareness-based interventions "do little to change the accumulated practices of social groups and social structures that systematically disadvantage those with mental ... problems".[83] I would go further in suggesting that they may contribute to those structures of disadvantage, as I will explicate in the next section. My overarching argument is that we can attend to the enacting and the feeling of stigma (drawing on well-established theorisations of stigma) as something that is fundamentally structured beyond the interpersonal level and that the neuropsychiatric biopolitics of dementia plays an important role in that structuring. A critical dementia studies approach to stigma must target the sociopolitical structuring of stigma, and by extension, a neurocritical dementia studies must deconstruct and resist the structuring of stigma in relation to neuropsychiatric biopolitics. In line with Stuart and Sartorius, one means of beginning that work is by attending to the othering capacities of the awareness economy.

6.5 Ageless Othering

The conceptualisation of stigma as discrimination stemming from prejudice and ignorance has informed anti-stigma approaches that seek to spread certain forms of awareness. As noted, this awareness typically manifests a neuropsychiatric biopolitics of dementia. It, therefore, reiterates core ideas regarding disease and ageing. This is evident in a collection of different approaches to dementia awareness. Some stakeholders have sought to remove the badness from dementia through the promotion of accounts of people living well with dementia. These types of initiatives often rely on the expertise-by-experience of people who have been diagnosed with a dementia but who maintain sufficient cognitive abilities to be able to effectively act as spokespeople, a role that would be highly demanding for many of us without dementia. I have met several such people, and their existence certainly undermines exclusively negative depictions of dementia. For instance, Wendy Mitchell is now a household name in dementia studies, having co-authored two books about her experiences of living with dementia. She has stated that her ability to articulate her experiences through writing poses a direct challenge to readers who might otherwise stigmatise people with dementia by assuming that they are inherently incapable.[84]

To understand the recent emergence of these dementia role models, we have to return once more to the shifting aetiological hypotheses of dementia. As discussed in various places throughout this book, repeated drug trial failures have led to a slight reconfiguration of dominant ideas about what causes dementia. The result is a lifecourse model of dementia, wherein pathological processes begin decades before symptoms first become evident. The thinking goes that if we intervene once symptoms have developed, then it is already too late. This shifting of dementia into earlier life has been coupled with drives for increasing early diagnosis rates.[85] Indeed, in 2014, the Department of Health sought to pay GPs in England £55 per diagnosis, which proved unpopular and was swiftly abandoned.[86] The overall expansion of diagnosis, at least up until the COVID pandemic, is evident in data published in the *Lancet*. Between 2005 and 2015, the number of people living in the UK who were diagnosed with dementia doubled.[87] COVID likely undermined these efforts, but in late 2022 the NHS launched a new dementia diagnosis drive to proactively screen care home residents, beginning with a £900,000 pilot scheme.[88] Targeted diagnostic transformations of this kind inevitably have an impact on the nature of the diagnosed population. Somewhat predictably, that population now contains people who are younger, more cognitively able and generally more well than one might anticipate of a person with dementia based on historic stereotypes. To some extent, these people are seeking to challenge those stereotypes through their own existence. Their very lives showcase an unorthodox, and perhaps more palatable, dementia.

Intriguingly, this development has catalysed a sort of identity-politics contestation of dementia, played out across academic publications, social media, conference presentations and workshops.[89] Again, this contestation revolves around the questions of legitimacy that seem to perpetually dog dementia. Prominent advocates manifest a version of living well with dementia. In response, a coalition of medical professionals and carers of people with advanced dementia accuse those people of misrepresenting dementia, being misdiagnosed, or even pretending to have dementia. Retaliating, various stakeholders berate these "dementia doubters" for attacking prominent advocates and questioning their diagnoses.[90–93] These arguments are emblematic of wider struggles within disability politics to attend to notions of representation and legitimacy, whereby figureheads with any disability will usually tend to be unrepresentatively capable and privileged simply by virtue of the demands placed upon them.

This situation evidently causes great anger and upset to many people. It also serves to underline the high stakes of dementia biopolitics as it continues to evolve. Relationally negotiated and personally important identities, be they carer, clinician, patient or person living with dementia, are imperilled on both sides, though the power dynamics are evidently unbalanced. Here we can see the ultimate risk of tying ourselves too absolutely to any specific normative commitments regarding dementia. It is a concept which has been transformed several times over the past two centuries and will undoubtedly be unrecognisable in another two. For the time being, it is probably unwise to commit steadfastly to specific prescriptions of what dementia is and what it is not. As outlined in the previous chapter, we must be mindful of "dementia heterogeneity" and the tendency for abstractions to represent a lot of people poorly and no person well.

One of the major tensions within this dementia identity politics is the question of positivity versus negativity. On the one hand, a core rationale of "living well" advocacy is to challenge negative perceptions of dementia, but, on the other hand, to emphasise the positive aspects of life with dementia risks sanitising circumstances that, for many people, are terrible. At worst, critics have claimed that it promotes a blame-laden ethic of wellness, whereby not living well with dementia is a personal failure. This debate often focuses on "living well" versus "suffering" depictions, but another interesting example of potential sanitation is the de-ageing of dementia. As noted, prominent advocates with dementia are not only well-er than the average person with dementia, but they are also typically younger. In a recent survey of social media personalities diagnosed with dementia, the average age was 59,[94] whereas the average age of onset for dementia in the general population is 80.[95] At the time of writing, the Alzheimer's Society lists 12 ambassadors who have dementia. Of those, seven were diagnosed in their fifties and four in their early sixties,[96] while around 95% of people with dementia in the UK are aged 65 and above.[97] Hence, dementia advocacy is not only sanitised in terms of cognition, albeit understandably so, but it is also stripped of its characteristic agedness, perhaps somewhat intentionally as a counter to focusing on late-stage dementia. It is important to note that the same trend is evident in dementia research. A recent meta-analysis of dementia research published in 2018–2019 found that participants were typically unrepresentatively young, likely because dementia in younger people is often more phenotypically pure and, therefore, easier to study.[98]

Again, the problematic relationship between dementia and ageing rears its head, accompanied by attempts to separate the two. It has been widely noted that negative imaginaries of ageing and dementia are often intimately entwined.[99, 100] To this end, gerontologists Paul Higgs and Chris Gilleard have explored the role of dementia within wider negative beliefs about advanced old age that centre on "fears of mental and physical decay".[101] These fears emphasise the danger that the oldest old lose all agency, an idea by which later life comes to be defined. Nothing represents this loss more than dementia. To this end, Higgs and Gilleard have argued that "the prospect of becoming demented represents a major fourth age fear more profoundly than any other infirmity".[102] Beliefs regarding the negative nature of dementia are among the most predominant manifestations of wider fears regarding the situation of extreme agedness. A wealth of material exists across critical gerontology documenting the many negative ways in which older age is generally viewed. Indeed, there is a flourishing tradition of critical scholarship attending to notions of *ageism*.[103, 104]

With the attitudinal relations between ageing and dementia in mind, it is easy to see why anti-stigma campaigners might seek to decouple the two entities, a strategy that echoes the wider neuropsychiatric pulling apart of ageing and dementia. As discussed in Chapter 4, the claim that "dementia is not a normal part of ageing" is a core message of the neuropsychiatric biopolitics of dementia and one that encompasses a complicated collection of ideas and interests. The tensions are somewhat comically evident in ARUK's *Dementia Statistics Hub*, which claims that, "It is a common misconception that dementia is a condition of older age" alongside statistics showing that around 95% of people with dementia in the UK are aged 65 and above.[97] The historian Jesse Ballenger has argued that the medicalisation of senility and senile dementia through the 20th century was partly an attempt to reduce the stigmas associated with ageing and dementia that effectively contaminated and amplified one another.[105]

To some extent, it makes sense that bracketing out a widely feared illness like dementia would make ageing more palatable. If you are not necessarily going to get dementia when you get older, then getting older might be less scary. The parallel line of argument is less intuitive because by removing "normal ageing" from dementia, awareness campaigns essentially demarcate dementia as the abnormal other category. We find ourselves in the perplexing position of emphasising abnormality as an anti-stigma strategy. This is evident in various institutional claims regarding stigma, dementia and ageing:

The British Psychological Society: Negative attitudes towards dementia can be perpetuated by the false belief that dementia is caused by normal ageing.[106]

NHS: All across the country dementia friends sessions, run by dementia champions, are disseminating awareness about dementia. Largely that it's not part of normal ageing, it is caused by brain diseases such as Alzheimer's disease … This is one way in which the stigma around dementia will be lessened.[107]

London School of Economics: Results from the world's largest survey on dementia related stigma reveal a lack of knowledge about the condition, with two-thirds of people thinking dementia is a part of normal ageing.[108]

Here, the conflation of stigma with misunderstanding, coupled with the conflation of understanding with biopolitics, leads us to a counterintuitive argument that the normalisation of dementia in terms of ageing is stigmatising. This underpins an argument for awareness interventions, whereby denormalisation is cast as a means of destigmatisation. Here, yet again, the matter of ageing causes significant difficulties for the neuropsychiatric biopolitics, leading to an unsettled de-ageing of dementia.

6.6 Abnormal Othering

Biopolitically, the denormalisation of dementia by distinguishing it from normal ageing is largely realised through appeals to brain disease and the abnormality of pathology. To reiterate the discussion in Chapter 4, appeals to pathophysiological disease entities rely on quantified notions of normality and abnormality as meaningfully distinct things. At the basic molecular and cognitive scales, this binary is difficult to sustain, but biopolitically it has proved successful. The aforementioned Dementia Friends scheme is indicative of this approach to destigmatisation via the biopolitical denormalisation and pathologisation of dementia. The first two of its five core messages are that "dementia is not a normal part of ageing" and "dementia is caused by diseases of the brain". The explicit aim of Dementia Friends is to foster social environments that are more conducive to the well-being of people affected by dementia, whereby the public is more understanding and therefore acts in better ways. The implication is that a society in which the public views dementia not as a normal phenomenon of later life but rather as a pathological entity is a society that is more dementia-friendly in attitude and practice.

The appeal to normal/abnormal divisions as a basis for social enablement echoes an established biogenic approach to illness-related stigma. The biogenesis of psychiatric disorder has long been championed by advocates as a means of extending sick role allowances to people whose behaviours are deemed problematic by others (and often themselves). The premise of such arguments is that if mental illness is the same type of thing as other diseases, then the people affected by it are equally beyond reproach and equally deserving of our sympathy, understanding, care and resources. People are absolved from the moral badness that would be attributed to their behaviours were it not for the underlying disease.[109] The badness is shifted to pathophysiologies, beyond individual control or responsibility, as opposed to personal moral failings. This enhanced social acceptability of abnormal behaviour when it is attributed to a disease entity can make psychiatric diagnoses incredibly valuable, affording those affected greater public sympathy[110]. We find similar arguments in relation to dementia. Troublesome behaviours are beyond reproach because they stem from people's brains, and you cannot blame people for what their brains do. For instance, when responding to challenging behaviour by people with dementia, the Alzheimer Society Canada recommends that we "Assure them that this is not their fault or intentional, but a result of the disease".[111]

There has been a lot of debate over the efficacy of biogenic messaging as an anti-stigma strategy.[112] The evidence does indicate that there is likely some reduction in the moral attribution of responsibility and hence blame, with the public deeming physiologically diseased people to be less morally accountable for their behaviour than if it were not rooted in a biological disease entity.[113] Unfortunately, reviews of empirical studies suggest that biogenic accounts of psychiatric disorder might actually exacerbate negative public attitudes. This is partially because a person whose behaviours are beholden to a disease rather than to him/herself is often seen as dangerously unpredictable and beyond control.[114, 115] Biogenic aetiology also emphasises the otherness of those affected because it points to the tangible physical differences between them and us,[113, 116] and individualises the problems that "stigma" encompasses by appealing to decontextualised ideals of *an-illness-like-any-other*.[112] This latter observation is particularly concerning, given contemporary sociological work on structural stigma. Felt stigma does not arise ex nihilo but instead represents what Stuart and Sartorius have articulated as the trickling down of structural stigma into people's personal lives. Structural stigma is the amalgamation of sociopolitical circumstances that collectively constitute inequalities, from laws that differentiate legal rights based on diagnoses to stereotypes that render some people less likely to be employed than others.[83] Awareness-raising appeals to biogenesis emphasise the influence of disease entities as fundamental causative agents underpinning the badness experienced by those affected. Such arguments risk attributing a wide array of extrinsic problems to an ill individual.[112]

Appeals to biogenic pathology as a means of destigmatising dementia are complicated because dementia has been widely conceptualised as a normal feature of later life for a lot of history by a lot of people. Indeed, it is only really under the contemporary influence of neuropsychiatric biopolitics that this general conception has started to shift, and even now, the normalisation of dementia as a component of ageing remains relatively commonplace worldwide. Where it has taken hold, there is debate regarding the (anti-)stigmatising effects of this denormalising biopolitics. Some have argued, in line with biogenic anti-stigma arguments more broadly, that the contemporary attribution of cognitive impairment in later life to disease processes has effectively reduced stigma by attributing behaviours to neuropathology and thereby removing the personal moral blame that was historically attributed to people with dementia.[117] Others have contended the opposite, that the rise of our contemporary disease-based notions of dementia has exacerbated stigma because what was traditionally a natural feature of human life is increasingly depicted as a highly prevalent incurable disease, stoking public fear, particularly among older people.[118] Ultimately, the state of contemporary anti-stigma scholarship and associated awareness-raising endeavours under the influence of neuropsychiatric biopolitics means that it is difficult to assess these claims. Moreover, the effects are likely heterogeneous and subtle.

What is clear is that, once again, despite a lack of robust evidence regarding stigma, awareness and the effects of intervention, neuropsychiatric biopolitics continues to pursue related strategies. These strategies are typically aligned with the interests of key stakeholders. To repeat Robert Butler's earlier-quoted admission, the dementia economy relies on generating and amplifying a "health politics of anguish".[119] In this manner, stigma can be a lucrative medium for resource accumulation if it motivates publics to act to change the entity that is stigmatised.[120] In particular, fear of dementia translates into funding for organisations, initiatives and individuals that are positioned as working toward defeating dementia. Hence, despite the complicated circumstances detailed in this chapter, we must not shy away from recognising the real material interests that are at stake in the anti-stigma economy. Felt stigma, while deeply personal for those affected, is but a manifestation of overarching biopolitical machinations, normatively driven, often in lieu of evidence, and serving stakeholder interests at the expense of those affected by dementia.

There is certainly a great deal of good intention underpinning a lot of the associated awareness-raising activity. However, good intentions do not necessarily entail good outcomes. There is a risk that anti-stigma and awareness-raising endeavours inadvertently contribute to something resembling the felt stigma described above by emphasising neuropsychiatric claims regarding the distinction between normal ageing and abnormal dementia, the gravity of this highly prevalent disease entity and the importance that we all engage appropriately with it. Reflecting on the neuropsychiatric biopolitics of awareness-raising around psychiatric disorders generally, the sociologist Nikolas Rose has questioned the ramifications of "all the anti-stigma campaigns, the fun runs, the celebrities speaking out, the argument that mental ill-health is, on the one hand, part of everyday experience and, on the other, just an illness like any other".[3] He points to the danger of benevolent othering.[121] This is a phenomenon wherein particular populations, such as people with psychiatric disorders, are subject to targeted public attention as a means of generating sympathy, which unintentionally singles them out by pointedly indicating their otherness. Hence, it is perhaps unsurprising that evidence suggests that more than two decades of major international anti-stigma campaigns regarding mental illness have not reduced purportedly stigmatising public attitudes.[122] This observation supports the idea that the awareness economy itself is a key structural determinant of stigma.

There is a well-known quote, attributed to French surgeon René Leriche, that, "Health is life lived in the silence of the organs".[123] By this, he meant that we are often only truly well when we are ignorant of our wellness and/ or illness altogether. Attentiveness to illness, even if couched in positivity, is inherently suggestive of an experience of illness. There is some merit to this observation, but it is not as if we can overcome ill health simply by ignoring it. Dementia would not go away if the awareness campaigns stopped. As noted throughout this book, the neuropsychiatric biopolitics of dementia cannot be characterised as either a good or a bad thing outright. The spread of dementia through public consciousness since the late 20th century has undoubtedly generated some positive effects, but it has simultaneously cultivated a dementia economy predicated on the othering of cognitive impairment in later life. Echoing this latter sentiment, professor of psychology Patrick Corrigan has strongly rebuked educational anti-stigma campaigns generally, arguing that, "education, at least for adults, is an overrated, mostly feckless approach to erasing stigma. In some ways, the educational zeal of the Western world is the biggest example of the stigma effect".[124] Different stakeholders reap different rewards from this economy. Biopolitical stakeholders such as research charities reap donations, and people affected by dementia reap stigma.

Despite having only been popularised over the past half-century, echoed and upheld in popular culture,[125–127] dementia now ranks among the public's most feared conditions and is consistently the most feared illness among older people.[128] It is probably no coincidence that the emergence of this fear has coincided with attempts to make dementia "a household word", to use the phrase of NIA founder Robert Butler. In this context, it is probably also no coincidence that I have encountered so much felt stigma among people affected by dementia. The constant disambiguation from normal ageing, coupled with an emphasis on disease and its grave epidemiological implications, provides copious fodder for stigma. Whether these developments have led to corresponding declines in something akin to enacted stigma and how such decline compares to the impact of felt stigma is unknown and perhaps unknowable. The limited dedicated research that exists suggests relatively little effect.[82] Across psychiatric disorder generally, the imposition of institutionalised knowledges into public thought has provided new means for dividing "us" from "them".[122] What is clearly observable is the uncritical complicity of much dementia studies scholarship in neuropsychiatric biopolitics, manifest in dementia awareness and anti-stigma.

* * *

Before ending this chapter, I want to be particularly explicit in rearticulating some of the arguments that I have made because the issues that I have covered can be contentious. First, a lot of bad feeling has been generated by arguments regarding the status of dementia advocacy. I am in no way contesting the nature of specific people's diagnoses and experiences that are in the public domain. Indeed, given the nebulousness of contemporary defi-nitions of dementia, as explicated throughout this text, it is actually rather difficult to see how anybody can make definitive statements about who does and who does not have dementia. After all, if we are to follow the latest diag-nostic guidance from the NIA and Alzheimer's Association workgroup, then most of us have AD.

Importantly, and perhaps surprisingly, I also have sympathy for the people who attack this form of dementia activism. For some clinicians, articulate advocates with dementia represent a new iteration of continuously evolving dementia classifications that may seem alien and hence alienating. From this perspective, those whose professional identities are tied to older notions of dementia face a similar existential challenge to the one experienced by the advocates whom they publicly denigrate. Similarly, people who are expe-riencing profound suffering due to dementia can look at those who seem to be prospering with a bitterness that is entirely understandable given the situations in which many people affected by dementia find themselves. The ill-tempered nature of the debate is regrettable, but emotional responses are entirely understandable and can easily be exacerbated by social media plat-forms. We could have some sympathy for those with painful experiences who are alienated by the evolving nature of dementia. A more neurocritical stance toward the biopolitics of dementia, as it influences the anti-stigma landscape, could enable us to do so by revealing the shaky nature of the knowledge claims upon which the debates are based and the power that those claims can exert over people's lives. This would encourage us to move beyond the moralisations of individuals' actions and to instead understand them in terms of structured stigma – enacted and felt.

Second, I am in no way suggesting that dementia is not subject to vari-ous derogatory attitudes. Neither am I suggesting that people affected by dementia are not judged detrimentally by others, that they do not face real-world mistreatment or that their own perceptions of this negativity are, in some sense, hyperbolic. I have repeatedly emphasised that a person's own perception of such phenomena is a sincerely grave issue that can have pro-foundly damaging effects on their own life and the lives of those around them. Ultimately, discussions of stigma too often individualise and psychol-ogise structural forces that are extrinsic to individuals but might be expe-rienced personally and potently as felt stigma, that is, the context-driven expectation that something stigma-esque and fundamentally undesirable will happen (or be done) to the person with dementia. My criticisms herein are not centred on the existence of stigma altogether or the undesirability of its effects, but rather on the manner in which a neuro-agnostic dementia studies often engage with it in line with neuropsychiatric biopolitics. A more critical dementia studies, particularly one inspired by critical psychiatry and critical gerontology, can pursue more robust conceptualisations of such phenomena and problematise the relations between neuropsychiatric awareness endeavours and the manifestations of stigma it purportedly addresses.

Stigma is repeatedly approached as something people do to other people at the level of human interaction. Conceptually, this interpersonal stigma echoes the shortcomings of psychosocial dementia studies scholarships that centre on relational selves. On the one hand, it downplays the importance of felt stigma, which can have a profound impact on the lives of those affected. On the other hand, it obscures structural manifestations of stigma that constitute contexts wherein felt stigma is a reasonable response. In an ironic twist, well-intentioned stakeholders in the awareness-economy risk exacerbating stigma by perpetuating the neuropsychiatric biopolitics of dementia through their various initiatives. The two facets of stigma relating to dementia – felt stigma and biopolitical othering – are resonant with one another. Both are likely worsened by interpersonal approaches predicated on a conviction that if publics can be made sufficiently aware, then good citizens will somehow stop doing stigma. Meanwhile, the dementia research economy simultaneously supports anti-stigma work and accrues resources by spreading certain forms of "awareness", e.g. that people with dementia are abnormal and that their brains resemble decomposing oranges.

In lieu of therapeutics or related progress, it is understandable that awareness raising as a response to dementia has a certain appeal. When a problem is very difficult, and we are largely at a loss for solutions, anti-stigma and awareness-spreading endeavours can sometimes be comforting because at least we are doing something rather than nothing.[129] However, uncritically applying ourselves to the promotion of an ageless disease is not inherently going to improve the lives of people who do suffer the consequences of stigma. As I have argued in this chapter, it may even exacerbate a pervasive felt stigma by cultivating the structural conditions of stigma that we have paid too little attention to. Moreover, there is even a risk that by promoting awareness as the solution to stigma, we are inadvertently contributing to a culture of victim blaming that characterises the neuropsychiatric biopolitics of dementia. It is to this danger that I will turn my attention to in Chapter 7.

Notes

1 I use the word "awareness" a lot, meaning efforts to engage with (measure and/or alter) what is known by X population, to draw attention to the biopolitical work that is being done and the resonances with trends across mental illness more broadly. In practice, the field is replete with alternative terms, e.g. "knowledge", "attitudes", "understanding", "literacy" and "beliefs". In the case of dementia, there is also the added terminology of "friendliness", which I unpack in Chapter 8. I am particularly cautious of "knowledge" and "belief" due to their function in racialising dementia, which I discuss at length in Chapter 7.
2 According to each respective study.
3 Note *attitudes*, *knowledges* and *thoughts* all in one sentence.

4 Diana Rose has argued that the proliferation of stigma-focused academia has been driven by its considerable capacity for bibliometric impact. For concerned scholars, stigma-related publication can be a productive strategy.[54]
5 "Brian" is not his real name. I have used a pseudonym to protect his identity.

References

1. Basu, A., and Wang, J. (2009). The role of branding in public health campaigns. *Journal of Communication Management 13*, 77–91. doi: 10.1108/136325409 10931409.
2. Bernhardt, J.M. (2004). Communication at the core of effective public health. *American Journal of Public Health 94*, 2051–2053.
3. Rose, N. (2018). *Our Psychiatric Future*. Polity.
4. BBC (2019). Jesy Nelson: "Odd one out." *BBC iPlayer*. https://www.bbc.co.uk/iplayer/episode/p07lsr4d/jesy-nelson-odd-one-out.
5. PHE (2020). HRH Duke of Cambridge and football legends champion mental health. GOV.UK. https://www.gov.uk/government/news/hrh-duke-of-cambridge-and-football-legends-champion-mental-health.
6. Demi Lovato (2021). Losing control : Dancing with the devil. *YouTube*. https://www.youtube.com/watch?v=uZmXF50Yx7I.
7. DoHSC (2009). Living well with dementia: A national dementia strategy. GOV.UK. https://www.gov.uk/government/publications/living-well-with-dementia-a-national-dementia-strategy.
8. Scotland's National Dementia Strategy: 2017–2020 (2017). http://www.gov.scot/publications/scotlands-national-dementia-strategy-2017-2020/.
9. Dementia Action Plan for Wales: 2018–2022 (2021). GOV.WALES. https://www.gov.wales/dementia-action-plan-2018-2022.
10. ARUK (2019). Samuel L. Jackson stars in powerful dementia campaign to challenge misunderstanding of condition. Alzheimer's Research UK. https://www.alzheimersresearchuk.org/samuel-l-jackson-share-the-orange/.
11. Alzheimer's Society (2022). Creating a global dementia friendly movement. Alzheimer's Society. https://www.alzheimers.org.uk/about-us/policy-and-influencing/global-dementia-friends-network.
12. ARUK (n.d.). #ShareTheOrange. Alzheimer's Research UK. https://www.alzheimersresearchuk.org/orange/.
13. ARUK (2018). Bryan Cranston confronts misunderstanding of dementia…using an orange. Alzheimer's Research UK. https://www.alzheimersresearchuk.org/bryan-cranston-confronts-misunderstanding-dementiausing-orange/.
14. Fletcher, J.R., and Maddock, C. (2021). Dissonant dementia: Neuropsychiatry, awareness, and contradictions in cognitive decline. *Humanities and Social Sciences Communications 8*, 1–11. doi: 10.1057/s41599-021-01004-4.
15. Alzheimer's Society Dementia Friends. https://www.dementiafriends.org.uk/.
16. Alzheimer's Society (2019). 3 million dementia friends. Dementia Friends. https://www.dementiafriends.org.uk/WEBNewsStory?storyId=a0B0J00000taEV1UAM#.YgYxZd_P2Uk.
17. Baker, J.R., Goodenough, B., Jeon, Y.-H., Bryden, C., Hutchinson, K., and Low, L.-F. (2019). The Kids4Dementia education program is effective in improving children's attitudes towards dementia. *Dementia 18*, 1777–1789. doi: 10.1177/1471301217731385.

18. Parveen, S., Robins, J., Griffiths, A., and Oyebode, J. (2015). Dementia detectives: Busting the myths. *Journal of Dementia Care 23*, 12.

19. Morano, C.L., and King, M.D. (2010). Lessons learned from implementing a psycho-educational intervention for African American dementia caregivers. *Dementia 9*, 558–568. doi: 10.1177/1471301210384312.

20. Valle, R., Yamada, A.-M., and Matiella, A.C. (2006). Fotonovelas. *Clinical Gerontologist 30*, 71–88. doi: 10.1300/J018v30n01_06.

21. Fletcher, J.R., Zubair, M., and Roche, M. (2021). The neuropsychiatric biopolitics of dementia and its ethnicity problem. *The Sociological Review*, 00380261211059920. doi: 10.1177/00380261211059920.

22. Lee, J.-Y., Park, S., Kim, K.W., Kwon, J.E., Park, J.H., Kim, M.D., Kim, B.-J., Kim, J.L., Moon, S.W., Bae, J.N., et al. (2016). Differences in knowledge of dementia among older adults with normal cognition, mild cognitive impairment, and dementia: A representative nationwide sample of Korean elders. *Archives of Gerontology and Geriatrics 66*, 82–88. doi: 10.1016/j.archger.2016.04.013.

23. Willis, R., Zaidi, A., Balouch, S., and Farina, N. (2020). Experiences of people with Dementia in Pakistan: Help-seeking, understanding, stigma, and religion. *The Gerontologist 60*, 145–154. doi: 10.1093/geront/gny143.

24. Andrews, S., McInerney, F., Toye, C., Parkinson, C.-A., and Robinson, A. (2017). Knowledge of dementia: Do family members understand dementia as a terminal condition? *Dementia 16*, 556–575. doi: 10.1177/1471301215605630.

25. Graham, C., Ballard, C., and Sham, P. (1997). Carers' knowledge of dementia and their expressed concerns. *International Journal of Geriatric Psychiatry 12*, 470–473. doi: 10.1002/(SICI)1099-1166(199704)12:4<470::AID-GPS503>3.0.CO;2-N.

26. Hinton, L., Franz, C.E., Yeo, G., and Levkoff, S.E. (2005). Conceptions of dementia in a multiethnic sample of family caregivers. *Journal of the American Geriatrics Society 53*, 1405–1410. doi: 10.1111/j.1532-5415.2005.53409.x.

27. Fessey, V. (2007). Patients who present with dementia: Exploring the knowledge of hospital nurses. *Nursing Older People (through 2013) 19*, 29–33.

28. Pathak, K.P., and Montgomery, A. (2015). General practitioners' knowledge, practices, and obstacles in the diagnosis and management of dementia. *Aging & Mental Health 19*, 912–920. doi: 10.1080/13607863.2014.976170.

29. Turner, S., Iliffe, S., Downs, M., Wilcock, J., Bryans, M., Levin, E., Keady, J., and O'Carroll, R. (2004). General practitioners' knowledge, confidence and attitudes in the diagnosis and management of dementia. *Age and Ageing 33*, 461–467. doi: 10.1093/ageing/afh140.

30. Cahill, S., Pierce, M., Werner, P., Darley, A., and Bobersky, A. (2015). A systematic review of the public's knowledge and understanding of Alzheimer's disease and dementia. *Alzheimer Disease & Associated Disorders 29*, 255–275. doi: 10.1097/WAD.0000000000000102.

31. Glynn, R.W., Shelley, E., and Lawlor, B.A. (2017). Public knowledge and understanding of dementia—Evidence from a national survey in Ireland. *Age and Ageing 46*, 865–869. doi: 10.1093/ageing/afx082.

32. McParland, P., Devine, P., Innes, A., and Gayle, V. (2012). Dementia knowledge and attitudes of the general public in Northern Ireland: An analysis of national survey data. *International Psychogeriatrics 24*, 1600–1613. doi: 10.1017/S1041610212000658.

33. Smith, B.J., Ali, S., and Quach, H. (2014). Public knowledge and beliefs about dementia risk reduction: A national survey of Australians. *BMC Public Health 14*, 661. doi: 10.1186/1471-2458-14-661.
34. Cations, M., Radisic, G., Crotty, M., and Laver, K.E. (2018). What does the general public understand about prevention and treatment of dementia? A systematic review of population-based surveys. *PLOS ONE 13*, e0196085. doi: 10.1371/journal.pone.0196085.
35. Van Patten, R., and Tremont, G. (2020). Public knowledge of late-life cognitive decline and dementia in an international sample. *Dementia 19*, 1758–1776. doi: 10.1177/1471301218805923.
36. Sullivan, K.A., and Mullan, M.A. (2017). Comparison of the psychometric properties of four dementia knowledge measures: Which test should be used with dementia care staff? *Australasian Journal on Ageing 36*, 38–45. doi: 10.1111/ajag.12299.
37. Ayalon, L., and Areán, P.A. (2004). Knowledge of Alzheimer's disease in four ethnic groups of older adults. *International Journal of Geriatric Psychiatry 19*, 51–57. doi: 10.1002/gps.1037.
38. Connell, C.M., Roberts, J.S., McLaughlin, S.J., and Akinleye, D. (2009). Racial differences in knowledge and beliefs about Alzheimer disease. *Alzheimer Disease and Associated Disorders 23*, 110–116. doi: 10.1097/WAD.0b013e318192e94d.
39. Jang, Y., Kim, G., and Chiriboga, D. (2010). Knowledge of Alzheimer's disease, feelings of shame, and awareness of services among Korean American elders. *Journal of Aging and Health 22*, 419–433. doi: 10.1177/0898264309360672.
40. Dieckmann, L., Zarit, S.H., Zarit, J.M., and Gatz, M. (1988). The Alzheimer's disease knowledge test. *The Gerontologist 28*, 402–408. doi: 10.1093/geront/28.3.402.
41. Spector, A., Orrell, M., Schepers, A., and Shanahan, N. (2012). A systematic review of 'knowledge of dementia' outcome measures. *Ageing Research Reviews 11*, 67–77. doi: 10.1016/j.arr.2011.09.002.
42. ADI (2019). *World Alzheimer Report 2019: Attitudes to dementia.* Alzheimer's Disease International. https://www.alzint.org/resource/world-alzheimer-report -2019/.
43. ADI (2019). World's largest dementia study reveals two thirds of people still incorrectly think dementia is a normal part of ageing, rather than a medical condition. https://www.alzint.org/news-events/news/worlds-largest-dementia -study-reveals-two-thirds-of-people-still-incorrectly-think-dementia-is-a -normal-part-of-ageing-rather-than-a-medical-condition/.
44. Andrews, M. (2019). Challenging the Alzheimer's stigma. Medical Xpress. https://medicalxpress.com/news/2019-09-alzheimer-stigma.html.
45. Templeton, L. (2019). 95% of people think they could develop dementia with age. Medical News Today. https://www.medicalnewstoday.com/articles /326492.
46. WHO (2017). WHO global action plan on dementia. Alzheimer's Disease International. https://www.alzint.org/what-we-do/partnerships/world-health -organization/who-global-plan-on-dementia/.
47. Kivipelto, M., Mangialasche, F., Snyder, H.M., Allegri, R., Andrieu, S., Arai, H., Baker, L., Belleville, S., Brodaty, H., Brucki, S.M., et al. (2020). Worldwide FINGERS network: A global approach to risk reduction and prevention of dementia. *Alzheimer's & Dementia 16*, 1078–1094. doi: 10.1002/alz.12123.

48. Fahey, M., Tinker, A., and Fletcher, J.R. (2023). Dementia's preventative futures: Researcher perspectives on prospective developments in the UK. Working with Older People. doi: 10.1108/WWOP-10-2022-0049.

49. Thornicroft, G., Rose, D., Kassam, A., and Sartorius, N. (2007). Stigma: Ignorance, prejudice or discrimination? *The British Journal of Psychiatry 190*, 192–193. doi: 10.1192/bjp.bp.106.025791.

50. Mulligan, C. (2016). Creating a world where every person in every corner of the globe is Dementia-Aware. HuffPost UK. https://www.huffingtonpost.co.uk/carey-mulligan/dementia-carey-mulligan_b_12101992.html.

51. Mittelman, M., and Batsch, N. (2012). *World Alzheimer Report 2012: Overcoming the stigma of dementia*. Alzheimer's Disease International. https://www.alzint.org/resource/world-alzheimer-report-2012/.

52. Alzheimer's Association (2022). Overcoming Stigma. Alzheimer's Association. https://alz.org/help-support/i-have-alz/overcoming-stigma.

53. Alzheimer's Society (2019). 5 ways dementia stigma must be challenged. Alzheimer's Society. https://www.alzheimers.org.uk/blog/dementia-stigma.

54. BSA (2022). *Critical Mental Health Seminar Series – 2022/2023*. British Sociological Association. https://www.britsoc.co.uk/groups/medical-sociology-groups/sociology-of-mental-health-study-group/events/.

55. Werner, P., and Kim, S. (2021). A cross-national study of dementia stigma among the general public in Israel and Australia. *Journal of Alzheimer's Disease 83*, 103–110. doi: 10.3233/JAD-210277.

56. Blay, S.L., and Peluso, É.T.P. (2010). Public stigma: The community's tolerance of Alzheimer disease. *The American Journal of Geriatric Psychiatry 18*, 163–171. doi: 10.1097/JGP.0b013e3181bea900.

57. Chan, P.A., and Chan, T. (2009). The impact of discrimination against older people with dementia and its impact on student nurses professional socialisation. *Nurse Education in Practice 9*, 221–227. doi: 10.1016/j.nepr.2008.05.005.

58. Gove, D., Small, N., Downs, M., and Vernooij-Dassen, M. (2017). General practitioners' perceptions of the stigma of dementia and the role of reciprocity. *Dementia 16*, 948–964. doi: 10.1177/1471301215625657.

59. Herrmann, L.K., Welter, E., Leverenz, J., Lerner, A.J., Udelson, N., Kanetsky, C., and Sajatovic, M. (2018). A systematic review of dementia-related stigma research: Can we move the stigma dial? *The American Journal of Geriatric Psychiatry 26*, 316–331. doi: 10.1016/j.jagp.2017.09.006.

60. Kirkman, A.M. (2006). Dementia in the news: The media coverage of Alzheimer's disease. *Australasian Journal on Ageing 25*, 74–79. doi: 10.1111/j.1741-6612.2006.00153.x.

61. Van Gorp, B., and Vercruysse, T. (2012). Frames and counter-frames giving meaning to dementia: A framing analysis of media content. *Social Science & Medicine 74*, 1274–1281. doi: 10.1016/j.socscimed.2011.12.045.

62. Peel, E. (2014). 'The living death of Alzheimer's' versus 'Take a walk to keep dementia at bay': Representations of dementia in print media and carer discourse. *Sociology of Health & Illness 36*, 885–901. doi: 10.1111/1467-9566.12122.

63. Gerritsen, D.L., Kuin, Y., and Nijboer, J. (2014). Dementia in the movies: The clinical picture. *Aging & Mental Health 18*, 276–280. doi: 10.1080/13607863.2013.837150.

64. Swaffer, K. (2014). Dementia: Stigma, language, and dementia-friendly. *Dementia 13*, 709–716. doi: 10.1177/1471301214548143.

65. Cheng, S.-T., Lam, L.C.W., Chan, L.C.K., Law, A.C.B., Fung, A.W.T., Chan, W., Tam, C.W.C., and Chan, W. (2011). The effects of exposure to scenarios about dementia on stigma and attitudes toward dementia care in a Chinese community. *International Psychogeriatrics 23*, 1433–1441. doi: 10.1017/S1041610211000834.

66. Woo, B.K.P., and Chung, J.O.P. (2013). Public stigma associated with dementia in a Chinese-American immigrant population. *Journal of the American Geriatrics Society 61*, 1832–1833. doi: 10.1111/jgs.12472.

67. Piver, L.C., Nubukpo, P., Faure, A., Dumoitier, N., Couratier, P., and Clément, J.-P. (2013). Describing perceived stigma against Alzheimer's disease in a general population in France: The STIG-MA survey. *International Journal of Geriatric Psychiatry 28*, 933–938. doi: 10.1002/gps.3903.

68. Werner, P. (2014). Stigma and Alzheimer's disease: A systematic review of evidence, theory, and methods. In: P. W. Corrigan (ed.), *The Stigma of Disease and Disability: Understanding Causes and Overcoming Injustices*. American Psychological Association, pp. 223–244. doi: 10.1037/14297-012.

69. Nguyen, T., and Li, X. (2020). Understanding public-stigma and self-stigma in the context of dementia: A systematic review of the global literature. *Dementia 19*, 148–181. doi: 10.1177/1471301218800122.

70. Kim, S., Richardson, A., Werner, P., and Anstey, K.J. (2021). Dementia stigma reduction (DESeRvE) through education and virtual contact in the general public: A multi-arm factorial randomised controlled trial. *Dementia 20*, 2152–2169. doi: 10.1177/1471301220987374.

71. Phillipson, L., Hall, D., Cridland, E., Fleming, R., Brennan-Horley, C., Guggisberg, N., Frost, D., and Hasan, H. (2019). Involvement of people with dementia in raising awareness and changing attitudes in a dementia friendly community pilot project. *Dementia 18*, 2679–2694. doi: 10.1177/1471301218754455.

72. Goffman, E. (1963). *Stigma: Notes on the Management of Spoiled Identity*. Simon and Schuster.

73. Fletcher, J.R. (2020). Distributed selves: Shifting inequities of impression management in couples living with dementia. *Symbolic Interaction 43*, 405–427. doi: 10.1002/symb.467.

74. Fletcher, J.R. (2019). Discovering deviance: The visibility mechanisms through which one becomes a person with dementia in interaction. *Journal of Aging Studies 48*, 33–39. doi: 10.1016/j.jaging.2018.12.003.

75. Fletcher, J.R. (2021). Situational expectations and surveillance in families affected by dementia: Organising uncertainties of ageing and cognition. *Health Sociology Review 0*, 1–17. doi: 10.1080/14461242.2021.1888653.

76. Ashworth, R. (2020). Perceptions of stigma among people affected by early- and late-onset Alzheimer's disease. *Journal of Health Psychology 25*, 490–510. doi: 10.1177/1359105317720818.

77. O'Sullivan, G., Hocking, C., and Spence, D. (2014). Dementia: The need for attitudinal change. *Dementia 13*, 483–497. doi: 10.1177/1471301213478241.

78. O'Connor, D., Mann, J., and Wiersma, E. (2018). Stigma, discrimination and agency: Diagnostic disclosure as an everyday practice shaping social citizenship. *Journal of Aging Studies 44*, 45–51. doi: 10.1016/j.jaging.2018.01.010.

79. Scambler, G., and Hopkins, A. (1986). Being epileptic: Coming to terms with stigma. *Sociology of Health & Illness 8*, 26–43. doi: 10.1111/1467-9566.ep11346455.

80. Scambler, G. (1989). *Epilepsy*. Routledge.
81. Fletcher, J.R. (2021). Destigmatising dementia: The dangers of felt stigma and benevolent othering. *Dementia 20*, 417–426. doi: 10.1177/1471301219884821.
82. Werner, P., and Kermel Schiffman, I. (2018). Exposure to a national multimedia Alzheimer's disease awareness campaign: Assessing stigmatic beliefs towards persons with the disease. *International Journal of Geriatric Psychiatry 33*, e336–e342. doi: 10.1002/gps.4814.
83. Stuart, H., and Sartorius, N. (2022). *Paradigms Lost, Paradigms Found: Lessons Learned in the Fight Against the Stigma of Mental Illness*. Oxford University Press.
84. Mitchell, W. (2018). How Society Labels Each and Everyone of Us…….. Which me am I today? https://whichmeamitoday.wordpress.com/2018/11/21/how-society-labels-each-and-everyone-of-us/.
85. Brayne, C., and Kelly, S. (2019). Against the stream: Early diagnosis of dementia, is it so desirable? *BJPsych Bulletin 43*, 123–125. doi: 10.1192/bjb.2018.107.
86. Bell, S., Harkness, K., Dickson, J.M., and Blackburn, D. (2015). A diagnosis for £55: What is the cost of government initiatives in dementia case finding. *Age and Ageing 44*, 344–345. doi: 10.1093/ageing/afu205.
87. Donegan, K., Fox, N., Black, N., Livingston, G., Banerjee, S., and Burns, A. (2017). Trends in diagnosis and treatment for people with dementia in the UK from 2005 to 2015: A longitudinal retrospective cohort study. *The Lancet Public Health 2*, e149–e156. doi: 10.1016/S2468-2667(17)30031-2.
88. NHS England (2022). NHS launches new dementia diagnosis drive. https://www.england.nhs.uk/2022/12/nhs-launches-new-dementia-diagnosis-drive/.
89. Fletcher, J.R. (2019). Dementia is changing. Social media arguments show us how. International Network for Critical Gerontology. https://criticalgerontology.com/dementia-changing-media/.
90. Murphy, D. (2020). Please Hold. Innovations in Dementia. http://www.innovationsindementia.org.uk/2020/05/please-hold/.
91. Swaffer, K. (2018). The reliability and meaning of a dementia diagnosis. *Australian Journal of Dementia Care 7*, 21–24.
92. Howard, R. (2017). Doubts about dementia diagnoses. *The Lancet Psychiatry 4*, 580–581. doi: 10.1016/S2215-0366(17)30150-5.
93. Hu, W.T. (2017). No doubts about dementia advocacy. *The Lancet Psychiatry 4*, 830. doi: 10.1016/S2215-0366(17)30373-5.
94. Talbot, C., O'Dwyer, S., Clare, L., Heaton, J., and Anderson, J. (2020). Identifying people with dementia on Twitter. *Dementia 19*, 965–974. doi: 10.1177/1471301218792122.
95. Nussbaum, R.L., and Ellis, C.E. (2003). Alzheimer's disease and Parkinson's disease. *The New England Journal of Medicine 348*, 1356–1364. doi: 10.1056/NEJM2003ra020003.
96. Alzheimer's Society (2022). Our Ambassadors. Alzheimer's Society. https://www.alzheimers.org.uk/about-us/our-people/ambassadors.
97. ARUK (2018). Prevalence by age in the UK. Dementia Statistics Hub. https://www.dementiastatistics.org/statistics/prevalence-by-age-in-the-uk/.
98. Mooldijk, S.S., Licher, S., and Wolters, F.J. (2021). Characterizing demographic, racial, and geographic diversity in dementia research: A systematic review. *JAMA Neurology 78*, 1255–1261. doi: 10.1001/jamaneurol.2021.2943.

99. Phillipson, L., Magee, D.C., Jones, S., Skladzien, D.E., and Cridland, E. (2012). *Exploring Dementia and Stigma Beliefs: A Pilot Study Of Australian Adults Aged 40 to 65 Years*. Alzheimer's Australia.

100. Gilleard, C., and Higgs, P. (2014). Studying dementia: The relevance of the fourth age. *Quality in Ageing and Older Adults 15*, 241–243. doi: 10.1108/QAOA-10-2014-0027.

101. Higgs, P., and Gilleard, C. (2014). Frailty, abjection and the 'othering' of the fourth age. *Health Sociology Review 23*, 10–19. doi: 10.5172/hesr.2014.23.1.10.

102. Higgs, P., and Gilleard, C. (2016). *Personhood, Identity and Care in Advanced Old Age*. Policy Press.

103. Cavaliere, G., and Fletcher, J.R. (2021). Age-discriminated IVF access and evidence-based ageism: Is there a better way? *Science, Technology, & Human Values*, 01622439211021914. doi: 10.1177/01622439211021914.

104. Fletcher, J.R. (2021). Chronological quarantine and ageism: COVID-19 and gerontology's relationship with age categorisation. *Ageing & Society 41*, 479–492. doi: 10.1017/S0144686X20001324.

105. Ballenger, J. (2006). The biomedical deconstruction of senility and the persistent stigmatization of old age in the United States. In: A. Leibing and L. Cohen (eds.), *Thinking About Dementia Culture, Loss, and the Anthropology of Senility*. Rutgers University Press, pp. 106–120. doi: 10.2307/j.ctt5hjbhp.9.

106. Hassan, E. (2021). Ageism in dementia. *The Psychologist*. https://thepsychologist.bps.org.uk/ageism-dementia.

107. Burns, A. (2014). The importance of dementia friendly communities. NHS England. https://www.england.nhs.uk/blog/alistair-burns-10/.

108. LSE (2019). World's largest dementia study reveals lack of understanding about the condition. London School of Economics and Political Science. https://www.lse.ac.uk/News/Latest-news-from-LSE/2019/i-September-2019/Worlds-largest-dementia-study-reveals-lack-of-understanding-about-the-condition.aspx.

109. Rosenberg, C.E. (2006). Contested boundaries: Psychiatry, disease, and diagnosis. *Perspectives in Biology and Medicine 49*, 407–424. doi: 10.1353/pbm.2006.0046.

110. Nettleton, S. (2006). 'I just want permission to be ill': Towards a sociology of medically unexplained symptoms. *Social Science & Medicine 62*, 1167–1178. doi: 10.1016/j.socscimed.2005.07.030.

111. ASC (2022). Understanding how your relationship may change. Alzheimer Society of Canada. http://alzheimer.ca/en/help-support/i-have-friend-or-family-member-who-lives-dementia/understanding-how-your-relationship.

112. Tyler, I., and Slater, T. (2018). Rethinking the sociology of stigma. *The Sociological Review 66*, 721–743. doi: 10.1177/0038026118777425.

113. Rüsch, N., and Xu, Z. (2017). Strategies to reduce mental illness stigma. In: W. Gaebel, W. Rössler, and N. Sartorius (eds.), *The Stigma of Mental Illness - End of the Story?* Springer International Publishing, pp. 451–467. doi: 10.1007/978-3-319-27839-1_24.

114. Angermeyer, M.C., Holzinger, A., Carta, M.G., and Schomerus, G. (2011). Biogenetic explanations and public acceptance of mental illness: Systematic review of population studies. *The British Journal of Psychiatry 199*, 367–372. doi: 10.1192/bjp.bp.110.085563.

115. Kvaale, E.P., Gottdiener, W.H., and Haslam, N. (2013). Biogenetic explanations and stigma: A meta-analytic review of associations among laypeople. *Social Science & Medicine 96*, 95–103. doi: 10.1016/j.socscimed.2013.07.017.

116. Rüsch, N., Todd, A.R., Bodenhausen, G.V., and Corrigan, P.W. (2010). Biogenetic models of psychopathology, implicit guilt, and mental illness stigma. *Psychiatry Research 179*, 328–332. doi: 10.1016/j.psychres.2009.09.010.

117. Lock, M. (2013). *The Alzheimer Conundrum: Entanglements of Dementia and Aging*. Princeton University Press.

118. Whitehouse, P.J., and George, D.R. (2008). *The Myth of Alzheimer's: What You Aren't Being Told About Today's Most Dreaded Diagnosis*. St. Martin's Griffin.

119. Fox, P. (1989). From senility to Alzheimer's disease: The rise of the Alzheimer's disease movement. *The Milbank Quarterly 67*, 58–102. doi: 10.2307/3350070.

120. Paton, K. (2018). Beyond legacy: Backstage stigmatisation and 'trickle-up' politics of urban regeneration. *The Sociological Review 66*, 919–934. doi: 10.1177/0038026118777449.

121. Grey, F. (2016). Benevolent othering: Speaking positively about mental health service users. *Philosophy, Psychiatry, & Psychology 23*, 241–251. doi: 10.1353/ppp.2016.0025.

122. Walsh, D.A.B., and Foster, J.L.H. (2021). A call to action. A critical review of mental health related anti-stigma campaigns. *Frontiers in Public Health 8*.

123. Fantuzzi, G. (2014). The sound of health. *Frontiers in Immunology 5*, 1–3.

124. Corrigan, P.W. (2018). *The Stigma Effect: Unintended Consequences of Mental Health Campaigns*. Columbia University Press.

125. Swinnen, A., and Schweda, M. (2015). *Popularizing Dementia: Public Expressions and Representations of Forgetfulness*. transcript Verlag.

126. Wearing, S. (2013). Dementia and the biopolitics of the biopic: From Iris to The Iron Lady. *Dementia 12*, 315–325. doi: 10.1177/1471301213476703.

127. Wearing, S. (2017). Troubled men: Ageing, dementia and masculinity in contemporary British crime drama. *Journal of British Cinema and Television 14*, 125–142. doi: 10.3366/jbctv.2017.0359.

128. Alzheimer's Society (2016). Over half of people fear dementia diagnosis, 62 per cent think it means "life is over." Alzheimer's Society. https://www.alzheimers.org.uk/news/2018-05-29/over-half-people-fear-dementia-diagnosis-62-cent-think-it-means-life-over.

129. de Montellano, P.M.O. (2017). The viewpoint of GAMIAN*-Europe. In: W. Gaebel, W. Rössler, and N. Sartorius (eds.), *The Stigma of Mental Illness - End of the Story?* Springer International Publishing, pp. 173–189. doi: 10.1007/978-3-319-27839-1_10.

7 Moralising Ethnicity
Governance through the Racialisation of Outcomes

In this chapter, I consider how the neuropsychiatric biopolitics of dementia is bound up with a recent problematisation of ethnicity facilitated by an uncritical dementia studies. I begin by charting the 21st-century escalation of interest in ethnicity across the dementia economy. In the context of wider political sensitivities to race and ethnicity, a range of dementia-related ethnic inequalities have become a major concern for charities, governments and researchers. This turn toward ethnicity as a dementia-related issue encompasses a collection of developments that should be of concern for dementia scholars, from the operationalisation of social difference (i.e. how we collate and compare people) to the attribution of blame for bad outcomes. After outlining dementia's ethnic turn generally, I unpack core representations of inequality, whereby a range of different dementia-related outcomes, such as diagnosis rates and medication use, are normatively evaluated as either good or bad. I argue that these normative appraisals of select outcomes are not based on evidence. Instead, they are grounded in intuition, convention and the wider influence of neuropsychiatric biopolitics, with which they are broadly aligned and hence serve to substantiate.

Once I have assessed the biopolitical nature of outcome measures in appeals to ethnic inequalities, I then consider the operationalisations of ethnicity used in such appeals. The extent to which ethnicity functions as a category fallacy in social scientific analyses has long been debated, and problems in this vein continue to undermine appeals to dementia-related ethnic inequalities. More than this, I argue that the use of ethnicity (however it is conceived) as a means of stratifying outcomes implicitly positions those inequalities as intrinsically ethnic in nature. Hence, it racialises them, irrespective of differences and similarities within and between the categories that are used. This leads to a problematisation of ethnicity, particularly minoritised ethnicity,[1] as a causal factor, itself contributing to the bad outcomes with which it is associated. From this position, arguments centring on notions of cultural inadequacy are commonly presented as explaining the observed ethnic inequalities. I contend that such arguments echo historic racialisations of psychiatric disorder to position minoritised ethnic people as

DOI: 10.4324/9781003398523-7

victims of ethnically distinct characteristics that are intrinsic to them rather than extrinsic structural constraints.

Following my discussion of the mechanics of this problematisation of ethnicity, I argue that the ethnic turn, within which dementia studies itself plays an important role, actively supports a neuropsychiatric biopolitics of dementia. I suggest that it does so by linking the "badness" of minoritised ethnicity with a failure to comply with neuropsychiatric biopolitics through the self-governance of personal conduct. Minoritised ethnicity becomes a cautionary tale of how not to be, showcasing the importance of neuro-compliance. The imagined ethnic other does not think right, does not act right, and is therefore doomed to suffer. In response, I argue that a more critical dementia studies should reflect on how it engages with ethnicity, particularly by asking whose interests are best served by that engagement, and to especially consider the extent to which such engagements might be considered racist. Rather than developing educational interventions to somehow improve minoritised ethnic people, we could pursue more pluralistic approaches to dementia that recognise the value commitments at stake in various perspectives and resist the tendency to position some ideas as inherently superior.

7.1 The Ethnic Turn

In this first section, I want to characterise the ethnic turn across the dementia economy, including dementia studies. This begins with some contextualisation because the making of ethnicity into a particular type of problem in relation to dementia can only be understood within a wider methodological and political landscape of race and ethnicity. The health-related social sciences have for a long time pursued the stratification of health outcomes in reference to demographic categories as a form of analysis, typically relying on class and gender. Historically, ethnicity has been comparably absent in these approaches. This is partly because people from minoritised ethnic backgrounds were simply considered less important as foci for research. It is also because ethnicity and race have traditionally been more contentious sociological concepts, subject to ongoing debates about the biological-ness and cultural-ness of such categorisations.[1] Indeed, I will consider the nature of what is contained within and what is excluded from ethnic categorisations later in this chapter. For now, suffice to say that ethnic categories are not natural entities with fixed boundaries and intrinsic properties, but instead reflect an attempt to highlight some specificities and obscure others in much the same way as was discussed at length in Chapter 5.

Race, in its old biological uses, has steadily fallen out of fashion in much health research, given its associations with the 19th- and 20th-century beliefs that all people could be allocated to a handful of physiologically, and often psychologically, distinct races. This operationalisation of race has proved scientifically and politically problematic, making little biological sense and often manifesting assumptions of white supremacy. Ethnicity complicates biologised notions by leaning heavily on culture, partly as a means of escaping the dubious history of race. Contemporary critical sociological uses of race largely echo this complexified ethnicity. However, ethnic and cultural groupings are typically used distinctively. Ethnicity retains a reliance on semi-biological ideas of descent and heritage that are far less prominent in discussions of non-racialised cultural groups.[2] As we will see, attempts to operationalise ethnicity via these blended racial–cultural ascriptions are fraught with difficulties. They ultimately produce rather nebulous methodological engagements with the relations between ethnicity and dementia.

Concerns regarding ethnicity have played a notable role in 21st-century British politics, from Islamophobia in the wake of 9/11 and concerns with segregation following the northern race riots to the Windrush scandal and anti-Eastern European sentiment during the Brexit referendum and contemporary discourses regarding refugees crossing the English Channel. Ethnic discordance, the very idea of which relies on ethnicities being potently distinct, has repeatedly been articulated as a core social pathology.[1] In line with culture-centred notions of ethnicity, much of this pathologisation has focused on the cultural differences between ethnic groups, particularly emphasising problematic features of minoritised ethnic cultures. This is evident in the contemporary promotion of British values in ethnicity-related policy, beginning in the 2000s, which represented a shift from late 20th-century liberal commitments to tolerance of diversity.[3] Latterly, reverberations of the Black Lives Matter (BLM) movement in the US have swept across the UK, perhaps most publicly manifest in debates regarding statues and policing.

In the US, the significant contemporary public status of BLM and affiliates has rearticulated race as a core point of contention in American society. The now familiar "black lives matter" phrase emerged following the 2012 killing of Trayvon Martin and the media attention dedicated to a recording of his killer's phone call to the police. At the time, the killing received the most media coverage of any race-related news story in US history, and in its wake, viral media clips of violence against minoritised ethnic victims have regularly garnered public attention. In particular, videos of police brutality have catalysed political sentiment regarding race and racism, leading to high-profile protests and even counter-protests on the grounds that BLM is itself racist.[4] Pew Centre research in 2021 revealed that racism and illegal immigration now rank among the most partisan issues in US politics.[5] Critical Race Theory[6] has become a contentious political issue, major sports stars kneel in anti-racist protest and widely documented discrepancies in COVID mortality have revealed the stark repercussions of racial inequalities. [7–9]

It is in this context that ethnicity has become another recent conceptual growth area in the dementia economy. Echoing the previous chapter's discussion of stigma, a constellation of social phenomena has contributed to an alertness to ethnicity within dementia studies and the neuropsychiatric biopolitics of dementia. Again, the topic was largely ignored during the 20th century but has suddenly attracted substantial interest during the 21st century. For example, in 2021, the Alzheimer's Society of Canada released its first organisational statement dedicated to race and dementia, which directly referenced BLM and associated protests:

> The assertive protests on systemic racism have made many Canadians and organizations realize they must do more to ensure representation, inclusion and, most of all, accountability. Black Lives Matter, and we are taking specific, measurable steps to deliver change.[10]

The race and dementia statement acknowledged that the organisation had focused too heavily on white Canadians. In response, the Society committed to a range of future activities targeting minoritised ethnic populations. Also in 2021, for the first time, the US Alzheimer's Association published a special report as an accompaniment to its annual *Facts and Figures* report, entitled *Race, Ethnicity and Alzheimer's in America*.[11] Indicating some of the contemporary political forces underpinning the ethnic turn in the dementia economy, the report notes that over recent years:

> Social justice movements sparked new conversations about endemic and long-standing health and health care disparities faced by non-White racial/ethnic populations.

The report argues that decades of dedicated policy initiatives have failed to address health disparities generally, including inequalities between ethnic groups. In it, a wide range of dementia-related metrics are stratified by ethnic categories to highlight inequalities. These include perceptions of service discrimination, proportions of populations involved in unpaid care, and knowledge about dementia, to name but a few. This metric-by-ethnicity analysis is a common manifestation of the newly racialised biopolitics of dementia, a development that I will unpack in this chapter.

While undoubtedly motivated by good intentions to some extent, dementia stakeholders also draw benefits from their pivot toward ethnicity. For instance, ethnic inequality has recently become a means of argument for the Alzheimer's Association when defending its interests. Broadly, if dementia impacts minoritised populations, then a failure to support the Alzheimer's Association's initiatives equates to a failure to support those populations. When the CMS announced its draft decision that aducanumab would only be eligible for Medicare funding when prescribed as part of a clinical trial, the Alzheimer's Association launched a scathing attack based on ethnicity. Their statement began:

> Today's draft decision by the Centers for Medicare & Medicaid Services (CMS) is shocking discrimination against everyone with Alzheimer's

disease, especially those who are already disproportionately impacted by this fatal disease, including women, Blacks and Hispanics.[12]

In this manner, the linking of dementia with ethnicity can furnish new strategies for depicting stakeholder interests as important matters of social justice. Critics were quick to note that the Alzheimer's Association had not shown similar concern when it was revealed that a tiny number of minoritised ethnic participants had been recruited into the phase-III trials for aducanumab. Overall, the combined trial samples were 0.6% Black, 3% Hispanic, 0.03% American Indian or Alaska Native and 0.03% Native Hawaiian or Pacific Islander.[13] The Alzheimer's Association's use of ethnic inequalities as a means of furthering their interests is partly indicative of the rationales behind and manifestations of a wider ethnic turn in the neuropsychiatric biopolitics of dementia. Olúfẹ́mi Táíwò has termed this process *elite capture*, pointing to a pervasive tendency for powerful groups to appropriate radical political concepts, strip them of their political substance and deploy them in service of their own interests.[14] An analysis of underlying motivations is beyond the scope of this chapter, but suffice to say that the laudable and the manipulative are likely entangled.

In the UK, the ethnic turn is similarly evident in the activities of associated charities. Over the past few years, the Alzheimer's Society has dedicated £2.4million to developing a "BAME" (Black, Asian and Minority Ethnic) research programme, so far comprised of four studies[15]. The Alzheimer's Society is seeking to expand its BAME research portfolio and actively encourages grant applications focussing on ethnicity. Dementia advocacy has also entered the ethnicity space at a more local level. The *Meri Yaadain*[2] project was established in 2006 in the North of England and became a Community Interest Company in 2019. It aims to explore the impact of dementia on minoritised ethnic families, raise awareness and provide support.[16] In 2019, project founder Mohammed Akhlak Rauf gave a keynote speech at the Alzheimer Europe conference, focusing on intercultural care amongst minoritised ethnic communities.[17]

The recent bringing of ethnicity into the dementia economy as a salient consideration is also evident in institutional politics. In 2012, the All Party Parliamentary Group (APPG) on Dementia announced an inquiry into the experiences of minoritised ethnic people affected by dementia. This announcement coincided with a report dedicated to increasing diagnosis rates, which, as we will see, is an important strand of the racialised biopolitics of dementia. The APPG aims to make dementia a policy priority and prides itself on highlighting related issues that it believes have not received sufficient attention from policymakers. The resulting report, entitled *Dementia Does Not Discriminate*, was published in 2013. It called for greater government, service and community efforts to raise awareness of dementia among minoritised ethnic populations, which has subsequently become a core aim of many ethnicity-focused endeavours.[18] In 2020, as the COVID situation drew greater attention to health inequalities intersecting ethnicity, ageing and dementia, the Department of Health and Social Care funded the Race Equality Foundation to support a range of dementia-related projects across England.[19]

The ethnic turn is also evident in dementia studies literature. In a similar manner to the publication trends regarding dementia awareness and stigma discussed in the previous chapter, ethnicity and race have become major areas of dementia research in the 21st century. Indeed, the contemporary ethnic turn in dementia studies is even more recent, having only really taken off over the past 10–15 years, coinciding with projections of increased minoritised ethnic population ageing in the coming decades.[20, 21] There has been a 500% increase in publications referring to "dementia" and either "ethnicity" or "race" as a proportion of overall research publications since 2007. In real terms, the use of both terms has increased tenfold, from roughly 20 publications in 2007 to nearly 200 in 2021. By decade, combined publication numbers rose from 159 in 1991–2000, to 503 in 2001–2010, and 1564 in 2011–2020, with most of that growth coming in the past 5 years. As mentioned, such statistical depictions are crude and must be interpreted accordingly, but the sheer scale of increase is indicative of the rapidly growing salience of ethnicity in dementia studies. Moreover, bibliometrics are essential to understanding the contemporary academic economy.

The emergence of ethnicity as a distinct issue in dementia research is manifest in several sub-traditions of associated work. Researchers have attended to educational and awareness-raising initiatives,[22–24] diagnosis rates,[25, 26] engagement with services[27–29] and participation in research.[30–32] Across this collection of work, there is a shared depiction of ethnicity as a particular type of problem in dementia based on the observation that a range of outcomes, typically deemed to be bad, can be associated with populations that are demarcated in terms of minoritised ethnic categories.[33] Below, I show that there is a great deal of normatively determined conceptual work at play in this literature, particularly in relation to culture. More specifically, I argue that the articulation of ethnicity in relation to culture, as outlined above, and particularly the idea that minoritised ethnicities are bound up with somewhat problematic cultures, is integral to the problematisation of ethnicity in dementia. For instance, scholars regularly claim that a certain group of people, defined via ethnicity, believes a certain thing (e.g. that dementia is associated with witchcraft) and then argues that said belief is bad. Hence, at its core, the ethnic turn is a matter of what things we imagine to be problematic and how we express those problems. This making of problems begins with the measurement of outcomes and their stratification in terms of inequality.

7.2 Weaponising Inequalities

Appeals to inequality are central to the making of an ethnicity problem in dementia. This typically entails selecting a specific outcome measure, for instance, "age at diagnosis", and stratifying that measure in reference to ethnic categories[3], for instance, "white" and "black". In this scenario, imagine that our results reveal that the average age of diagnosis in the white category is 78, while the average age of diagnosis in the black category is 82. Here, we have discovered an ethnic inequality in dementia. By itself, this example might seem rather underwhelming. To make the inequality more important, or at least interesting, we can consider whether the inequality is good or bad. Imagine that we decide that it is better to be diagnosed earlier; now, our inequality has a moral component that is more deserving of our attentions and perhaps interventions. We can go further by considering the reasons that the bad thing happens, perhaps concluding that a lack of recognition of dementia is contributing to black people not seeking a diagnosis. Now we have moved from having a correlation to having both a problem and a cause. We move from statement A: "there is, on average, a four-year disparity in age of diagnosis between white and black people" to statement B: "black people with dementia experience worse outcomes" to statement C "a lack of dementia awareness among black people leads to worse outcomes". We have taken that rather mundane inequality and made it into a basis for action. If there is a problem and there is a cause, then there is potentially something good that we can do in response.

A good deal of research in this area attends to inequalities in service use. The following are a few examples from recent research papers:

> People from minority ethnic groups are under-represented in dementia diagnosis, treatment, and care.[34]
>
> Despite the rapidly ageing population and a predicted sevenfold increase in the prevalence of dementia in minority ethnic communities, people from these communities remain under-represented in specialist dementia services.[35]
>
> South Asian older adults are represented less frequently in mainstream mental health services or those for people with dementia.[36]

The proliferation of appeals to service inequalities is also evident in the wider dementia economy. For instance, the Alzheimer's Society's BAME portfolio justifies itself in relation to the research literature on ethnic inequalities in dementia. It states that "research suggests BAME communities often face delays in dementia diagnosis and barriers in accessing services".[15] These service inequalities are typically operationalised in terms of diagnosis rates and stages, use of institutional services, participation in research and receipt of medication. Supporting the existence of ethnic inequalities across all these metrics, a systematic review of the literature in 2010 concluded that minoritised ethnic people with dementia were, on average, when compared with the majority ethnic population, diagnosed less frequently and with more advanced dementias, less likely to transfer to institutional care, less likely to take part in research and less likely to receive some form of related medication.[37] In line with the wider tradition of ethnicity-focused dementia research, this review positions the inequalities as problematic for the minoritised ethnic groups. In response, it advocates for interventions to bring the outcomes in line with majority ethnic metrics.

In light of the first paragraph of this section, it should be fairly apparent that the badness of these inequalities is not inherent. Nonetheless, each is repeatedly treated as bad per se, with little reflection on how or why this is the case. Let us consider each in turn, beginning with diagnosis. It is relatively orthodox for comparative research on diagnosis rates to position diagnosis as a net positive phenomenon. Put simply, the more the diagnosis and the earlier it happens, the better. The arguments in favour of diagnosis are often regurgitated in an uncritical manner. Proponents contend that diagnosis leads to services, treatment and support, facilitates planning and can be empowering. These rationales were embedded in the National Service Framework for Older People:

> For older people with suspected dementia, early diagnosis gives access to treatment, allows planning of future care, and helps individuals and their families come to terms with the prognosis.[38]

The same justifications were carried through into the UK's National Dementia Strategy:

> Making the diagnosis early on in the illness means that there is the chance to prevent future problems and crises and to benefit more from positive interventions.[39]

Each of the component arguments in favour of diagnosis warrants independent examination. Let us begin with treatment options. As noted in Chapters 2 and 5, drug development in dementia has, to date, been an underwhelming and increasingly problematic field. Putting aside the aducanumab and lecanemab controversies, the treatments that most people diagnosed with dementia will be offered are cholinesterase inhibitors. There is debate regarding the timeliness of cholinesterase inhibitors. Some argue that, from a preventative perspective, earlier intervention is more effective. However, cholinergic deficits are greatest in more advanced Alzheimer's disease, and people with more advanced disease show a greater response to treatment.[40] More broadly, as discussed, cholinesterase inhibitors offer relatively minor positive effects and their cost–benefit is increasingly contested, to the extent that France discontinued funding in 2018.[41]

Turning to the argument that diagnosis leads to service access, it is somewhat intuitive that a person is more likely to receive dedicated services if they have a diagnosis. If nothing else, it seems unlikely that people would receive dementia services if they did not have a dementia diagnosis. However, as noted in Chapter 3, the institutionalisation and administration of dementia as a social problem rather than a health problem means that, in practice, dementia is largely an informal affair. Most people with dementia are supported by family and friends, with little formal service contact beyond irregular GP visits. That said, it is important to note that a diagnosis can entitle people to less obvious forms of institutional support. People affected by dementia can qualify for perks such as disabled parking, rapid-response vehicle breakdown assistance or even prioritisation for local authority pavement maintenance.[42]

Another common argument in favour of diagnosis is the idea that it enables planning for the future. The importance of planning is often advocated in relation to putting one's affairs in order, authorising a power of attorney and documenting any advance decisions. These ideals are, to a large extent, reliant on prognostic assumptions that are at odds with the realities of dementia. In practice, a newly diagnosed person might be severely impaired within 6 months or relatively able after 5 years. Moreover, decline can be characterised by sudden instances of deterioration interspersed by longer periods of relative stability, particularly in vascular dementia, influenced by events and conditions beyond the cause of the dementia itself. As an extreme example of prognostic uncertainty, I once interviewed a lorry driver who gave up his driving licence when diagnosed with dementia in expectation of forthcoming decline. Ten years later, this man was still fairly independent and regretted his decision to stop driving. Prognostic variability is exacerbated by the imprecision of diagnoses. For all the hype around biomarker-based diagnostic precision, most dementia diagnoses are still dependent on cognitive assessment and family testimony. The majority of diagnoses are broad brush and technically provisional.[43] Ultimately, the real-world experience of dementia is often one of profound uncertainty.[44]

Finally, there is an argument that diagnosis can be psychologically beneficial, empowering people to make sense of their experiences and take steps to improve their circumstances. Research has suggested that most people would wish to know if they had dementia. However, a sizeable minority do not, and around half of people who receive a positive screening result do not seek any diagnostic confirmation for fear of repercussions.[43] Unsurprisingly, a dementia diagnosis can be deeply distressing, both for the person and for loved ones. As mentioned in the previous chapter, research has shown that dementia is now the most feared diagnosis among older adults, bound up with negative assumptions about a loss of agency and even self. This can lead to depression and even elevated suicide risk.[45] That said, a review of diagnostic disclosure found that negative psychological implications were typically short-lived and that there was scant evidence of long-term negative effects.[46]

While the evidence base is inconclusive, my own experience of working with people with dementia is that the potential for a diagnosis to be empowering is somewhat dependent on the individual. I have encountered some people who have been relieved to have a medical explanation for their troubling experiences and have used that diagnosis to conduct their own research and pursue strategies for living well with dementia. This dependency on the idiosyncrasies of an individual's character and his/her circumstances reminds us that it is important not to conflate *early* diagnosis with *timely* diagnosis. The former is a diagnosis as chronologically early as possible, while the latter is a diagnosis at the time most suited to the needs and circumstances of the individual.[47] The promotion of a timely approach to diagnosis has potential in principle because, by definition, it is a diagnostic approach that centres on the person's unique interests. However, it is difficult to envision how such ideals could be realised in practice, that is, how we could practically determine who would benefit from a diagnosis, how so, and at what point in their trajectory. Logically, "timeliness" can only be judged retrospectively and can never be known for certain. Indeed, for some individuals, the timeliest diagnosis might be never at all.

Besides questioning the purported positives of diagnosis, critics have also highlighted the potential harms. Greater emphasis on diagnosis can lead to more false positives, risky medications, reduced treatment of concurrent mental illness, overstretching specialist services, emotional distress, experiences of negative treatment by others, isolation, increased insurance premiums, driving restrictions, reduced legal rights and family attempts to control finances and assets.[48] Again, these arguments are ultimately open to debate, and many of the risks of diagnosis can be mitigated against. Regardless of the relative merits of different arguments for and against the expansion of diagnosis, it is a core commitment within the neuropsychiatric biopolitics of dementia. To some extent, this makes sense because it is a particularly obvious manifestation of the expansion of dementia as a personal, public and political concern. More diagnosis equals more dementia. This commitment to diagnosis feeds into the ethnic turn as a means of problematising ethnicity, while the ethnic turn simultaneously provides another justification for extolling the importance of diagnosis. To this end, the Prime Minister's Challenge on Dementia 2020 explicitly advocated for "improving the diagnosis of dementia for people of Black, Asian and Minority Ethnic origin and other seldom heard groups".[49] The emphasis on diagnosis largely preceded the emphasis on ethnic inequalities, the latter serving to substantiate the former commitment.

Uncritical appeals to diagnosis as a positive thing, both generally and in relation to ethnicity specifically, are grounded in a wider neuropsychiatric biopolitics of diagnostic expansion more than a corresponding evidence base. Ultimately, we lack sophisticated and robust evidence from longitudinal multi-measure studies that would enable us to make sound assessments of the relative pros and cons of diagnostic expansion. As a result, such arguments are largely rooted in a mix of presumption and convention.[50, 51] Of course, that does not necessarily entail that such arguments lack merit absolutely. My point here is not that diagnosis is good or bad per se, but rather that we cannot say this with any guise of empirical or moral justification. As such, strong appeals in either direction are essentially biopolitical manifestations of select normative commitments. They serve some interests and do a disservice to others.

Moving on from the major issue of diagnosis, inequalities in the uptake of residential care, wherein minoritised ethnic people are underrepresented in these institutions, are another area in which research has positioned outcomes as bad. This problematisation of low institutionalisation often appeals to two things: (1) the motivations behind it and (2) the potential implications for caregivers. The first of these concerns is that the motivations behind low uptake are themselves somehow negative or at least indicative of something negative. A review of the research literature on ethnic inequalities across many dementia-related metrics found that lower service uptake was typically attributed to minoritised ethnic people being "too proud to accept supportive services" and having an "aversion to institutionalization of relatives" and a "distrust of outsiders".[52] Here, the problematic nature of the inequality is not so much the outcome itself but rather the implication that bad psychologies (explicitly racialised) underpin those inequalities. However, in practice, Sahdia Parveen and Jan Oyebode have observed that stereotypes regarding minoritised ethnic group's aversion to service use (stereotypes that are often not supported by survey data) have led to services not being offered to those groups.[53] This self-fulfilling prophecy again reveals the dangers of ethnicity-based classifications.

As well as negatively appraising the psychological motivations behind low institutional care uptake, this outcome has also been problematised for having undesirable repercussions for family carers. This argument seems intuitive, i.e. that having a relative cared for by other people in a different location could feasibly reduce carer stress compared to personally caring for that person. The equation is that less proximity and instrumental involvement begets less stress. However, while intuitive, the assumption is questionable. Research indicates that caregivers can experience considerable emotional turmoil, particularly feelings of guilt and shame, leading up to and following the institutionalisation of a loved one. Reviewing existing studies, Afram and colleagues have concluded that pre- and post-institutionalisation are typically misinterpreted as two distinct caregiving periods when, in practice, the difficulties experienced by carers often continue throughout.[54] Hence, the logic that greater institutionalisation fosters lower carer stress is appealing but potentially misleading.

A great deal of the work on institutionalisation focuses on carers. Often missing from these discussions is any consideration of the desirability of institutional care from the perspectives of the care recipients themselves. Research around the world consistently indicates that most people would prefer not to be institutionalised in later life.[55–57] Indeed, an Alzheimer's Society study found that around 70% of British older adults feared being admitted to a care home with dementia. The substantial gerontological field of "ageing in place" scholarship has largely been predicated on a recognition that people typically want to remain in their own homes,[58] a commitment shared by the WHO.[57] This anti-institution sentiment has been exacerbated by the COVID pandemic, which was characterised by high death rates and heavy lockdowns in care homes.[59] Of course, personal preferences for a particular outcome do not necessarily mean that the outcome is positive, but such preferences do at least warrant sincere acknowledgement and reflection. When it comes to more objective empirical assessments, review evidence suggests that there is little difference across various health outcomes when comparing domiciliary and institutional care settings.[60] Again, we find a situation in which an outcome associated with minoritised ethnic populations is problematised in lieu of evidence. To reiterate, I am not saying that the outcome is good or even neutral. Rather, again, the purported badness of the outcome does not answer to a corresponding evidence base.

Another outcome that is used in this manner is medication receipt. Again, research shows that minoritised ethnic people with dementia are less likely to receive associated medications than their majority ethnic counterparts. This lower medication use is typically articulated as a bad outcome, with corresponding appeals to develop targeted interventions to increase medication uptake among minoritised ethnic populations. The following concluding statements, taken from recent research publications that stratified medication use by ethnicity, are indicative of this trope:

> Targeted efforts to improve treatment of dementia in under-represented populations are urgently needed.[61]
>
> Policy guidelines need to take account of these inequalities by ethnicity and education and potentially support the financial uptake of anti-dementia medication better to address and reduce social inequalities.[62]

The argument here is that (1) medication is good, (2) minoritised ethnic people consume less medication than majority ethnic people, therefore (3) we need to make minoritised ethnic people take more medication.

As discussed in Chapters 2 and 5, the dementia medication landscape can charitably be described as underwhelming. In Europe, only four treatments are typically used, the most recent of which was approved in 2003. These are all short-term symptom-modifying medications with substantial side effect profiles, including gastrointestinal and cardiac problems.[63, 64] All but one of these drugs are cholinesterase inhibitors, the value of which is subject to continued debate, with France having revoked public funding for them in recent years. Cholinesterase inhibitors are effective in around two-thirds of patients for between two and five months on average.[65] These figures may feel somewhat disappointing, but it is always important to remember that dementia medication is not a case of cure or nothing. Even slightly enhanced cognition for a few months can mean more precious moments with a loved one.

Beyond specific anti-dementia medications, people with dementia are also often prescribed anti-psychotics and other psychotropic medications, including antidepressants, anti-convulsants and sedatives. These are typically used to manage behavioural symptoms, such as "agitation". Such medications are associated with increased mortality, and their use is generally not advised, especially in instances where non-pharmacological interventions could similarly address behavioural symptoms.[66–68] Significant steps have been taken over recent years to address the over-prescription of harmful behaviour-managing medications, with some success. However, it is feared that the locking down of care institutions during COVID reversed this trend and led to new increases.[69, 70] This is one area where the data is quite clear. The use of these medications, which is sadly all too common, should be avoided wherever possible.

We also must not forget that, in the US at least, aducanumab and lecanemab are now officially licensed disease-modifying treatments. Indeed, as noted above, the Alzheimer's Association has made strong claims regarding the moral imperative of getting this medication to more minoritised ethnic people with dementia. However, the data that has been made available suggests negligible clinical efficacy. Moreover, around 40% (aducanumab) and 20% (lecanemab) of recipients develop brain abnormalities, and despite extremely limited uptake so far, the treatments have already been linked to several deaths. With this in mind, it is unsurprising that aducanumab has been rejected by European regulators and is now restricted to clinical trials in the US (at the time of writing, lecanemab is under review by the EMA). As noted, white Americans have so far been substantially over-represented in aducanumab use, showing a continuation of ethnic inequalities in relation to new medications. Again, this is repeatedly identified as a bad thing,[12] but considering the evidence regarding effectiveness and safety, or the lack thereof, the under-representation of minoritised ethnic people in aducanumab uptake seems difficult to frame as a disadvantage.

Again, increased medication uptake is cast as a good outcome in discussions of ethnic inequalities, but it is not clear that this normative appraisal can be sustained in relation to the existing evidence base on medication use in dementia. The normative positioning of medication is perhaps even more questionable than similar arguments relating to diagnosis and institutional care because there is ample evidence highlighting its dangers. In the cases of aducanumab and lecanemab, relatively few people would consider the increased risk of brain damage to be a positive outcome. Throughout all of these measures of ethnic inequality, we see outcomes that are normatively appraised as inherently bad being associated with minoritised ethnic populations. In many cases, there is little reflection on the extent to which the purported badness of the outcome is based on convention, intuition or evidence. Too often, the latter is missing. These biopolitical credos are absorbed and regurgitated by an uncritical tradition of ethnicity-focused dementia studies, which lends an unwarranted authority to those claims. This is not dissimilar, albeit less sensational, to the mass media hyperbole discussed in Chapter 5.

7.3 BAME Blame

Having shown how inequalities are made into a particular type of normative schema so as to associate certain groups with bad outcomes, I now want to turn to the making up of those groups themselves. The crudeness of social categorisation across much social science has long been recognised. As discussed in Chapter 5, regarding the notion of reductionism, it is sometimes useful in empirical analyses of research problems to develop crude representations of phenomena to enable us to conduct an analysis in a feasible manner. We are aware of the shortcomings, but it is a case of either doing the research with said shortcomings or not at all. For example, a complex concept such as social class might be operationalised in terms of income level because this is far easier to gather data on. The work required to produce a truly conceptually robust dataset representing social class might extend well beyond funding timelines or imperil the technical requirements of an analytic strategy. Of course, the difficulty here is that while income might enable us to do the work, it simultaneously undermines the quality of that work because our data does not speak directly to social class and likely loses a lot of the important considerations that make up that concept. Ethnicity is similar in this respect. Ethnicity is not a naturalistic entity. Despite common assumptions, there is no genetic, geographic, skin colour, lingual, religious or any other direct analogue for a distinct type of ethnic group. This means that the groups themselves are based on value judgements, which is not to say that ethnicity is not a meaningful entity, but rather that it is inseparable from our value commitments.

Regarding dementia studies specifically, the use of ethnicity as a means of social stratification was critiqued as long ago as 2004. Steve Iliffe and Jill Manthorpe argued that dementia studies paid too little attention to ethnicity as a category fallacy that was so abstracted from the real world that its use risked actively concealing many of the phenomena that were of interest to such research. For instance, they observed that ethnicity was often used to stratify data without recourse to economic or educational correlates, which might better explain findings than ethnicity itself. They argued that intra-ethnic differences in dementia-related phenomena could likely be more significant than inter-ethnic differences but that much ethnicity-focused research would obscure this by its very design.[71] If you recall the discussion of circularity in Chapter 5, you may recognise here a danger that the answers are embedded in the questions. Ethnicity-focused dementia studies was relatively undeveloped in the early 2000s. Almost 20 years later, Iliffe and Manthorpe's observations regarding ethnicity as a category fallacy have proved to be prescient. Unfortunately, they are seemingly unheeded to a large extent.[4]

Today, the sizeable body of dementia studies research that attends directly to ethnicity is typified by a vast proliferation of idiosyncratic operationalisations. For example, research in the US includes groups defined as White,[76] Anglo,[77] Anglo European American, [78]Latino,[76] Hispanic,[79] Black,[76] African American,[80] Asian,[77] Asian-American,[78] Asian Indian American,[81] Vietnamese American,[82] Hmong American,[83] Chinese American,[84] Chinese,[85] Korean American[86] and Pacific Islander.[87] These categories differ in the UK context, encompassing White,[88] East European,[89] East and

Central European,[35] African-Caribbean,[90] Black African and Caribbean,[91] Asian,[90] South Asian,[92] South Asian (Indian),[93] British Indian,[35] Hindi and Punjabi South Asian[94] and Sikh.[92] Throughout, we see little standardisation across definitions that variably draw on country, (sub)continent, religion and skin colour to delineate supposedly coherent types of people, with scant consideration of what such categories really contain, exclude, reveal and conceal. Inevitably, these categories lack sensitivity when it comes to almost all other factors that might constrain experiences of dementia. There is little reflection on the racialisation of datasets that likely represent a diversity of experiences at the intersection of social, political and economic circumstances.

Moreover, research shows that the majority of dementia research on minoritised ethnic people is conducted by majority ethnic researchers.[95] This ethnic discordance reflects the broader historic problem in dementia research of scholars making claims about populations on their behalf rather than engaging with lived experiences and distinct positionalities as legitimate research considerations. Exemplifying the pitfalls of this approach, Maria Zubair has described her experience of accompanying a senior white colleague to a patient and public involvement meeting with a South Asian community group to prepare some dementia research.[96] Her colleague begins by explaining the research problem to the group, focusing on low diagnosis and low rates of service use. This colleague goes on to clarify that the issue is not racism but is instead attributable to more complex cultural barriers, in particular, a lack of awareness among minoritised ethnic groups. Zubair's anecdote exemplifies how the parameters of engagement with ethnicity are embedded in dementia research from the beginning, often by majority ethnic stakeholders with a predilection for identifying "complex cultural factors" rather than racism.

The questionable methodological approaches used to categorise ethnicity further undermine the already dubious claims regarding the badness of certain dementia-related outcomes as they relate to ethnic groupings. To an extent, this is by itself a regrettable route for dementia studies to progress down, racialising dementia in a manner that substantiates neuropsychiatric biopolitics. Unfortunately, the ethnic turn becomes even more dubious when it comes to subsequent attempts to articulate the underlying causes of ethnic inequalities. Often, when it comes to accounting for the observed "bad" inequalities, causation is attributed to minoritised ethnic people themselves. To some extent, this is predictable. If we approach a problem as somehow ethnic in nature, then we are likely to interpret its causes as similarly rooted in matters of ethnicity. In much dementia research, rather than attending to institutional and other extrinsic determinants of inequality, notions of minoritised culture are highlighted as a leading culprit. For example, when services are poorly suited to certain people's requirements, responsibility is attributed to inadequate help-seeking by those people. Similarly, when diagnosis rates are low among a certain group, that group is positioned as having an inadequate understanding of dementia. As an example of this approach to attributing cultural blame, the current Social Care Institute for Excellence (SCIE) advice for professionals when working with minoritised ethnic carers states the following:

> There is evidence that minority ethnic carers are more likely to be isolated from mainstream services. Some may view using a service as a source of shame. In Islam, Hinduism and Sikhism the duty of care is apparent or is regarded as a 'test from God'. There is stigma around dementia in some cultures; it may be regarded as a punishment for past misdemeanours or a family member with dementia may damage the marriage prospects of a young relative.
>
> There's evidence that people from BME communities are not sure where or how to find information about dementia. This is exacerbated by language barriers or when people have lost cognitive skills, or if online information is not available in community languages. People may confuse the symptoms of dementia with "normal ageing" and not seek the support that is available.[97]

The phrasing positions the cultures of minoritised ethnic people as barriers to support so that those cultures, and the people who participate in them, become the problem. The influence of and concordance with a neuropsychiatric biopolitics of dementia is evident in familiar warnings of "stigma" and "normal ageing". The appeal to "evidence" reveals the dangers that come from a neuro-agnostic dementia studies, because much of this evidence is supplied by dementia scholarship that has too readily absorbed that biopolitics and subsequently fed back into its self-justification. The answer is embedded in the question. A confluence of biopolitical commitments constitutes a particular type of ethnicity problem in relation to dementia that manifests and perpetuates the neuropsychiatric biopolitics of dementia from which it originates. At worst, the problematisation of ethnicity in relation to dementia allows stakeholders to simultaneously belittle minoritised ethnic people while advertising their social justice credentials, as the Alzheimer's Association did in its aforementioned response to the CMS decision on aducanumab.

Perhaps nowhere is this problematisation of minoritised ethnicity in dementia more evident than at the intersection of dementia's ethnicity problem and the awareness economy discussed in the previous chapter. Again, a host of bizarre true/false statement surveys are a key tool for stratifying knowledge in terms of ethnicity. The following examples, which you might recall from the previous chapter, are all taken from ethnicity-focused dementia awareness research, exemplifying the cross-fertilisation of the awareness economy and the ethnicity problem:

> Alzheimer's disease is a normal process of aging, like graying of hair or wrinkles.[77]

> Significant loss of memory and mental ability, commonly known as senility, is a normal part of aging.[80]
>
> All humans if they live long enough, will probably develop Alzheimer's disease.[86]

As discussed in Chapter 6, there is no robust basis in molecular, cognitive or clinical science for treating any of these claims as true or false. We have not run a randomised control trial on the effects of "living long enough". The statements represent the peculiar normative commitments of a neuropsychiatric biopolitics of dementia. Nonetheless, they are used to make explicit and authoritative claims about the inferiority of minoritised ethnic people.

One common manifestation of the attribution of inferiority and superiority is evident in the binary terminology of "belief" and "knowledge". In critical psychiatry, the use of a belief versus knowledge binary in these types of awareness discussions has long been recognised as a rhetorical trick for demeaning the group who have beliefs in relation to the people who have knowledge. Unsurprisingly, the knowledgeable people are typically the same people applying the terms, while the people with beliefs are usually the subject of the analysis. Anti-colonial critiques of global psychiatry have extended this observation to highlight the way in which the mental health practices of various people defined in terms of ethnicity are couched in terms such as "cultural" or "traditional" as a means of distinguishing them from proper science and hence establishing an ethnic divide between legitimate and illegitimate thought.[98] Minoritised ethnic people *believe* things; neuropsychiatric stakeholders *know* things.

The above SCIE example is indicative of the manner in which a substantial body of material across academia, government, media and the third sector promotes an idea that the (supposedly) poor outcomes experienced by (crudely operationalised) minoritised ethnic people affected by dementia are attributable to the illegitimacy of their dementia *beliefs*, which differ from legitimate dementia *knowledge*. For example, the APPG on Dementia concluded that minoritised ethnic people "are unlikely to recognise the early symptoms of the condition or perceive them as a health problem" and that "the lack of a concept of cognitive impairment or dementia can make it difficult to provide a coherent account of symptoms".[118] The critical reader might rightly wonder: "coherent" according to who? This line of argument is also pervasive in the research literature. Consider the following examples:

> People from ethnic and cultural backgrounds who view dementia as a "normal" part of ageing may be less likely to request support for family members with dementia until a crisis point is reached, because they do not think they have an illness.[99]
>
> Ethnic minority families may lack the necessary information or hold culturally influenced beliefs about dementias that can delay necessary help-seeking. Unfortunately, the increased understandings of

dementia resulting from medical/scientific advances are not commonly held among members of various ethnic minority groups.[79]

Here, the drawing of distinctions between the normal and the pathological, a core component of neuropsychiatric biopolitics, facilitates the problematisation of minoritised ethnic cultures as anti-scientific. Hence, the failure of minoritised ethnic culture is a failure to accept and comply with the truth, and that truth is neuropsychiatric biopolitics. In other words, this is a failure to comply with particular normative commitments, but it is articulated as a failure to comply with science. This logic transforms minoritised ethnic people into a tool for biopolitical self-substantiation. By linking the bad outcomes attributed to minoritised ethnic people with their lack of compliance with neuropsychiatric biopolitics, those people are implicitly made into a sort of ethnic antagonist. Their purported inadequacies act as a cautionary tale, highlighting the dangers of a failure to engage appropriately with the neuropsychiatric biopolitics of dementia. The moral of the story is that we do not want to be like those problematic others, so we should be neuro-compliant instead. We are presented with a bad ethnic way of being and a good scientific way of being. This manifests Nikolas Rose's observation that biopolitics inspires continuous self-governance of one's conduct in pursuit of idealised forms of being, which are often defined in opposition to bad forms of being.[100]

This self-governance through correct beliefs guiding correct conduct is perhaps most explicitly manifest in the concurrent tradition of educational intervention that has been built upon the ethnicity problem. The governance of populations deemed non-compliant is a key feature of neuropsychiatric biopolitics more broadly,[101] and dementia is no different. Lamentations of poor minoritised ethnic outcomes, owing to their cultural inadequacies, often end with appeals to develop educational interventions that will improve their ways of thinking and thereby improve their ways of being. A recent review found 25 ethnicity-targeted awareness-raising interventions that have been developed as part of a published research project.[102] Such initiatives also extend beyond research and into third-sector activities at national and local levels. Several of the aforementioned community projects funded by the Race Equality Foundation and the Department of Health and Social Care had a belief-altering component.[19] The underlying logic is largely the same as that described in Chapter 6 regarding stigma and awareness. However, in the ethnicity tradition, such arguments attend to notions of culture and cultural beliefs more specifically as the source of the problem. It is telling that the awareness tradition typically speaks directly to "culture" only when it is focusing on minoritised ethnic groups, as though culture, and by extension ethnicity itself, is limited to those people specifically. Here, what is "cultural" is set up as the opposite of what is "natural" and, therefore, what is "right" (in both a moral and an empirical sense).

As well as reflecting on the biopolitical nature of the ethnic turn as an imposition of normative commitments onto publics at the expense of science, dementia studies could also consider the extent to which this new ethnicity problem relies on and perpetuates historic racist representations of psychiatric illness and mental capability. Notions of racial inferiority and psychological inferiority have long been entwined as a means of enforcing political projects. In the US, enslaved people were widely considered to be predisposed to the madness of escaping; in Nazi Germany, Jewish people were commonly depicted as mentally weak and prone to various psychiatric disorders; today, the IQ movement repeatedly casts minorities as cognitively lesser.[103–105] Charity press officers and dementia researchers are by no means comparable with slavers and Nazis, but the substantive heritage of racialised neuropsychiatric truth claims, and their conduciveness to the governance of specific modes of being, should give us pause for thought. In practical terms, blaming things like insufficient support on minoritised cultures obscures structural determinants of health by attributing blame to individuals and their ways of life.

* * *

The development of an ethnicity problem within the neuropsychiatric biopolitics of dementia should be of particular concern to us because a neuroagnostic dementia studies has been integral to its fruition. The ethnic turn represents a confluence of several questionable phenomena. A greater attentiveness to the circumstances of minoritised ethnic people is laudable, but it is too often opportunistic, being principally accountable to biopolitical aims. Moreover, the laudable and the opportunistic cannot necessarily be neatly disaggregated. As discussed, representations of the goodness and badness of select outcomes are enmeshed with particular normative commitments. These commitments are fundamentally biopolitical in nature, having little grounding in robust evidence bases. Normatively defined outcomes are then attributed to crudely operationalised notions of ethnic category, with the bad outcomes being delegated to the minoritised groups. Having established these associations, the mechanics of the problem are then attributed to the illegitimate forms of being of those minoritised groups, defined in terms of unscientific beliefs, stigmatisation, distrust and aversions to help. The ethnicity problem substantiates the neuropsychiatric biopolitics of dementia. Echoing longstanding racialised depictions of psychiatric disorder, it positions minoritised ethnic people as a cautionary tale, showcasing the negative repercussions of a failure to conduct oneself accordingly. To be clear, I am not suggesting that minoritised ethnic groups should be excluded from services. Rather, people should have access to evidence-based services, tailored to their circumstances if and when they need them.

The ethnic turn is also highly relevant to developing a more critical dementia studies because it furnishes opportunities for us to nurture the types of pluralism that may ultimately help us to move beyond narrow normative commitments. The problematisation of ethnicity in relation to dementia is typically manifest in the attribution of badness to things such as outcomes and cultures. Since the 1990s, dementia studies has successfully changed how people with dementia are viewed and treated in research. We can similarly challenge the ethnicity problem by engaging with people's experiences as legitimate, irrespective of assumptions made about them by virtue of ethnicity, rather than as mistakes to be rectified. For instance, consider the claim, often attributed to minoritised ethnic people, that dementia is a white person's problem.[91] This tends to be presented in a belittling fashion as evidence of their poor understanding. However, from Alois Alzheimer to Robert Katzman, dementia has historically been developed by white people, and it is largely white people who have profited from the development of the dementia economy. Indeed, the ethnic turn is characterised by white people doing work on, and on behalf of, minoritised ethnic people.[95] Sociologically, dementia has always been very white, and its contemporary racialisation remains a largely white project.

In a similar manner, commentators have repeatedly noted that some South Asian languages do not have a word for dementia.[106] Again, this observation is used to indicate the problematic nature of those cultures. However, there is a rich tradition of scholarship examining the generative capacities of language. For instance, the philosopher Ian Hacking famously described dynamic nominalism, wherein defining a group of people as somehow problematic leads to circumstances which make it more likely that those people will live up to the definition.[107] Indeed, Margaret Lock has argued that people with AD are "an excellent example of this process", having only recently emerged as a distinct and culturally meaningful group of people by virtue of late-20th-century classification.[108] Building on Lock's work, Jonathan Yahalom has observed that the dynamic nominalism of AD has not yet spread worldwide, citing various societies around the globe where AD is yet to be realised.[109] Similarly, the longstanding sociological tradition of labelling theory has documented the manner in which being defined as having a specific behavioural condition changes the way that people and institutions act toward that person, with the effect that the person is guided toward manifesting the attributes typically associated with the label.[110] Laurence Cohen noted that scholars who used the word "dementia" were themselves complicit in the pathologisation of later life. Words can be potently generative, so not using a word can be a form of resistive social action. To be clear, I am not arguing that a person who says "dementia is a white problem" is making a claim about the political nature of disease, nor that a language not having a word for dementia is a form of linguistic resistance. Rather, my point is that the use of such phenomena as examples of cultural inadequacy is not an apolitical representation of facts. It is a normative depiction that serves a specific biopolitics.

In response, we could pursue a range of parallel, and more equitable, engagements that respect the heterogeneity of experiences of later-life cognitive decline and acknowledge that nobody has an absolute solution to the associated problems. We could challenge claims that some approaches are inherently better than others, as well as ideas that they are mutually exclusive. In practice, people's understandings of illness often blend seemingly opposed categories to cultivate meaningful composite conceptions.[111] There are examples of research that engage with the preferences of local communities and draw on those experiences to advocate for support structures. For instance, researchers in the US have gathered rich accounts of the role of spirituality as a form of emotional support for Alaskan Natives affected by dementia and have subsequently used those accounts to advocate for the funding of spiritual support as a form of dementia service.[112] In Australia, researchers have documented the importance of communal art projects as a form of spiritual support for Aboriginal people affected by dementia in remote areas. Again, rather than interpreting people's accounts as indicative of an anti-science illegitimacy rooted in a problematic culture, scholars have used this evidence to argue for more support for spiritually engaged communal art projects as a form of dementia support.[113] Sincere engagement with these initiatives offers opportunities for supporting well-being. This does not mean turning our backs on the neuropsychiatric biopolitics of dementia. Rather, it is a case of acknowledging that said biopolitics encompasses a set of values that sit alongside many alternative values, none of which are inherently superior.

An awareness of the ethnic turn should also draw our attention to the capacities of the neuropsychiatric biopolitics of dementia to obscure the political economies within which our experiences of dementia are realised. Highlighting the purported deficiencies of the ethnic other is a familiar form of diverting attention away from the structural determinants of social problems.[114] Every indication and implication, however subtle and/or well-intentioned, that a person's belief system is causing their dementia-related problems can effectively pull our attention away from the more pervasive structural issues that constrain our collective experiences of dementia. It is to these determinants, and the wider political economy of dementia, that I turn my attention in Chapter 8.

Notes

1 I use "minoritised ethnic" throughout as an established means of referring to racialised and minoritised people and groups in general, but I recognise that this phrase is not without its problems. As will become clear in the chapter, the terminology used in reference to race and ethnicity is fraught, and almost inherently perpetuates many of the problems that I critique herein. I prefer "minoritised ethnic" for two reasons: (1) to encompass people who identify as ethnically different from the majority white populations of the high-income countries that I write about and (2) to represent the active, processual and socially contingent nature of ethnic categorisation that various people are subject to.
2 Translates as "my memories".

3 I will attend more critically to this categorisation of ethnicities below.
4 It is worth acknowledging a growing body of intersectional research attending to dynamic and interrelated manifestations of multiple social locations in the lives of people with dementia, though this literature is dominated by work on disability, gender and sexuality.[72–75]

References

1. Bradby and, H., and Nazroo, J.Y. (2021). Health, ethnicity, and race. In: W. C. Cockerham (ed.), *The Wiley Blackwell Companion to Medical Sociology*. John Wiley & Sons, Ltd, pp. 258–278. doi: 10.1002/9781119633808.ch13.
2. Fenton, S. (2013). *Ethnicity*. Polity Press.
3. Kundnani, A. (2007). *The End of Tolerance: Racism in 21st Century Britain*. Pluto Press.
4. Leach, C.W., and Teixeira, C.P. (2022). Understanding sentiment toward "black lives matter." *Social Issues and Policy Review* 16, 3–32. doi: 10.1111/sipr.12084.
5. Pew Research Center (2021). Americans' views of the problems facing the nation. Pew Research Center. https://www.pewresearch.org/politics/2021/04/15/americans-views-of-the-problems-facing-the-nation/.
6. Delgado, R., Stefancic, J., and Harris, A. (2017). *Critical Race Theory*, 3rd edition. NYU Press.
7. Krumholz, H.M., Massey, D.S., and Dorsey, K.B. (2022). Racism as a leading cause of death in the United States. *BMJ 376*, o213. doi: 10.1136/bmj.o213.
8. Nazroo, J., and Becares, L. (2020). Evidence for ethnic inequalities in mortality related to COVID-19 infections: Findings from an ecological analysis of England. *BMJ Open 10*, e041750. doi: 10.1136/bmjopen-2020-041750.
9. Public Health England (2020). COVID-19: Review of disparities in risks and outcomes. GOV.UK. https://www.gov.uk/government/publications/covid-19-review-of-disparities-in-risks-and-outcomes.
10. ASC (2022). Race and dementia. Alzheimer Society of Canada. http://alzheimer.ca/en/take-action/change-minds/race-dementia.
11. Alzheimer's Association (2021). New Alzheimer's association report examines racial and ethnic attitudes on Alzheimer's and dementia. Alzheimer's Association. https://alz.org/news/2021/new-alzheimers-association-report-examines-racial.
12. Alzheimer's Association (2022). Alzheimer's association statement on CMS draft decision. Alzheimer's Association. https://alz.org/news/2022/alzheimers-association-statement-on-cms-draft-deci.
13. Manly, J.J., and Glymour, M.M. (2021). What the Aducanumab approval reveals about alzheimer disease research. *JAMA Neurology 78*, 1305–1306. doi: 10.1001/jamaneurol.2021.3404.
14. Táíwò, O.O. (2022). *Elite Capture: How the Powerful Took Over Identity Politics (And Everything Else)*. Haymarket Books.
15. Alzheimer's Society (2019). Black, Asian and minority ethnic communities and dementia research. Alzheimer's Society. https://www.alzheimers.org.uk/for-researchers/black-asian-and-minority-ethnic-communities-and-dementia-research.
16. Meri Yaadain BAME Dementia. http://www.meriyaadain.co.uk/.

17. Meri Yaadain (2019). Keynote speech on 'Intercultural care' at Alzheimer Europe Conference 2019. Meri Yaadain BAME Dementia. http://www.meriyaadain .co.uk/2019/10/23/keynote-speech-on-intercultural-care-at-alzheimer-europe -conference-2019/.

18. APPG (2013). Dementia does not discriminate: The experiences of black, Asian and minority ethnic communities. Alzheimer's Society. https://www.alzheimers .org.uk/2013-appg-report.

19. REF (2021). Dementia and BAME communities. Race Equality Foundation. https://raceequalityfoundation.org.uk/project/dementia-and-bame -communities/.

20. Centre for Policy on Ageing (2020). The future ageing of the ethnic minority population of England and Wales. http://www.cpa.org.uk/BMEprojections/ BMEprojections.html.

21. Lievesley, N. (2010). *The Future Ageing of the Ethnic Minority Population of England and Wales*. Centre for Policy on Ageing.

22. Morano, C.L., and King, M.D. (2010). Lessons learned from implementing a psycho-educational intervention for African American dementia caregivers. *Dementia 9*, 558–568. doi: 10.1177/1471301210384312.

23. Valle, R., Yamada, A.-M., and Matiella, A.C. (2006). Fotonovelas. *Clinical Gerontologist 30*, 71–88. doi: 10.1300/J018v30n01_06.

24. Lam, N.H.T., and Woo, B.K.P. (2018). Exploring the role of YouTube in delivering dementia education to older Chinese. *Asian Journal of Psychiatry 31*, 25–26. doi: 10.1016/j.ajp.2017.12.022.

25. Nielsen, T.R., Vogel, A., Phung, T.K.T., Gade, A., and Waldemar, G. (2011). Over- and under-diagnosis of dementia in ethnic minorities: A nationwide register-based study. *International Journal of Geriatric Psychiatry 26*, 1128–1135. doi: 10.1002/gps.2650.

26. Schrauf, R.W., and Iris, M. (2012). Very long pathways to diagnosis among African Americans and Hispanics with memory and behavioral problems associated with dementia. *Dementia 11*, 743–763. doi: 10.1177/1471301211416615.

27. Haralambous, B., Dow, B., Tinney, J., Lin, X., Blackberry, I., Rayner, V., Lee, S.-M., Vrantsidis, F., Lautenschlager, N., and LoGiudice, D. (2014). Help seeking in older Asian people with dementia in Melbourne: Using the cultural exchange model to explore barriers and enablers. *Journal of Cross-Cultural Gerontology 29*, 69–86. doi: 10.1007/s10823-014-9222-0.

28. Low, L.-F., Anstey, K.J., Lackersteen, S.M.P., and Camit, M. (2011). Help-seeking and service use for dementia in Italian, Greek and Chinese Australians. *Aging & Mental Health 15*, 397–404. doi: 10.1080/13607863.2010.536134.

29. Sun, F., Mutlu, A., and Coon, D. (2014). Service barriers faced by Chinese American families with a dementia relative: Perspectives from family caregivers and service professionals. *Clinical Gerontologist 37*, 120–138. doi: 10.1080/07317115.2013.868848.

30. Mooldijk, S.S., Licher, S., and Wolters, F.J. (2021). Characterizing demographic, racial, and geographic diversity in dementia research: A systematic review. *JAMA Neurology 78*, 1255–1261. doi: 10.1001/jamaneurol.2021.2943.

31. Gallagher-Thompson, D., Solano, N., Coon, D., and Areán, P. (2003). Recruitment and retention of latino dementia family caregivers in intervention research: Issues to face, lessons to learn. *The Gerontologist 43*, 45–51. doi: 10.1093/geront/43.1.45.

32. Hinton, L., Guo, Z., Hillygus, J., and Levkoff, S. (2000). Working with culture: A qualitative analysis of barriers to the recruitment of Chinese–American family caregivers for dementia research. *Journal of Cross-Cultural Gerontology 15*, 119–137. doi: 10.1023/A:1006798316654.

33. Fletcher, J.R., Zubair, M., and Roche, M. (2021). The neuropsychiatric biopolitics of dementia and its ethnicity problem. *The Sociological Review*, 00380261211059920. doi: 10.1177/00380261211059920.

34. Nielsen, T.R., Nielsen, D.S., and Waldemar, G. (2020). Barriers to post-diagnostic care and support in minority ethnic communities: A survey of Danish primary care dementia coordinators. *Dementia 19*, 2702–2713. doi: 10.1177/1471301219853945.

35. Parveen, S., Peltier, C., and Oyebode, J.R. (2017). Perceptions of dementia and use of services in minority ethnic communities: A scoping exercise. *Health & Social Care in the Community 25*, 734–742. doi: 10.1111/hsc.12363.

36. Giebel, C.M., Worden, A., Challis, D., Jolley, D., Bhui, K.S., Lambat, A., Kampanellou, E., and Purandare, N. (2019). Age, memory loss and perceptions of dementia in South Asian ethnic minorities. *Aging & Mental Health 23*, 173–182. doi: 10.1080/13607863.2017.1408772.

37. Cooper, C., Tandy, A.R., Balamurali, T.B.S., and Livingston, G. (2010). A systematic review and meta-analysis of ethnic differences in use of dementia treatment, care, and research. *The American Journal of Geriatric Psychiatry 18*, 193–203. doi: 10.1097/JGP.0b013e3181bf9caf.

38. DoHSC (2001). National service framework: Older people. GOV.UK. https://www.gov.uk/government/publications/quality-standards-for-care-services-for-older-people.

39. DoHSC (2009). Living well with dementia: A national dementia strategy. GOV.UK. https://www.gov.uk/government/publications/living-well-with-dementia-a-national-dementia-strategy.

40. Small, G., and Bullock, R. (2011). Defining optimal treatment with cholinesterase inhibitors in Alzheimer's disease. *Alzheimer's & Dementia 7*, 177–184. doi: 10.1016/j.jalz.2010.03.016.

41. Walsh, S., King, E., and Brayne, C. (2019). France removes state funding for dementia drugs. *BMJ 367*, l6930. doi: 10.1136/bmj.l6930.

42. Fletcher, J.R. (2019). *A Problem Shared: The Interacted Experience of Dementia within Care.* King's College London.

43. Milne, A. (2010). Dementia screening and early diagnosis: The case for and against. *Health, Risk & Society 12*, 65–76. doi: 10.1080/13698570903509497.

44. Samsi, K., and Manthorpe, J. (2014). Care pathways for dementia: Current perspectives. *Clinical Interventions in Aging 9*, 2055–2063. doi: 10.2147/CIA.S70628.

45. Erlangsen, A., Zarit, S.H., and Conwell, Y. (2008). Hospital-diagnosed dementia and suicide: A longitudinal study using prospective, Nationwide register data. *The American Journal of Geriatric Psychiatry 16*, 220–228. doi: 10.1097/01.JGP.0000302930.75387.7e.

46. Robinson, L., Gemski, A., Abley, C., Bond, J., Keady, J., Campbell, S., Samsi, K., and Manthorpe, J. (2011). The transition to dementia – Individual and family experiences of receiving a diagnosis: A review. *International Psychogeriatrics 23*, 1026–1043. doi: 10.1017/S1041610210002437.

47. Dhedhi, S.A., Swinglehurst, D., and Russell, J. (2014). 'Timely' diagnosis of dementia: What does it mean? A narrative analysis of GPs' accounts. *BMJ Open* 4, e004439. doi: 10.1136/bmjopen-2013-004439.

48. Harding, R. (2017). *Duties to Care: Dementia, Relationality and Law.* Cambridge University Press.

49. GOV.UK (2015). Prime Minister's challenge on dementia 2020. GOV.UK. https://www.gov.uk/government/publications/prime-ministers-challenge-on -dementia-2020/prime-ministers-challenge-on-dementia-2020.

50. Fox, C., Lafortune, L., Boustani, M., and Brayne, C. (2013). The pros and cons of early diagnosis in dementia. *British Journal of General Practice 63*, e510– e512. doi: 10.3399/bjgp13X669374.

51. Watson, R., Bryant, J., Sanson-Fisher, R., Mansfield, E., and Evans, T.-J. (2018). What is a 'timely' diagnosis? Exploring the preferences of Australian health service consumers regarding when a diagnosis of dementia should be disclosed. *BMC Health Services Research 18*, 612. doi: 10.1186/s12913-018-3409-y.

52. Napoles, A.M., Chadiha, L., Eversley, R., and Moreno-John, G. (2010). Reviews: Developing culturally sensitive dementia caregiver interventions: Are we there yet? *American Journal of Alzheimer's Disease & Other Dementias® 25*, 389–406. doi: 10.1177/1533317510370957.

53. Parveen, S., and Oyebode, J.R. *Dementia and Minority Ethnic Carers.* Race Equality Foundation.

54. Afram, B., Verbeek, H., Bleijlevens, M.H.C., and Hamers, J.P.H. (2015). Needs of informal caregivers during transition from home towards institutional care in dementia: A systematic review of qualitative studies. *International Psychogeriatrics 27*, 891–902. doi: 10.1017/S1041610214002154.

55. Stones, D., and Gullifer, J. (2016). 'At home it's just so much easier to be yourself': Older adults' perceptions of ageing in place. *Ageing & Society 36*, 449–481. doi: 10.1017/S0144686X14001214.

56. Kendig, H., Gong, C.H., Cannon, L., and Browning, C. (2017). Preferences and predictors of aging in place: Longitudinal evidence from Melbourne, Australia. *Journal of Housing for the Elderly 31*, 259–271. doi: 10.1080/02763893.2017.1280582.

57. Mah, J.C., Stevens, S.J., Keefe, J.M., Rockwood, K., and Andrew, M.K. (2021). Social factors influencing utilization of home care in community-dwelling older adults: A scoping review. *BMC Geriatrics 21*, 145. doi: 10.1186/s12877-021-02069-1.

58. Lewis, C., and Buffel, T. (2020). Aging in place and the places of aging: A longitudinal study. *Journal of Aging Studies 54*, 100870. doi: 10.1016/j.jaging.2020.100870.

59. The King's Fund (2022). Social care 360: Providers. The King's Fund. https://www.kingsfund.org.uk/publications/social-care-360/providers.

60. Boland, L., Légaré, F., Perez, M.M.B., Menear, M., Garvelink, M.M., McIsaac, D.I., Painchaud Guérard, G., Emond, J., Brière, N., and Stacey, D. (2017). Impact of home care versus alternative locations of care on elder health outcomes: An overview of systematic reviews. *BMC Geriatrics 17*, 20. doi: 10.1186/s12877-016-0395-y.

61. Zhu, C.W., Neugroschl, J., Barnes, L.L., and Sano, M. (2022). Racial/ethnic disparities in initiation and persistent use of anti-dementia medications. *Alzheimer's & Dementia.* doi: 10.1002/alz.12623.

62. Giebel, C., Cations, M., Draper, B., and Komuravelli, A. (2020). Ethnic disparities in the uptake of anti-dementia medication in young and late-onset dementia. *International Psychogeriatrics*, 1–10. doi: 10.1017/S1041610220000794.

63. Valenzuela, M., Sachdev, P., and Brodaty, H. (2021). Concerns about cholinesterase inhibitor recommendations. *Neurology*. https://n.neurology.org/content/concerns-about-cholinesterase-inhibitor-recommendations.

64. Petersen, R.C., Lopez, O., Armstrong, M.J., Getchius, T.S.D., Ganguli, M., Gloss, D., Gronseth, G.S., Marson, D., Pringsheim, T., Day, G.S., et al. (2018). Practice guideline update summary: Mild cognitive impairment: Report of the Guideline Development, Dissemination, and Implementation Subcommittee of the American Academy of Neurology. *Neurology 90*, 126–135. doi: 10.1212/WNL.0000000000004826.

65. Vaci, N., Koychev, I., Kim, C.-H., Kormilitzin, A., Liu, Q., Lucas, C., Dehghan, A., Nenadic, G., and Nevado-Holgado, A. (2021). Real-world effectiveness, its predictors and onset of action of cholinesterase inhibitors and memantine in dementia: Retrospective health record study. *The British Journal of Psychiatry 218*, 261–267. doi: 10.1192/bjp.2020.136.

66. Maust, D.T., Kim, H.M., Seyfried, L.S., Chiang, C., Kavanagh, J., Schneider, L.S., and Kales, H.C. (2015). Antipsychotics, other psychotropics, and the risk of death in patients with dementia: Number needed to harm. *JAMA Psychiatry 72*, 438–445. doi: 10.1001/jamapsychiatry.2014.3018.

67. Kales, H.C., Gitlin, L.N., and Lyketsos, C.G. (2019). When less is more, but still not enough: Why focusing on limiting antipsychotics in people with dementia is the wrong policy imperative. *Journal of the American Medical Directors Association 20*, 1074–1079. doi: 10.1016/j.jamda.2019.05.022.

68. Ballard, C., and Corbett, A. (2020). Reducing psychotropic drug use in people with dementia living in nursing homes. *International Psychogeriatrics 32*, 291–294. doi: 10.1017/S1041610219001455.

69. Howard, R., Burns, A., and Schneider, L. (2020). Antipsychotic prescribing to people with dementia during COVID-19. *The Lancet Neurology 19*, 892. doi: 10.1016/S1474-4422(20)30370-7.

70. Suárez-González, A., Rajagopalan, J., Livingston, G., and Alladi, S. (2021). The effect of COVID-19 isolation measures on the cognition and mental health of people living with dementia: A rapid systematic review of one year of quantitative evidence. *EClinicalMedicine 39*. doi: 10.1016/j.eclinm.2021.101047.

71. Iliffe, S., and Manthorpe, J. (2004). The debate on ethnicity and dementia: From category fallacy to person-centred care? *Aging & Mental Health 8*, 283–292. doi: 10.1080/13607860410001709656.

72. Thomas, C., and Milligan, C. (2018). Dementia, disability rights and disablism: Understanding the social position of people living with dementia. *Disability & Society 33*, 115–131. doi: 10.1080/09687599.2017.1379952.

73. Baril, A., and Silverman, M. (2022). Forgotten lives: Trans older adults living with dementia at the intersection of cisgenderism, ableism/cogniticism and ageism. *Sexualities 25*, 117–131. doi: 10.1177/1363460719876835.

74. Watchman, K. (2018). The intersectionality of intellectual disability and ageing. In: S. Westwood (ed.), *Ageing, Diversity and Equality*. Routledge.

75. Hulko, W. (2016). LGBT* individuals and dementia: An intersectional approach. In: S. Westwood and E. Price (eds.), *Lesbian, Gay, Bisexual and Trans* Individuals Living with Dementia*. Routledge.

76. Ayalon, L. (2013). Re-examining ethnic differences in concerns, knowledge, and beliefs about Alzheimer's disease: Results from a national sample. *International Journal of Geriatric Psychiatry 28*, 1288–1295. doi: 10.1002/gps.3959.

77. Ayalon, L., and Areán, P.A. (2004). Knowledge of Alzheimer's disease in four ethnic groups of older adults. *International Journal of Geriatric Psychiatry 19*, 51–57. doi: 10.1002/gps.1037.

78. Hinton, L., Franz, C.E., Yeo, G., and Levkoff, S.E. (2005). Conceptions of dementia in a multiethnic sample of family caregivers. *Journal of the American Geriatrics Society 53*, 1405–1410. doi: 10.1111/j.1532-5415.2005.53409.x.

79. Gray, H.L., Jimenez, D.E., Cucciare, M.A., Tong, H.-Q., and Gallagher-Thompson, D. (2009). Ethnic differences in beliefs regarding Alzheimer disease among dementia family caregivers. *The American Journal of Geriatric Psychiatry 17*, 925–933. doi: 10.1097/JGP.0b013e3181ad4f3c.

80. Connell, C.M., Roberts, J.S., McLaughlin, S.J., and Akinleye, D. (2009). Racial differences in knowledge and beliefs about Alzheimer disease. *Alzheimer Disease and Associated Disorders 23*, 110–116. doi: 10.1097/WAD.0b013e318192e94d.

81. Otilingam, P., and Gatz, M. (2008). Perceptions of dementia among Asian Indian Americans. *AAPI Nexus: Policy, Practice and Community 6*, 45–66. doi: 10.17953/appc.6.2.e86kk514w8321304.

82. Lee, S.E., and Casado, B.L. (2019). Knowledge of Alzheimer's disease among Vietnamese Americans and correlates of their knowledge about Alzheimer's disease. *Dementia 18*, 713–724. doi: 10.1177/1471301217691616.

83. Gerdner, L.A., Tripp-Reimer, T., and Yang, D. (2005). [P-142]: Perception and care of elders with dementia in the Hmong American community. *Alzheimer's & Dementia 1*, S54–S55. doi: 10.1016/j.jalz.2005.06.123.

84. Diamond, A.G., and Woo, B.K. (2014). Duration of residence and dementia literacy among Chinese Americans. *International Journal of Social Psychiatry 60*, 406–409. doi: 10.1177/0020764013491742.

85. Mahoney, D.F., Cloutterbuck, J., Neary, S., and Zhan, L. (2005). African American, Chinese, and latino family caregivers' impressions of the onset and diagnosis of dementia: Cross-cultural similarities and differences. *The Gerontologist 45*, 783–792. doi: 10.1093/geront/45.6.783.

86. Jang, Y., Kim, G., and Chiriboga, D. (2010). Knowledge of Alzheimer's disease, feelings of shame, and awareness of services among Korean American elders. *Journal of Aging and Health 22*, 419–433. doi: 10.1177/0898264309360672.

87. Braun, K.L., and Browne, C.V. (1998). Perceptions of dementia, caregiving, and help seeking among Asian and Pacific Islander Americans. *Health & Social Work 23*, 262–274. doi: 10.1093/hsw/23.4.262.

88. Turner, S., Christie, A., and Haworth, E. South Asian and white older people and dementia: A qualitative study of knowledge and attitudes. *Diversity & Equality in Health and Care 2*.

89. Mackenzie, J. (2006). Stigma and dementia: East European and South Asian family carers negotiating stigma in the UK. *Dementia 5*, 233–247. doi: 10.1177/1471301206062252.

90. Jolley, D., Moreland, N., Read, K., Kaur, H., Jutlla, K., and Clark, M. (2009). The 'Twice a Child' projects: Learning about dementia and related disorders within the black and minority ethnic population of an English city and improving relevant services. *Ethnicity and Inequalities in Health and Social Care 2*, 4–9. doi: 10.1108/17570980200900024.

91. Berwald, S., Roche, M., Adelman, S., Mukadam, N., and Livingston, G. (2016). Black African and Caribbean British communities' perceptions of memory problems: "we don't do dementia." *PLOS ONE 11*, e0151878. doi: 10.1371/journal.pone.0151878.

92. Uppal, G., and Bonas, S. (2014). Constructions of dementia in the South Asian community: A systematic literature review. *Mental Health, Religion & Culture 17*, 143–160. doi: 10.1080/13674676.2013.764515.

93. Purandare, N., Luthra, V., Swarbrick, C., and Burns, A. (2007). Knowledge of dementia among South Asian (Indian) older people in Manchester, UK. *International Journal of Geriatric Psychiatry 22*, 777–781. doi: 10.1002/gps.1740.

94. La Fontaine, J., Ahuja, J., Bradbury, N.M., Phillips, S., and Oyebode, J.R. (2007). Understanding dementia amongst people in minority ethnic and cultural groups. *Journal of Advanced Nursing 60*, 605–614. doi: 10.1111/j.1365-2648.2007.04444.x.

95. Roche, M., Higgs, P., Aworinde, J., and Cooper, C. (2021). A review of qualitative research of perception and experiences of dementia among adults from black, African, and Caribbean background: What and whom are we researching? *The Gerontologist 61*, e195–e208. doi: 10.1093/geront/gnaa004.

96. Zubair, M. (2023). Reframing "ethnicity" in dementia research: Reflections on current whiteness of research and the need for an anti-racist approach. In: R. Ward and L. Sandberg, (eds.), *Critical Dementia Studies*. Routledge.

97. SCIE (2020). Understanding dementia. Social Care Institute for Excellence. https://www.scie.org.uk/dementia/after-diagnosis/communication/understanding-dementia.asp.

98. Cooper, S. (2016). Research on help-seeking for mental illness in Africa: Dominant approaches and possible alternatives. *Transcultural Psychiatry 53*, 696–718. doi: 10.1177/1363461515622762.

99. Botsford, J., and Dening, K.H.H. eds. (2015). *Dementia, Culture and Ethnicity: Issues for All*. Jessica Kingsley Publishers.

100. Rose, N. (2009). Normality and pathology in a biomedical age. *The Sociological Review 57*, 66–83. doi: 10.1111/j.1467-954X.2010.01886.x.

101. Rose, N. (2018). *Our Psychiatric Future*. Polity.

102. Huggins, L.K.L., Min, S.H., Dennis, C.-A., Østbye, T., Johnson, K.S., and Xu, H. (2022). Interventions to promote dementia knowledge among racial/ethnic minority groups: A systematic review. *Journal of the American Geriatrics Society 70*, 609–621. doi: 10.1111/jgs.17495.

103. Pickens, T.A. (2019). *Black Madness: Mad Blackness*. Duke University Press.

104. Gilman, S.L., and Gilman, S.L. (1985). *Difference and Pathology: Stereotypes of Sexuality, Race, and Madness*. Cornell University Press.

105. Fernando, S. (2010). *Mental Health, Race and Culture*, Third Edition. Red Globe Press.

106. Hossain, M.Z., and Khan, H.T.A. (2019). Dementia in the Bangladeshi diaspora in England: A qualitative study of the myths and stigmas about dementia. *Journal of Evaluation in Clinical Practice 25*, 769–778. doi: 10.1111/jep.13117.

107. Hacking, I. (2006). Making up people. *London Review of Books*. https://www.lrb.co.uk/the-paper/v28/n16/ian-hacking/making-up-people.

108. Lock, M. (2007). Biosociality and susceptibility genes: A cautionary tale. In: S. Gibbon and C. Novas (eds.), *Biosocialities, Genetics and the Social Sciences*. Routledge.

109. Yahalom, J. (2019). *Caring for the People of the Clouds: Aging and Dementia in Oaxaca.* University of Oklahoma Press.
110. Scheff, T.J. (1999). *Being Mentally Ill: A Sociological Theory.* Aldine Transaction.
111. Fletcher, J.R. (2020). Mythical dementia and Alzheimerised senility: Discrepant and intersecting representations of cognitive decline in later life. *Social Theory & Health 18,* 50–65. doi: 10.1057/s41285-019-00117-w.
112. Fife, B., Brooks-Cleator, L., and Lewis, J.P. (2021). "The world was shifting under our feet, so I turned to my devotionals as his dementia worsened": The role of spirituality as a coping mechanism for family caregivers of Alaska Native elders with dementia. *Journal of Religion, Spirituality & Aging 33,* 252–270. doi: 10.1080/15528030.2020.1754995.
113. Lindeman, M., Mackell, P., Lin, X., Farthing, A., Jensen, H., Meredith, M., and Haralambous, B. (2017). Role of art centres for Aboriginal Australians living with dementia in remote communities. *Australasian Journal on Ageing 36,* 128–133. doi: 10.1111/ajag.12443.
114. Karlsen, S., and Nelson, R. (2021). Staying "one step ahead of a racist": Expanding understandings of the experiences of the covid-19 pandemic among people from minoritized ethnic groups living in Britain. *Frontiers in Sociology 6.*

8 The Political Economy of Dementia

Post-2008 Financialisation, Awareness-as-Welfare and Speculative Demographic Alarmism

Building on the previous chapter's critique of blaming under-supported people affected by dementia for institutional inadequacies, in this chapter, I explore aspects of the wider political economy of dementia that warrant critical social scientific attention. I argue that the contemporary political economy of dementia has not been sufficiently critiqued by dementia studies because of its lack of attention to neuropsychiatric biopolitics. This biopolitics supports a political economy centred on well-informed and correctly acting publics. The result is a political economy that is characterised by transformations of social support that are partially at odds with the interests of people affected by dementia. It is here that dementia studies has considerable scope for developing forms of resistance. To do so, I suggest that critical gerontological scholarship on the political economy of ageing can provide a basis for dementia studies to generate more robust analyses of political economy and the role of biopolitics in manifesting it.

To begin, I argue that the contemporary political economy of dementia, particularly following the 2008 financial crisis, is characterised by two transformations: (1) social support into information and (2) prospective dementia incidence into capital accumulation. First, there is a revitalisation of traditional anti-institution and pro-community care sentiment, operating under familiar moral and fiscal imperatives, with the latter proving particularly potent in the context of austerity politics. In practice, idealised notions of community care are too readily devolved to lone family members, often women, in distressing circumstances. This devolution is assisted through the provision of information and awareness, disciplining people into becoming individual sources of support. Second, there is a transformation of dementia into a speculative investment to facilitate capital accumulation. This relies heavily on the promissory technoscientific claims that characterise the neuropsychiatric biopolitics of dementia. Over recent years, such claims have cast traditional demographic alarmism in a new light as a financial opportunity, emphasising the size of the prospective market for curative therapeutics.

DOI: 10.4324/9781003398523-8

Having outlined the contemporary political economy of dementia, I then consider the position of dementia studies as a component of this political economy. As I have noted throughout the book, much dementia studies occupies an ambiguous position in relation to the dementia economy more broadly. The success of a neuropsychiatric biopolitics of dementia since the 1970s has been both politically and economically integral to the prosperity of dementia studies over recent decades. To some extent, this existential dependency undermines the capacity for dementia studies to develop robust critiques of political economy. This political economy can often serve a range of stakeholders within dementia studies more than it serves people affected by dementia. In response, I argue that dementia studies could learn from the successes of promissory technoscience in creating futures that materially transform the present. Dementia studies could pursue a promissory biopolitics of social support that presents desirable, feasible and inevitable alternatives to contemporary forms of welfare-as-awareness and cure-as-lucrative.

8.1 Anti-Institutional Familialism

As noted, dementia care is mostly informal, provided by friends and families, with little involvement from formal services. This is true both nationally and internationally and has largely always been the case. In the UK, around two-thirds of people with dementia live outside of institutions with the support of more than 700,000 unpaid carers.[1] A 2019 report from the London School of Economics estimated that unpaid care accounted for around £14.6 billion of dementia care's total £36.7 billion cost.[2] The remaining cost is largely attributed to privately funded social care, so that people with dementia and their families contribute, directly or indirectly, about two-thirds of total dementia care costs.[3] Some caution is required here because the monetary value of informal relations, and which of those relations count as care, is far from clear. For instance, what is the £ value of making an older relative a cup of tea or helping them to get dressed? Are both of those things care? Moreover, costings are often used to represent the value of care, which in people's real lives can far transcend money. Hence, the headline monetary valuations are crudely indicative of the scale of informal involvement in dementia care, but we must remain alert to the ambiguous nature of personal relations as a site of social reproduction, their emotional and social vitalities and their irreconcilability with financial operationalisations.

The indebtedness of dementia care to unpaid informal support is largely attributable to the anti-institution, pro-community sentiment that typifies the British political economy of care. As mentioned in the previous chapter, surveys consistently indicate that most older people have an aversion to institutional care, and these public preferences for life in the community are written into national and international policy (e.g. the WHO's Global Strategy and Action Plan on Ageing and Health[4]) as well as a large body of scholarship (e.g. the "ageing in place" research field[5]). The ubiquity of notions of community as the paramount site of care is largely a feature of the past 50 years, which was preceded by a century of mass institutionalisation. Following the 1845 Asylums Act, older people and those with mental illnesses[1] experienced high rates of institutionalisation during the 19th and early 20th centuries, principally via workhouses (subsequently "Public Assistance Institutions") and asylums (subsequently "mental hospitals").[6-8]

During the mid-20th century, public and government sentiment shifted against mass institutionalisation for several reasons, to the effect that deinstitutionalisation became a major policy impetus.[6] Sensational accounts of poor conditions and ill-treatment within increasingly decrepit Victorian-era institutions stirred public condemnation. Such accounts, combined with a burgeoning anti-psychiatry movement, as discussed in Chapter 3, cast doubts on several facets of institutional psychiatric practice. Another potentially important contributing factor was the development of effective psychopharmacological agents such as chlorpromazine, haloperidol and imipramine, which enabled people to manage their symptoms outside of institutions. In 1962, the Hospital Plan pledged to close down mental hospitals, instigating a pronounced anti-institution/pro-community care policy trajectory that has been supported by every subsequent government. The transition from institutional to community care was initially subtle and largely driven by falling admissions, but from the 1980s onward, this intensified toward active discharge and closure.[6, 8, 9]

Besides the oft-cited moral imperatives and therapeutic facilitators of deinstitutionalisation, it is also important to recognise the concurrent economic and fiscal rationales. The closure of state-run institutions has repeatedly been championed as a financially conservative initiative.[10-12] Put simply, it costs a lot more (at least upfront) to house, feed and support people than it does to set them free. This fiscal tightening manifests underlying ideological concerns with notions of deservingness. The intensification of deinstitutionalisation through the 1980s echoed the wider anti-welfare sentiment that characterised Margaret Thatcher's governments from 1979 onward. She argued that the problems of individuals, such as psychiatric disorder, should not be borne by the state. In this spirit, the withdrawal of institutional support was also an effort to foster personal responsibility. Subsequent governments of various flavours have largely emulated this scepticism toward institutional provision, albeit with less abrasive rhetoric. For many scholars, other arguments concerning the rationales behind deinstitutionalisation are largely retrospective reappraisals of a political endeavour that has always been financially conservative, ideologically motivated and fundamentally anti-welfarist.[13]

Irrespective of the rationales, the resulting deinstitutionalisation was significant. The number of general hospital beds in England decreased from 299,000 in 1988 to 141,000 in 2020, at the same time as the general population grew by 10 million.[14] Institutional geriatric and psychiatric places have been especially impacted by this trajectory. In the UK, specialist mental health beds declined from 150,000 in 1955[15] to 18,000 in 2021,[16] while long-stay geriatric capacity fell from 53,000 in 1987 to 21,000 in 2010.[17] Private institutional care provision for older people actually increased up until the mid-1990s. A cottage industry of small providers flourished as state provision declined amidst population ageing and a desire to dedicate state funding to private services. However, this began to change with falling profits and tighter regulation.[18–20] While there is significant regional variation, as a proportion of the British population generally and the older population specifically, nursing and residential home places have fallen consistently since the mid-1990s.[21, 22]

Given the economic rationales that have contributed to deinstitutionalisation, it is unsurprising that one of the major shortcomings has been a lack of comparable support for people outside of institutions. As institutions closed, there was relatively little development of non-institutional services. In 1986, The Audit Commission warned that community care had failed to materialise because, while people had been transferred from institutions to local authorities, there had not been a corresponding transfer of financial support or formal responsibility.[8, 23] These concerns led to a report, then a white paper, and eventually the *National Health Service and Community Care Act 1990*, which set out a programme for marketising care. The care market was created by making local authorities responsible for assessing people's needs, creating a corresponding care package made up of various services (the majority of which were to be purchased from external providers) and regulating care provision.[8] These reforms were intended to stimulate a competitive market that was sensitive to consumer choice. As a result, private and charity non-institutional care provision increased dramatically relative to in-house local authority services.[24]

Establishing a market is not the same thing as providing funding. In lieu of adequate financial support, local authorities regularly run care budget deficits, private providers complain that they cannot afford to fulfil local-authority contracts and care workers are chronically underpaid. Social care spending in England peaked at £18 million in 2010. Under the government's austerity programme, spending fell yearly in real terms until 2020, when it rose sharply in response to COVID. However, even accounting for dramatic COVID-related increases, adult social care spending per head remains slightly down compared with 2010.[25] In 2021, Unison warned that English local authorities responsible for social care provision were facing a combined £2.1 billion deficit in 2022/23.[26] The lack of public money allocated to social care feeds into provider pressures. A National Care Forum survey in 2022 found that 66% of providers were refusing new contracts, while 21% were handing existing contracts back to local authorities because they were no longer able to fulfil them.[27] Care staff are equally adversely affected by budgetary restrictions. A 2015 review by the House of Common Public Accounts Committee reported that roughly 220,000 care professionals were being paid less than the minimum wage.[24] In 2022, the staff vacancy rate across English social care hit a record 9.8%.[28] Overall, stakeholders across the care market struggle as demand increases and funding remains tightly restricted.

Those in need of care are not spared from the repercussions of this system. The challenging financial landscape of community care provision has impelled local authorities to limit expenditure. This has often been enacted by tightening eligibility criteria so that fewer people qualify for public funding. In 2019, more than half of 282 community care practitioners surveyed claimed that local authorities had rules for assessing service eligibility that were deliberately not written down. This was done because local authorities recognised that their cost-saving restrictions transgressed the minimum requirements stipulated in the Care Act 2014.[29] The problem appears to be growing. Year on year, requests for care among older adults are increasing while provision is declining.[30] The result of this restrictive approach is that the majority of social care recipients are fully self-funded, receiving no public assistance.[31] This means that the personal financial cost of dementia can be ruinous. The average cost is around £100,000, but some people can spend upwards of £500,000.[32] Unsurprisingly, a lot of people simply cannot afford care.

A lack of public funding, coupled with the prospects of astronomical private costs, feeds into the characteristic informality of dementia care. The tab for defunding dementia care, under the guise of "community" rhetoric, is picked up by a mix of unmet need and unpaid provision. Most dementia care is provided by family members in private homes. This family-reliant, non-institutional care is often framed in terms of "community" in a rather idealistic manner, but the realities can be grim. In practice, community care often entails a sleep-deprived wife relying on anti-depressants or a daughter quitting her job and struggling to balance childcare responsibilities. These are the invisible realities of care that is supposedly in and of an imagined community but which is instead often limited to a single family member and takes place within a single house. The extent to which there is any degree of community in such scenarios is debatable, and I often find myself reflecting on this question when entering the homes of people with dementia who are living most of their lives between a handful of rooms and interacting with one or two people. Hence, ideals of community care often conceal a stark familialism.

Familialism is a political ideology whereby families or private households are envisioned, and acted toward, as key producers of social welfare. Familialist states rely on assumptions that the family should and will provide care, typically for children, older people and the disabled, and develop policy accordingly. In principle, the British approach to dementia care since at least the 1990s can be characterised as a form of *optional* familialism. Here, the family is formally recognised by policy – e.g. the Care Act 2014 explicitly recognises the status, rights and responsibilities of informal carers[33] – and is assumed to provide some welfare within a broader mixed economy of various options. However, while there is technically a market offering alternatives to family care, that market has substantial barriers to access, heavily incentivising family involvement. In practice, British familialism has become more *implicit* than *optional*. Austerity has squeezed budgets and made non-familial options increasingly unrealistic for many people. Fiscally conservative approaches (e.g. tightening care eligibility criteria) have produced a welfare vacuum that families fill.[34, 35]

Familialist regimes traditionally rely heavily on, and hence perpetuate, gender norms. Under these conditions, welfare is principally produced by women, typically wives and daughters. To this end, around two-thirds of family dementia carers are female.[36]Moreover, almost 90% of the formal dementia care workforce is female.[33] The overrepresentation of women as carers generally and dementia carers specifically is well known and has traditionally been attributed to norms that position women as more naturally caring than men.[37–39] In my own research, I have witnessed the ways in which gender norms unconsciously shape the caregiving trajectories of family members. Women are subtly guided toward carer roles by shared assumptions regarding their unique personal suitability for those roles. Family members are structurally positioned in relation to one another before dementia. Their positions correspond to structural determinants, e.g. gender and age, but are articulated in reference to personal characteristics, e.g. a caring nature or being experienced. Those seemingly personal attributes function as analogues for structural determinants. When a need for care arises, pre-existing structural positioning can guide certain individuals (typically female, older, lower earner, etc.) toward main carer roles, largely unconsciously.[40] This concealed naturalisation of female welfare production in relation to dementia means that the consequences of familialism are more commonly visited upon women. Hence, when we speak of community care in the abstract, we obscure the circumstances of female family members and the complex political economic systems that act to position those women as sites of welfare extraction.[41]

8.2 The Big Friendly Society

Contemporary familism is manifest in the "Big Society" political philosophy, popularised by former prime minister David Cameron in the early 2010s. While the phrase has fallen out of favour, the vision is realised today in a substantial social enterprise economy. The notion of the Big Society articulates a sort of welfare utopia predicated on private-capital-backed personal relationships and third-sector stakeholders as an alternative to state provision. The Big Society centred on familiar notions of markets, decentralisation, dynamism and efficiency. Also familiar were its dual fiscal and moral concerns, based on the identification of two core societal problems: (1) government overspending, particularly in the wake of the 2008 financial crash and (2) declining social reproduction, with various commentators highlighting fashionable moral panics (violence, hedonism, etc.) to forecast the decay of civilisation. Not only does the Big Society offer to fix these problems, but it also reconstrues them as opportunities for capital accumulation through returns on socially conscious investments. The talisman policy of this platform was the creation of a £600 million social investment fund in 2012 to support intermediary financiers which in turn would support social sector initiatives. Its legacy of capital-stimulated community welfare remains evident in the UK's thriving social enterprise sector, which has been characterised by some commentators as the political economy of the Big Society.[42, 43]

Irrespective of the original intentions behind the Big Society, the fiscal constriction of the austerity agenda defined British politics through the 2010s. A decade of budgetary cuts leading up to the COVID pandemic resulted in dramatic welfare reductions, with the implicit assumption that *communities* (which typically entails *private households* (which typically entails *family carers*)) would fill the gaps. In this context, the Big Society was almost immediately co-opted as a cover story for austerity, reanimating earlier deinstitutionalisation sentiments along the lines that people financially must, and morally should, deal with their own problems to a greater extent as state service provision was withdrawn. As with 1980s deinstitutionalisation, appeals to imagined communities (or societies) as fiscal and moral saviours quickly reinforced familialism in lieu of community care service provision.[42, 43] In practice, the "Big Society", like the "community care" it subsumed, is too often a single person invisibly trampled by extraordinary pressures.

It was in this context of the Big Society's reinvigoration of familialism that the Prime Minister's Challenge on Dementia was published in 2012, replete with renewed appeals to community. In particular, the creation of dementia-friendly communities was one of three key focuses. This was to be achieved by raising awareness among members of the public and encouraging private businesses to pledge support, developed with the help of initial state investment[44]. The Alzheimer's Society and Dementia Action Alliance were to work together to define dementia-friendliness and regulate its implementation across up to 20 initial communities. A year later, the Alzheimer's Society launched its Dementia Friends scheme in conjunction with Public Health England, jointly funded by the Department of Health and the Office of Civil Society for an initial sum of £2.4 million.[45] In 2015, the successful recruitment of one million Friends was announced, and the government continues to encourage communities to become dementia friendly.[46]

The idea of dementia-friendliness rests on an application of social disability understandings to dementia. As discussed in Chapter 2, the social model of disability emphasises the extent to which disabilities that are typically considered to be inherently biological and problematic are socially determined. Here, physiological characteristics become disabling in disabling contexts. The classic example is two wheelchair users trying to access two buildings, one of which has a ramp and the other stairs. In one scenario, the person is disabled; in the other, the person is enabled.[47] Regarding dementia, this social dis/abling has been extended, albeit often implicitly, to policy (e.g.

mental capacity legislation undermining one's ability to enact legal rights[48]), relationships (e.g. malignant social psychology undermining one's ability to manifest oneself[49, 50]) and environments (e.g. poor signage undermining one's ability to navigate spaces[51]). At its heart, a disability-inspired dementia-friendliness suggests that not everything that is seemingly problematic about dementia is inherently derived from cognitive impairment. By transforming context, we can transform the experiences of dementia that are determined by that context.

As well as an intellectual indebtedness to the social model of disability, dementia-friendliness also channels the earlier popularity of the World Health Organisation's "age-friendly" programme. This programme has similarly sought to make communities more amenable to older people generally, albeit with a focus on cities in the context of global urbanisation. As with deinstitutionalisation, the Big Society, familialism and the like, a significant motivation behind age-friendliness is a dual fiscal-moral argument for reduced service dependency and an idealised notion of community filling the resulting gaps. Indeed, the age-friendly agenda has similarly been critiqued as a medium of austerity and governmentality, encouraging "communities" and individuals to take on greater responsibility for limiting the state costs supposedly associated with population ageing.[52]

In the context of global financial anxiety and public austerity, it is unsurprising that fiscal concerns quickly came to dominate Big Society approaches. To this end, the dementia-friendly agenda has attended rather heavily to the relatively inexpensive task of adapting communities through awareness raising. Encouraging publics to think and act accordingly is typically a cheaper approach to public health than developing the practical institutional and infrastructural conditions that permit public health, at least in the short term. Self-governance is cheaper than governance. As we have seen throughout this book, the pursuit of appropriate conduct through the governance of thought is fundamental to the neuropsychiatric biopolitics of dementia. When we use the word "friendliness" to encompass a range of disability rights concerns, we depoliticise dementia in a manner befitting the Big Society and concealing the biopolitical determination of dementia. We situate the constitution of dementia-related problems in the (inter)personal realm, between friends and family, and within ourselves. Our moral relations and the ways that we act toward one another become the sites for change. Hence, the word "friend" does a lot of symbolic work.

As discussed in Chapter 2, for over a decade, citizenship scholars in dementia studies have warned against focusing too heavily on interpersonal relations at the expense of attentiveness to wider sociopolitical determinants. Ultimately, distributing an email telling care workers to treat care recipients more humanely is easier than altering the political economy of care within which those workers have 15-minute slots and are paid poverty wages. Helping people to help themselves is laudable, but when this focus on personal conduct functions as a smokescreen for otherwise worsening circumstances, it is actively harmful. Following years of decline, the number of carers receiving some type of formal support began to increase in 2018. However, that increase has been made up of advice and information provision, with funding and other instrumental services continuing to decline.[28] Here, the big dementia-friendly society is realised via the reformulation of welfare as awareness. As we have seen in previous chapters, this awareness is often a series of biopolitical commitments with questionable usefulness in real life. In line with its moral rationales, the big dementia-friendly society encourages forms of community and independence. Unfortunately, these ends are too often manifest as a lack of formal support, the promotion of awareness (i.e. neuropsychiatric biopolitics) and reliance on a family carer.

8.3 Financialising Futures

Beyond questions of friendliness, the biopolitics of promissory technoscience also catalyses similar combinations of government, private and third-sector initiatives in the dual interests of social welfare and investment returns. While the rearticulation of welfare as awareness under austerity has been driven by fiscal conservativeness, the prospects of high-return speculative ventures have been successfully leveraged in other areas of the dementia economy to great effect. Indeed, at the same time as formal social support systems for people affected by dementia were steadily eroded, the 2010s was actually a remarkably lucrative decade for the wider dementia economy. The British government increased dementia research funding from £28 million in 2009–2010 to £83 million in 2017–2018, and in 2019 the new government pledged to double this amount to £160 million per year for a further decade.[53] This impressive growth is indicative of the transformation of dementia into a type of post-financial-crash speculative market, achieved via the promissory technoscience biopolitics described in Chapter 4.

Since the early 2010s, successive British governments have developed a notable interest in dementia, or more specifically, in dementia research. During the UK's G8 presidency in 2013,[2] health ministers from the member states met in London for a conference dedicated to dementia. This meeting resulted in an international commitment to the development of a cure or a disease-modifying treatment by 2025.[54] The commitment was backed up with the creation of the Dementia Discovery Fund. This is a £250 million investment fund dedicated to supporting promising dementia drug discovery programmes. It encompasses investments from various pharmaceutical corporations and continues to target the 2025 goal.[55] At the same meeting, the World Dementia Council was established, a team of senior global figures in industry, academia and charities who would oversee progress toward the 2025 goal.[56] Echoing the Dementia Discovery Fund, G8 nations subsequently established comparable national initiatives with similar aims. In the UK, the government set up a collection of UK Dementia Research Institutes, combining public and third-sector money, largely via the Medical Research

Council, Alzheimer's Society and Alzheimer's Research UK, to the value of £290 million. Again, the aim is to expedite the development of promising curative or disease-modifying candidates, with a stated date of 2025.[57]

In 2019, the proliferation of these types of programmes led to the first meeting of the Dementia UK Ecosystem, an umbrella organisation encompassing the various large dementia-related organisations that now exist in the UK. The meeting was attended by Dementias Platform UK, ARUK Drug Discovery Alliance, European Prevention of Alzheimer's Dementia, NIHR National Director for Dementia Research Office, Alzheimer's Research UK, Alzheimer's Society, Medical Research Council, Wellcome Trust and Dementia Discovery Fund. The very existence of the Dementia UK Ecosystem, and the impressive capital that it encompasses, is emblematic of the growth of the dementia economy over recent years. Nonetheless, the meeting resulted in a call for "long-term funding commitment and increased investment in a field that remains considerably underfunded".[58] The Dementia UK Ecosystem is dedicated to drug discovery. However, one of the three core aims to emerge from the initial meeting was a commitment to public communication and destigmatising dementia, echoing the concerns of friendliness.[59] In such idiosyncrasies, we find indications of the indebtedness of seemingly dissimilar enterprises to a core neuropsychiatric biopolitics of dementia. Here, the organisation tasked with developing pharmaceutical cures nonetheless reiterates intuitively unrelated appeals to anti-stigma campaigns and awareness raising.

Building on the government's impressive record of increasing dementia research funding across the 2010s, the incumbent Conservative party entered the 2019 general election with a promise to double funding to £1.6 billion over the following decade. This manifesto pledge was termed the "dementia moonshot", using the familiar R&D-policy trope of drawing equivalence with the US administration's successful 1960s efforts to send astronauts to the moon. The stated aim of this moonshot was to "make finding a cure one of our Government's biggest collective priorities."[53] The 2021 report by the APPG on Dementia was dedicated to the moonshot. Produced with the Alzheimer's Society and based on testimony from dementia researchers, the report applauded sustained government commitment to research and maintained a heavy emphasis on biomarker development and drug discovery, with a familiar nod to raising public awareness of dementia.[60] In 2022, the prime minister reaffirmed the moonshot funding, this time dedicating it to Dame Barbara Windsor, an actress who had recently passed away with dementia.[61]

The moonshot is a speculative investment based on belief in a particular future. As discussed in Chapter 4, speculative futures and collective expectations can have formative consequences for our presents.[62, 63] Conviction in the likelihood of a given future can contribute to making that future seem more probable, and perhaps even making it more probable, by catalysing resources and using them to pursue that future. The financial potency of promissory futures is evident in the extraordinary valuations of technology companies relative to their actual revenue. At the time of writing, the cloud computing firm Snowflake has a market cap of $95.8 billion despite recording a $760.7 million loss over the past 12 months and most analysts predicting losses for years to come. This high-value, high-loss model is made possible via the power of technoscientific promise. Those seemingly ridiculous investments represent a staunch belief that, given the inevitability of technoscientific progress, such initiatives will eventually become profitable, or at least a belief that similar investments will keep accruing, swelling valuations. Indeed, in the post-2008 low-interest credit environment, profit has become increasingly irrelevant compared with valuation. Hype trumps end product. As well as making the imagined future more likely, belief in that future is already profoundly changing the present, e.g. by generating a $95.8 billion company. In a similar manner, the neuropsychiatric biopolitics of dementia has successfully leveraged the power of promissory technoscience to stimulate speculative investment in the future and hence reshape the present. This is manifest in the moonshot, Dementia Research Institutes, Dementia Discovery Fund, etc. As long as long-term profits (i.e. cures) remain believable, medium-term value (i.e. funding) can be cultivated.

Promissory technoscience does not solely transform the present in ways that make the favoured future more probable. Those present transformations simultaneously make alternative futures less likely, even where those alternatives may appear more desirable and attainable. In much the same way that the hype surrounding driverless cars can overshadow arguments for developing better public transport, dementia cures, particularly pharmaceuticals, can overshadow arguments for social support. That said, it is important to avoid slipping into zero-sum arguments regarding cure versus care expenditure. Such arguments imagine that a Chancellor or CEO. has a fixed pile of cash which he/she designates into several distinct pots. This is an argument often made in regard to care versus cure investment and is a little naïve. Rather, the extreme contrast between cure and care is indicative of the manner in which capital can be leveraged by certain stakeholders and for certain projects. The possibility of a dementia cure offers potential financial returns that £160 million worth of social care seemingly could never yield. Hence, much of what is invested only exists by virtue of the thing that it is invested in, that is, the promise. Rather than stealing resources from elsewhere, the promise is itself generative of resources.

Moreover, a cure seems likely because a host of respectable stakeholders say that it is so. Savvy investors typically seek out the most assured returns. The assuredness of returns on any speculative investment is based on a host of factors that contribute toward making a certain outcome appear more or less realistic. Again, importantly, this is not the end product per se, but rather the plausibility of sustained investment in that promissory future so as to ensure medium-term value growth. As a dementia researcher, my advice to an investor regarding the prospects of a dementia treatment would likely be valued more than the advice of a member of the public. However, the power of my advice to dictate the future of that treatment pales in comparison to the stance taken by major organisations and leading figures in the field. This is applicable not only to expert stakeholders and associated institutions but also to the investments themselves. If a government is putting a lot of money into a speculative endeavour, then the realisation of that endeavour becomes more likely, or at least the artificial maintenance of its value, irrespective of whether it eventually fails. Hence, big non-expert investments can make that investment more probable, encouraging further investment, and so on.

While major stakeholders have considerable power in the determination of probable and desirable futures, there are also notable subcultures doing similar work in relation to the financialisation of dementia. As a young white man, I am heavily exposed to the world of digital finance, an environment where the prospects and fates of biotech are continually negotiated. The likelihoods of various interventions succeeding, and therefore their stock prices increasing, are contested across Discord servers and subreddits. YouTube comment sections are targeted with "fake news" accusations when a drug's prospects are talked down. Twitter bots promote upcoming initiatives, tagging stocks. Biogen is "$BIIB"; Eisai is "$ESALY" (explore these tags at your own peril). This is a facet of the dementia economy that is rarely discussed in dementia studies, yet it has profound implications for intervention development and exemplifies the dangers of financialisation to generate perverse incentives. It can be tempting to dismiss financial social media as inconsequential, but in 2021 the r/WallStreetBets subreddit caused several major hedge funds to take billions of dollars in losses when users collectively squeezed hedge fund short positions on GameStop stock.[3] Dementia drug research has become a strong candidate for shorting because it can generate considerable value and has a high probability of ultimate failure, resulting in extremely large, sudden and predictable drops in value.[64] Coincidentally, in cryptocurrency slang, "to the moon" or "mooning" refers to a large spike in a valuation. Hence, a range of stakeholders, from prime ministers to shitposters, can work to make certain futures, and by extension investments in them, more or less appealing than they might otherwise be based on their own merits.

8.4 Shoot for the Orange

The appeal of financialising dementia's future is embedded in the normative commitments of a neuropsychiatric biopolitics of dementia that offers technoscientific solutions to technoscientific problems. Here, the task becomes one of enabling the appropriate experts to work out the problem sufficiently enough that they can then use that expertise to develop the corresponding (hopefully simple and efficient) fixes. This appeal is a potent force well beyond the world of dementia. Solar power and carbon capture technologies offer solutions to climate change rather than decreasing our energy consumption. Egg freezing and ectogenesis technologies offer solutions to declining fertility rather than legislating parental rights. Automation offers solutions to labour costs rather than limiting cheap consumption and corporate profiteering. At extremes, space colonisation offers solutions to many complex and sometimes seemingly insurmountable earthly problems. Throughout, promissory technoscience offers us a range of prospective fixes for problems that can be considered to have substantial sociopolitical facets, and in doing so, makes it seem as though those problems are intrinsically technoscientific in nature. The risk here is that technoscientific reimaginings of sociopolitical problems conceal their sociopolitical facets and dissuade us from pursuing sociopolitical solutions in tandem.

An example of this reimagining of dementia as a problem for promissory technoscience is ARUK's #ShareTheOrange initiative. The #ShareTheOrange campaign was launched in 2015 and surpassed two million social media shares in 2019. It is most well known for several high-production audiovisual advertisements, fronted by renowned actors Christopher Eccleston, Bryan Cranston and Samuel L Jackson. The core premise of each media segment is that, on average, AD is associated with a loss of brain mass equivalent to the weight of an orange. As noted in Chapter 4, the ageing brain can lose about 20% of its peak weight, so operationalising this orange-loss as AD is difficult, particularly given that associated protein aggregation will make up some of that variable weight.[65] Irrespective of its scientific difficulties, the orange analogy is instrumentally effective in simplifying and materialising the issue. Critically, the weight loss is interpreted as evidencing the inherent physicality of the problem. This inherent physicality is then similarly interpreted as evidence of its inherent amenability to technoscientific research and intervention. This argument is made explicitly in each of the campaign adverts:

Eccleston: While scary, this does prove it's a physical disease and not just part of ageing. Research has beaten diseases in the past and, with your help, research can defeat dementia.

Cranston: The shows us that Alzheimer's is a physical disease that we can fight. Research has already made great breakthroughs in other diseases, like cancer and AIDS, and with your support, Alzheimer's Research UK will breakthrough against dementia.

Jackson: This shows that Alzheimer's is a physical disease, and through research we know that disease can be slowed. They can be stopped. So lets change the conversation and help Alzheimer's Research UK make these breakthroughs possible for dementia.[66]

Each of these media segments uses the orange analogy to position dementia as a technoscientific problem with prospective technoscientific solutions that will be realised through dedicated technoscientific efforts. At an immediate level, the charity's motivation is the accrual of donations, which it depends on for its existence and to develop its work. If dementia does not have a technoscientific solution, then there is little reason for funding the pursuit of that solution. However, in summoning a version of dementia as a problem that is conducive to its own interests, ARUK contributes to the making of that problem into particular forms befitting the wider speculative economy of promissory technoscience. If that making involves somebody as notable as Samuel L Jackson in a polished video with the backing of a leading dementia research organisation, then the resulting product seems far more worthy of investment than if I was to simply ask for funding by myself.

The promissory biopolitics that typifies moonshots and oranges renders dementia more financially appealing. Consider the alternatives. On the one hand, approaching dementia as a complex disability that requires long-term social support renders it one more component of a gloomy political economy of ageing that devalues state welfare and equates demographic ageing with economic collapse. On the other hand, approaching dementia as a vast future health market renders it a fantastic investment opportunity and offers a means of replacing social reproduction (e.g. care) with consumption (e.g. drugs). Importantly, such an approach reinterprets the traditional demographic alarmism of big population ageing statistics and renders those big numbers financially appetising. Rather than representing escalating economic parasitism, those big numbers now represent the scale of a forthcoming market. Victoria Pitts-Taylor has argued that this generation of speculative potential typifies the political economic repercussions of neuroculture, presenting unenhanced brains as a form of unrealised value that warrants speculation:

> The value of biological materials in biocapitalism – or … *biovalue* – is often articulated in the hyped up language of future possibilities brought by current biological investment. That is, biovalue depends upon speculation. … In popular accounts of the brain's value as a bioresource, we are continually instructed that most people's brains are underutilized. Again and again, the brain's potential is presented as untapped.[67]

Reiterating these conceptual mechanics, moonshots and oranges depict a version of the future in which people with dementia are an economic net positive by virtue of the drugs they will purchase and the value that will be unlocked. Financial and political imperatives coalesce around the dementia that is depicted by promissory technoscience. Fund managers and fiscally conservative politicians alike can shoot for the orange because it simultaneously promises that there is much money to be saved and much money to be made.

While the transformation of dementia into an orange is amenable to certain political and economic interests, it is difficult to reconcile with what you, I or other people affected by it might recognise as dementia. It is a manifestation of circularity, befitting its wider political economic context, as a technoscientific problem that will have a technoscientific solution because it is a technoscientific problem, and such problems have technoscientific solutions. This is a tautological approach to dementia. It strips away challenging dementia-related considerations such as ageing and the associated idiosyn-crasies of neurological senescence and cognitive decline. It does away with the heterogeneous sociopolitical determination of experiences of dementia, questions of ecology and interpersonal relationships. To some extent, it is financially vital that it does this. Acknowledging the uncertainties and complexities of dementia risks undermining the neuropsychiatric biopolitics upon which the speculative economy of promissory dementia technoscience is built. As we saw in 2008, a dangerous implication of the large-scale financialisation of speculative futures is that a great deal of capital rests on the maintenance of belief in a particular future (house prices go up; research cures diseases). Any insult to that future risks undermining the present circumstances that are heavily leveraged against certainty in that future. At this point, for many stakeholders to re-engage with real-world dementia, replete with its many idiosyncrasies, would be akin to revealing to the bank that their newly mortgaged house is riddled with asbestos and built on an ex-mining site.

The fragility of such a position has latterly been exemplified. As the 2010s drew to an end, the big dementia-friendly society seemed relatively secure. Real-terms state care expenditure remained below 2010 levels, and at the 2019 general election, the Conservative party re-emphasised its decade-long devotion to dementia research with a manifesto commitment to further double funding, amounting to £1.6 billion across the next decade. Labelled the "dementia moonshot", this initiative was promoted as proof of the government's prioritisation of curing dementia.[53] The Conservatives won a landslide victory, and hence it seemed that the dementia economy would remain lucrative into the 2020s. We all know what happened next. Around the world, the COVID crisis halted government programmes as states redirected their administrations to dealing with the pandemic. There was little talk of the moonshot at the same time that charity finances were decimated.[60] In 2021, the APPG on Dementia dedicated its report to the moonshot, in partnership with the Alzheimer's Society.[60] The report lavished praise on the government's record of support for dementia research, including the moonshot pledge, and emphasised the need to fulfil that promise.

The report was indicative of growing uneasiness across the dementia economy that the moonshot would not be forthcoming. It opened with familiar appeals to higher levels of funding in cancer research and emphasised the detrimental effects of the pandemic on dementia research and the finances of associated charities.[53] By February 2022, the Alzheimer's Society and the APPG were more forthright, directly calling on the government to respect their manifesto pledge. During a newspaper interview a fortnight later, a minister admitted that the government was reneging on the moonshot and had, in fact, cut annual funding from £83 million to £75 million.[68] A series of media appearances and public statements followed from stakeholders calling for reconsideration. Then, in August 2022, the prime minister reanimated the moonshot in remembrance of Dame Barbara Windsor, committing to increase dementia research funding to £160 million annually by 2024.[69] Cue sighs of relief, but the underlying fragility remains. By embracing financialisation and leaning into speculation as a foundation for growth, the political economy of dementia has inevitably been opened up to the characteristic booms and busts of investment markets. It is unlikely to avoid the busts forever.

8.5 Gerontological Insights

In the final sections of the chapter, I want to do two things. First, I argue that Dementia Friends, #ShareTheOrange and their kin are united as particular manifestations of a neuropsychiatric biopolitics that collectively comprise a wider political economy of dementia. They materialise and institutionalise the neuropsychiatric biopolitics of dementia. The resulting political economy serves a range of interests, including those of researchers, investors and politicians, but not those of many people affected by dementia. Second, I critique the role of dementia studies in often failing to adequately hold to account, and hence being more or less complicit in, that neuropsychiatric biopolitics and concurrent political economy. In response, I will argue that a critical dementia studies should not only deconstruct neuropsychiatric biopolitics but also learn from its successes to develop an alternative biopolitics of social support, depicting promissory futures capable of generating investment.

First, let's consider the bigger picture and the affinities that run through it. Enterprises such as Dementia Friends and #ShareTheOrange are too often interpreted through the well-established lens of *cure versus care* as different, and perhaps even opposite, types of things. In practice, community awareness initiatives and promissory technoscience initiatives are more closely aligned than this binary would imply. They rely on and perpetuate a shared neuropsychiatric biopolitics of dementia as:

> A syndrome of cognitive decline caused by discrete neuropathologies that are distinct from ageing, and … not enough people are aware of this. Furthermore, because dementia is caused by disease, and biomedical sciences have cured some diseases, dementia is a technoscientific challenge that will be solved through technoscientific endeavours.[70]

This biopolitics dictates an imperative. Each member of the public must know it, comply with it and govern their personal conduct accordingly. With this imperative in mind, biopolitical enterprises are explicitly public facing. More than this, they are explicit in their aims to change public mentalities and, following on from this psychic transformation, to change public action. In manifesting this biopolitics, community and promissory initiatives comprise important components of a political economy of dementia that manifests the neuropsychiatric biopolitics of dementia as a structural force serving specific ends. These projects coalesce around the reallocation of social reproduction downwards, from the state to the community, which in practice means to family members. That reallocation also extends into the future in reference to promissory technoscience, marking the final replacement of social reproduction altogether with personal consumption. This is a story of progress toward a liberal capitalist utopia, whereby dementia care moves from the dank institutional oppressions of the asylum system to the consumer with dementia renewing their medication subscription. In this scenario, our contemporary situation becomes a prickly moment on the longer-term road to progress.

Dementia has evidently been a major area of focus for successive governments, undoubtedly due in large part to sincere concern for the well-being of those affected. It is no coincidence that, following his resignation as prime minister, David Cameron became the president of ARUK. There is considerable appetite and capacity for developing dementia-related enterprises. Unfortunately, the political commitment to addressing dementia has been pursued in line with particular ideological commitments that are difficult to reconcile with the practical realities of dementia. It is difficult to blend a commitment to improving experiences of dementia with an aversion to collective welfare and a predilection for capital accumulation. It is especially here, in response to ideology-led tensions, that we need to develop critical analyses of the political economy of dementia. The neurocritical dementia studies scholar should be wary of blindly championing research investment and awareness enterprises.

Critical gerontology has a rich heritage of critiquing the political economy of ageing. Indeed, such critique was foundational to the emergence of critical gerontological scholarship generally.[71] Amidst the political and economic upheaval of the late 1970s and early 1980s, critical gerontological work on the political economy of ageing began to unpack the various ways in which experiences of later life were constrained by economics and social policy. At that time, post-war welfare arrangements began to unravel as states responded to global economic crises with cutbacks. Based on pension and care expenditure, ageing populations were increasingly politicised as economically burdensome and, by extension, as society and economy became increasingly conflated, societally burdensome. This transformation of the meanings of agedness and the relations between ageing and the state alerted gerontologists to the political economic constitution of ageing.

At the forefront of these gerontologists was Carroll Estes.[72] She argued that post-industrial capital, states and sex/gender systems, all under the influence of ideology, determined the circumstances of citizens. Estes characterised capitalist states as those enshrining private property ownership, with state apparatuses financed by taxing privately generated wealth. Such states have dual roles, on the one hand, ensuring the conditions for private wealth growth and, on the other hand, ensuring social welfare. Balancing the two, both of which are costly, presents something of a bind. It is difficult to sustain low taxation and high expenditure. The trick, then, is to align private and public interests. Estes argued that, in the late 20th century, states were increasingly beguiled by hyper-mobile post-industrial capital investment into traditional state functions as a means of decreasing public expenditure and generating private growth while sustaining welfare.

Regarding this capital, Estes noted that the intensification of marketisation and vast transnational investment flows meant that the power of private capital often superseded the capacity of national governments and banks to act in the national interest when things went awry. Growing state reliance on being perceived favourably by speculative investment meant that states were increasingly tempted to marketise and deregulate social services in the interests of investors. This meant that states were subsequently forced to pick up the tab for resulting financial calamities because, in societies rendered dependent on private capital, the alternative to bailouts was societal collapse. Bear in mind, Estes was arguing this well before 2008, when the excesses of deregulated private speculation in a vital component of public welfare – housing – almost collapsed the global banking system so that states were forced to offer up huge public funds to replace capital losses and prevent potentially apocalyptic societal repercussions. At the same time, financialisation saps those funds. A 2019 report by the Centre for Health and the Public Interest revealed that several major care home providers were offshoring millions of pounds in funding through opaque company structures.[73]

Beyond traditional political economic concerns of state and capital, Estes also drew on feminist scholarship to argue that a sex/gender system similarly constrained later-life circumstances. This system denotes the many forms in which assumptions about sex are transformed into specific social functions through institutions such as the family, the labour market and policy. At the interpersonal level, these effects are manifest in the aforementioned structural positioning of family members in ways that render them more or less likely to become a main carer. Here, a person who earns less than others, is financially encouraged by labour policy to take time out of employment to provide care and is generally considered by others to be naturally caring, is more likely to become a carer. Within the sex/gender system, this person is far more likely to be a woman than a man.

Estes's work on ageing in the late 20th century remains remarkably applicable to the contemporary political economy of dementia, but much has changed since. Indeed, we have subsequently lived through the very crisis that her work foreshadowed. The 2008 financial crash catalysed concerns regarding social reproduction, public expenditure and capital accumulation.[43] As discussed in relation to the Big Society, state austerity programmes addressed public expenditure to some extent but simultaneously undermined welfare. The global turn to quantitative easing also intensified the accumulation problem because the abundance of cheap credit effectively devalued capital, lowering yields and forcing investors toward riskier prospects. Given the current state of dementia drug discovery, investment can appear to be a relatively bad bet, irrespective of the promises offered by charity campaigns. Nonetheless, as we have seen with aducanumab, even bad bets are now seemingly worth a punt. Echoing the discussion in Chapter 5, investors are not dependent on what you or I might consider to be research "success". Capital only has to accumulate for a certain period of time and can then be seized upon by speculators, even if the research appears to fail in terms of cognitive effects. The complexity of dementia research also means that failed trials can feasibly be presented as successes, leading to large value gains (at least short term). This happened with aducanumab and lecanemab's contentious trial results, resulting in 42% and 40% jumps in Biogen stock, respectively.[74–76] Profitability has been separated from research outcomes, and financialised dementia drug discovery has (d)evolved into a casino, often at the expense of robust science. The ultimate effect is a decoupling of the productive economy from investment markets, the former struggling while the latter prosper, and dementia expanded its slice of that prosperity through the 2010s.

The pandemic has further complicated the political economic landscape. On the one hand, the scale of state mobilisation in response to COVID showed the power of states to pursue transformative welfare programmes. Capital is available when the state so desires it. On the other hand, the sustained economic and fiscal repercussions, coupled with criticism of government responses and the linking of care homes with imprisonment and death, furnish fertile terrain for renewed appeals to state retrenchment. Ideologically, the political economy of ageing has long rested on a moralisation of the ageing population generally and older people specifically as economically, and therefore societally, problematic. This ideology has been furthered through the concentration of COVID morbidity and mortality in older populations and particularly those with dementia. Much public debate has centred on age–COVID relations, catalysing arguments regarding the extent to which disabled and older people deserve social support, as well as the extent to which institutional support is implicated in grim outcomes.[77]

Contemporary appeals to demographic ageing, especially in light of COVID, as evidence that institutional forms of care are fiscally untenable and morally unpalatable can be read as continuations of the political trends documented by Estes several decades ago. To some extent, the shift of post-1970s political consensus away from large-scale state welfare to a greater emphasis on privatisation and marketisation has struggled to come to terms with the practicalities of care as a form of social reproduction that is essential to our well-being, and indeed, our very existence. I am cautious of slipping into crude arguments regarding *neoliberalism* as some sort of nefarious monolith (not dissimilar to *(bio)medicalisation*), but suffice it to say that our contemporary political economy centres on notions of independence (or at least dependence on the labour market and personal consumption rather than on the care of others) that are difficult to reconcile with the material realities of human life. Promissory technoscience offers a means of addressing this tension through its radical reimagining of welfare as consumption. Estes argued:

State policies define and commodify the problems of aging. Policies define the problems as individual medical problems requiring medical services sold privately for profit. This approach is ideologically and practically consistent with the state's dual and contradictory roles in promoting the process of capital accumulation and in the legitimation of capitalist social relations through safety net and other provisions.[72]

Here, she could be directly describing government alignments with promissory technoscience over recent years to position dementia as a speculative investment and catalyst for capital accrual. The neuropsychiatric biopolitics of dementia feeds into this political economy because it takes a dementia that is ill-suited to capital accumulation – later-life cognitive decline requiring sustained social support to maximise well-being – and turns it into a dementia that promises financial reward – a disease requiring the purchase of biotech products to ensure independence and generate value.

Of course, a biopolitical remaking of dementia to suit a particular political economy does little to help those affected by dementia, at least in the present. Irrespective of how stakeholders pursue idealised imaginings of dementia both now and in the future, many people remain confronted with the practical realities of dementia as they are experienced today. You cannot yet consume your way out of dementia. In the meantime, the erosion of welfare has been pursued regardless. Above and beyond straightforward cuts, this erosion is manifest in outsourcing of care to communities under the guise of friendliness. Estes argued that the proliferation of information and communication technologies presented new opportunities for various political actors to bring publics into line. Notions of friendliness, enacted through online awareness courses and social media campaigns aimed at sharing neuropsychiatric claims, are contemporary forms of this biopolitical bringing into line.

Critical gerontological work on age-friendly programmes tells a familiar story of laudable aims relating to public well-being being implemented in an ideologically economised manner. This is manifest in chronic underfunding and reliance on information provision and volunteerism. The overall effect is reminiscent of the Big Society in as much as a utopian societal vision becomes something of a smokescreen for the nominal transfer of welfare from states to communities, which entails the practical transfer of welfare from states to either individuals (particularly women) or nowhere at all.[78] The demographic alarmism underpinning friendliness initiatives is often evident in policy documents that frame the problem to which they respond in terms of population ageing and associated costliness, rather than framing the problem as one of how to help people live well.[79] Dementia-friendliness operates under the influence of similar logics, whereby the problem to which associated initiatives respond is often framed as one of dread disease and associated costs. One recent analysis of dementia-friendly policy documents found that every one framed the problem in terms of increasing prevalence and growing costs and the solution in terms of knowledge dissemination.[80] Friendliness, aka awareness, responds to notions of demographic costliness.

8.6 Transforming Our Complicities

So far, I have argued that notions of community and promissory technoscience are essential to a political economy of dementia characterised by the reduction of shared (especially state) obligation toward dementia and the transformation of dementia into an opportunity for capital accrual. This political economy nurtures and benefits from a neuropsychiatric biopolitics of dementia that disciplines publics accordingly. I now want to focus on how a portion of dementia studies fits into this political economy. As with many of the issues covered throughout this text, I argue that there is too much uncritical dementia studies engagement with friendliness, promissory technoscience and other core tenets of the political economy of dementia. A recent "State of the Science Review" of friendliness, published in the *Dementia* journal, exemplifies some of the potential problems with these engagements.[81] It draws on the longstanding self-positioning language of dementia studies to define dementia-friendliness as a reaction against the (bio)medical model, instead promoting ideals of social inclusion and human rights. The review characterises dementia-friendly initiatives as fitting into the following philosophy:

> Alternative non-medical approaches in dementia studies have allowed us to move beyond the individual pathology of "symptoms and behaviour" to focus instead on broader concepts of well-being, human rights, and social inclusion, prompted through social and environmental solutions.[81]

Few dementia studies scholars would contest the overall approach developed here. Nonetheless, as with appeals to dementia research more broadly, researchers advocating for friendliness initiatives are attentive to the underlying cost imperatives and "communities", and actively engage corresponding arguments in support:

> The financial cost and potential savings of specific [dementia-friendly initiatives] must be quantified to determine economic feasibility of implementation. Information on the fiscal impact of DFIs could enhance the draw and adoption of evidence-based dementia-friendly practices on larger scales across settings. Preventing institutionalization through enactment of comprehensive DFIs has potential for cost savings multiplied across communities.[81]

This strategy is undoubtedly well intentioned, but perpetuates the idea that dementia is fundamentally a fiscal concern. As discussed earlier, emphasising the necessity of dementia-related initiatives is important to dementia studies. At a basic level, dementia studies relies on being perceived as responding to an important problem and therefore being financially worthwhile. This generates questions regarding how a truly critical dementia studies might fruitfully engage with matters of political economy and the fiscal logics that characterise contemporary public health generally. On the one hand, the development of supportive infrastructures of any kind requires an alertness to and engagement with economic constraints if anything is to be practically achieved. On the other hand, engaging with economic constraints as though they are intrinsic properties of the world risks bolstering restrictive circumstances by concealing their sociopolitical contingency. To be fair, it is important to note that a sizeable chunk of dementia studies scholarship actively resists naturalising representations of dementia as an economic burden, at least to some extent. This resistance should be nurtured throughout critical dementia studies. However, it is simultaneously a line of critique that eats away at its own material foundations if it fails to offer equally influential alternative visions with resource-generating capacities.

Another tricky issue with dementia-friendliness and similar social disability model schemas is that, as with deinstitutionalisation, many of the core ideals and associated moral imperatives are genuinely commendable. They are partly aligned with longstanding ideals in dementia studies, framed as resisting a (bio)medical model and re-humanising people through the development of salutogenic social contexts. There now exists a sizeable body of uncritical dementia studies work on dementia-friendliness that partly reiterates idealised appeals to "community" and "inclusion". The following examples are taken from the beginnings of recent research articles in the *Dementia* journal:

> A dementia friendly community is one that is informed about dementia, respectful and inclusive of people with dementia and their families, provides support, promotes empowerment, and fosters quality of life[82].
>
> [Dementia friendly communities] are one of a range of initiatives that aim to improve the lives of people living with dementia and their supporters and to reduce stigma. DFCs are defined as "a place or culture in which people with dementia and their carers are empowered, supported and included in society, understanding their rights and recognise their full potential". DFCs recognise the imperative of including people living with dementia as valued members of their local communities.[83]
>
> Dementia-friendly communities (DFCs) are one way in which people living with dementia can be supported to be active, engaged and valued citizens.[84]

Nominally, the ideals at stake here are laudable. However, there is little concern with the manner in which such ideals are leveraged in practice to achieve a different set of political and economic ends. As has been noted more generally in political science, well-meaning liberal commitments to humanism can easily facilitate deinstitutionalisation as a form of welfare dismantlement.[13] Here, we find another form of neuro-agnosticism at play. There is a lot of well-meaning work in dementia studies that is seeking to develop, extend and enhance dementia-friendliness. Scholars, including me, are busy planting community gardens, running dementia cafes and organising accessible performances, all under a banner of friendliness. When viewed outside of their political economic contexts, it is difficult to argue that such activities are anything other than a good thing. However, when we attend to the real-world political and economic implications of friendliness, that desirability becomes murkier.

In 2017, I conducted some research with a church, the congregation of which included people with dementia. The vicar was heavily involved in supporting these people in the community, checking in on them, organising activities and even running errands on their behalf. His efforts genuinely improved the lives of people in his community, but those same efforts had also been recognised by the local council, to the extent that they were increasingly asking him to perform certain supportive roles. In a conversation that has stayed with me, he said that he increasingly felt like a social worker with a dog collar. The more he did, the more the local authority could withdraw, increasing the need for his support, and so on. The problem here is one of substitution. Community support (which we must remember is often an over-stretched individual) can be a wonderful thing, but it is too often seized upon as an opportunity for removing formal support rather than as an addition. In health economics, the *crowding-out* hypothesis contends that when formal support increases, informal support decreases correspondingly, and vice versa. This zero-sum approach seems intuitive. However, comparative research across Europe reveals that increasing formal care can actually be associated with increasing informal care, with each form enabling the greater specialisation of the other so that overall support is both increased and improved.[85]

Through engagements with friendliness that are stripped of political economic context, these forms of dementia studies risk overlooking core tensions. As noted throughout, a failure to critically attend to these issues is essentially a form of complicity in them. It not only fails to foster robust scrutiny of systemic problems but also supports the perpetuation of those problems through the development and celebration of corresponding initiatives. At its worst, friendliness can become the promissory technoscience of dementia studies. Here, social science, if permitted to pursue sufficient future research and development, will refine increasingly sophisticated, friendly communities wherein awareness thrives and stigma is eliminated. This friendliness will eventually become so supportive that it will significantly alleviate the problems of dementia and the associated need for costly care. There is some merit to dementia studies articulating positive alternative futures to the mainstream promissory technoscience of moonshots and oranges, but those futures should be framed as fixing political economic problems rather than fiscal problems. We should certainly avoid playing any part in making aware-ness a substitute for support.

The same is broadly true of zero-sum critiques of dementia studies' rela-tionship with the promissory technoscience of neuropsychiatric biopolitics. The erosion of social support and growth of biotech speculation is a con-temporary manifestation of traditional hierarchies of care and cure that have long animated some critics within dementia studies. Scholars going right back to Lyman in the 1980s have complained that the (bio)medical model diverts resources into curative efforts at the expense of care.[86] At face value, this is a fair observation. There are over 30,000 projects registered in the International Alzheimer's Disease Research Portfolio database, and only 5% of those are about care, compared with 45% dealing with pathophysiology and drug discovery.[87] However, as noted above, these zero-sum care ver-sus cure funding arguments in dementia studies are naïve to the extent that promissory technoscience is able to leverage capital that simply does not exist in relation to care. This is not always a matter of money going to one thing instead of another. It speaks to the power of neuroscientific biopolitics to generate beneficial material conditions for itself. It creates a future that feels both sufficiently desirable and realistic to grant it productive power in the present.

In this respect, dementia studies scholarship that bemoans (bio)medicali-sation can be its own worst enemy in as much as it fails to offer an alternative promissory biopolitics complete with its own generative capacities. In lieu of such an alternative, social support is cast as an undesirable sticking plas-ter, the best bad option that we have until technoscience solves the problem properly. This is not an argument against the pursuit of technoscientific solu-tions; I am actually broadly supportive of such an approach. Instead, it is a dual argument, firstly for thoroughly explicating the problematic influence of neuropsychiatric biopolitics on the political economy of dementia, and sec-ondly for learning from the successes of promissory technoscience and trying to imbibe social support with some of that biopolitical artfulness. The great promise of critical dementia studies is to envisage a future in which social support is primarily guided by the well-being of people affected by dementia rather than political economic constraints that are too often at odds with those interests. That future is at least as attainable as popular technoscientific promises if only we can effectuate the same aura of investment potential.

* * *

The problematic relations between areas of dementia studies and the neu-ropsychiatric biopolitics of dementia are perhaps most pertinently real-ised in the contemporary political economy of dementia. Social support is devolved to individuals under the guise of friendliness, while particular ver-sions of dementia garner substantive investment in the interests of capital accumulation. Appeals to dementia as an inherently economic problem, pursued as a means of asserting the importance of dementia research generally, are indicative of the wider problem that institutionalised dementia studies can face when attending to dementia-related initiatives that garner substantial investment. Financially, that support is conducive to the flourishing of a lot of dementia studies itself, creating incentives to emulate the biopolitics that generate it. We should not be naïve to the embeddedness of institutionalised dementia studies within the contemporary political economy of dementia. The neuropsychiatric biopolitics of dementia have enabled various stakeholders to accrue a lot of capital over recent decades, and components of dementia studies have undoubtedly benefitted from that accrual, with funding for university groups, research initiatives and conferences. At worst, some areas of dementia studies risk translating neuro-agnosticism into forms of complicity in the erosion of social support.

I argue that scholars who identify with dementia studies should promote more critical responses to the neuropsychiatric biopolitics of dementia and the political economy that it contributes to. However, given the current state of that political economy, critical engagement poses dangers for dementia research and people affected by dementia, particularly if the house of cards abruptly comes down. The political economy of dementia is problematic, but it has resulted in real material gains for dementia research that we might partially seek to transform rather than do away with. In practice, withdrawn investment would simply equate to unemployed researchers. It would do little for people affected by dementia other than shutting down the few opportunities that the dementia research economy does offer them for involvement. We do not necessarily want to create conditions for further disinvestment without corresponding reinvestment. This is especially true given that the financialisaton of the dementia economy makes it more vulnerable to boom-and-bust cycles and therefore risks finding itself suddenly impoverished.

Here, the critical commitment to political transformation becomes especially pressing. An escape route out of the neuropsychiatric biopolitics of dementia, and the creation of a political economy more conducive to the well-being of people affected by dementia, needs to be carefully traced out and enacted if we are to minimise detrimental fallout and seek progress for as many stakeholders as possible. To this end, a critical dementia studies might rearticulate friendliness as robust social support within which institutions play a significant role, guided most prominently by the interests of people affected by dementia. Rather than raising awareness about normal ageing and the prospects of curative technologies, those same dementia studies efforts could instead raise awareness about the political economic constitution of the problems experienced by people affected by dementia and promote promissory visions of future political economies that address those problems. I am evidently not speaking to all dementia studies scholars here. Many are already doing this work, but too many are not, and they need to be brought on side. Ultimately, a critical dementia studies can only realise its full transformative potential when it coherently shows that another political economy of dementia is desirable, attainable and, better yet, perhaps even inevitable.

Notes

1 Before contemporary classifications of dementia were popularised, people with dementia would have typically been contained within these two categories in statistics.
2 The UK dedicated its presidency to promoting social enterprise generally.
3 "Shorting" entails borrowing a stock that you suspect will soon lose value, selling it at its current high price, buying it back at its lower future price, returning the original stock and keeping the difference. Hostile investors can "short squeeze" these short positions by buying that stock, keeping its value high. The original short sellers abandon their positions to limit their losses, and in doing so, further increase the value of the stock that the short squeezers have acquired.

References

1. SCIE (2020). Dementia: At a glance. *Social Care Institute for Excellence*. https://www.scie.org.uk/dementia/about/.
2. Wittenberg, R., Hu, B., Barraza-Araiza, L., and Rehill, A. (2019). Projections of Older People with Dementia and Costs of Dementia Care in the United Kingdom, 2019–2040. London School of Economics and Political Science.
3. Alzheimer's Society (2022). Facts for the media. Alzheimer's Society. https://www.alzheimers.org.uk/about-us/news-and-media/facts-media.
4. Mah, J.C., Stevens, S.J., Keefe, J.M., Rockwood, K., and Andrew, M.K. (2021). Social factors influencing utilization of home care in community-dwelling older adults: A scoping review. *BMC Geriatrics 21*, 145. doi: 10.1186/s12877-021-02069-1.
5. Lewis, C., and Buffel, T. (2020). Aging in place and the places of aging: A longitudinal study. *Journal of Aging Studies 54*, 100870. doi: 10.1016/j.jaging.2020.100870.
6. Turner, T. (2004). The history of deinstitutionalization and reinstitutionalization. *Psychiatry 3*, 1–4. doi: 10.1383/psyt.3.9.1.50257.
7. Sinclair, I. (1988). *Residential Care the Research Reviewed: Literature Surveys Commissioned by the Independent Review of Residential Care*. HMSO.
8. Means, R., Richards, S., and Smith, R. (2008). *Community Care: Policy and Practice*. Palgrave.
9. Taylor, B. (2011). The demise of the asylum in late twentieth-century Britain: A personal history. *Transactions of the Royal Historical Society 21*, 193–215.
10. Rose, S.M. (1987). Deinstitutionalization — A structurally generated opportunity for social work. *International Social Work 30*, 251–257. doi: 10.1177/002087288703000305.
11. Goldman, H.H., Adams, N.H., and Taube, C.A. (1983). Deinstitutionalization: The data demythologized. *Psychiatric Services 34*, 129–134. doi: 10.1176/ps.34.2.129.
12. Bachrach, L.L. (1983). Concepts and issues in deinstitutionalization. In: Barofsky and R. D. Budson (eds.), *The Chronic Psychiatric Patient in the*

Community: Principles of Treatment, I. Springer Netherlands, pp. 5–28. doi: 10.1007/978-94-011-6308-8_1.

13. Scull, A. (2021). UK deinstitutionalisation: Neoliberal values and mental health. In: G. Ikkos and N. Bouras (eds.), *Mind, State and Society: Social History of Psychiatry and Mental Health in Britain 1960–2010*. Cambridge University Press, pp. 306–314. doi: 10.1017/9781911623793.033.

14. The King's Fund (2021). NHS hospital bed numbers. The King's Fund. https://www.kingsfund.org.uk/publications/nhs-hospital-bed-numbers.

15. Green, B.H., and Griffiths, E.C. (2014). Hospital admission and community treatment of mental disorders in England from 1998 to 2012. *General Hospital Psychiatry 36*, 442–448. doi: 10.1016/j.genhosppsych.2014.02.006.

16. NHS (2022). Statistics taBed Availability and Occupancy Data – Overnight. National Health Service. https://www.england.nhs.uk/statistics/statistical-work-areas/bed-availability-and-occupancy/bed-data-overnight/.

17. Ewbank, L., Thompson, J., McKenna, H., Anandaciva, S., and Ward, D. (2021). NHS hospital bed numbers. The King's Fund. https://www.kingsfund.org.uk/publications/nhs-hospital-bed-numbers.

18. Macdonald, A., and Cooper, B. (2007). Long-term care and dementia services: An impending crisis. *Age and Ageing 36*, 16–22. doi: 10.1093/ageing/afl126.

19. Bartlett, H.P., and Phillips, D.R. (1996). Policy issues in the private health sector: Examples from long-term care in the U.K. *Social Science & Medicine 43*, 731–737. doi: 10.1016/0277-9536(96)00117-7.

20. Netten, A., Williams, J., and Darton, R. (2005). Care-home closures in England: Causes and implications. *Ageing & Society 25*, 319–338. doi: 10.1017/S0144686X04002910.

21. The King's Fund (2022). Social care 360: Providers. The King's Fund. https://www.kingsfund.org.uk/publications/social-care-360/providers.

22. Grant Thornton UK (2018). *Care Homes for the Elderly: Where Are We Now?*

23. Audit Commission (1986). *Making a Reality of Community Care: A Report by the Audit Commission*. Audit Commission.

24. Hudson, B. (2016). *The Failure of Privatised Adult Social Care in England: What is to be Done?* Centre for Health & Public Interest.

25. The King's Fund (2022). Social care 360: Expenditure. The King's Fund. https://www.kingsfund.org.uk/publications/social-care-360/expenditure.

26. Preston, R. (2021). Local authorities delivering social care facing £2.1bn black hole. *Community Care*. https://www.communitycare.co.uk/2021/08/27/local-authorities-delivering-social-care-facing-2-1bn-black-hole/.

27. National Care Forum (2022). Just grim, difficult and relentless. National Care Forum. https://www.nationalcareforum.org.uk/ncf-press-releases/just-grim-difficult-and-relentless/.

28. The King's Fund (2022). Social care 360: Workforce and carers. The King's Fund. https://www.kingsfund.org.uk/publications/social-care-360/workforce-and-carers.

29. Carter, R. (2019). Service users left isolated as councils fail to meet eligible social support needs, say social workers. *Community Care*. https://www.communitycare.co.uk/2019/05/29/service-users-left-isolated-councils-fail-meet-eligible-social-support-needs-say-social-workers/.

30. The King's Fund (2022). Social care 360: Access. The King's Fund. https://www.kingsfund.org.uk/publications/social-care-360/access.

31. Wenzel, L., Bennett, L., Bottery, S., Murray, R., and Sahib, B. (2018). Approaches to social care funding. The King's Fund. https://www.kingsfund .org.uk/publications/approaches-social-care-funding.
32. Alzheimer's Society (2021). How much does dementia care cost? Alzheimer's Society. https://www.alzheimers.org.uk/blog/how-much-does-dementia-care -cost.
33. Harding, R. (2017). *Duties to Care: Dementia, Relationality and Law.* Cambridge University Press.
34. Leitner, S. (2014). Varieties of familialism: Developing care policies in conservative welfare states. In: P. Sandermann (ed.), *The End of Welfare as We Know It? Continuity and Change in Western Welfare State Settings and Practices.* Verlag Barbara Budrich, pp. 37–52. doi: 10.3224/84740075.
35. Le Bihan, B., Da Roit, B., and Sopadzhiyan, A. (2019). The turn to optional familialism through the market: Long-term care, cash-for-care, and caregiving policies in Europe. *Social Policy & Administration 53*, 579–595. doi: 10.1111/ spol.12505.
36. Wimo, A., Reed, C.C., Dodel, R., Belger, M., Jones, R.W., Happich, M., Argimon, J.M., Bruno, G., Novick, D., Vellas, B., et al. (2013). The GERAS Study: A prospective observational study of costs and resource use in community dwellers with Alzheimer's disease in three European countries--Study design and baseline findings. *Journal of Alzheimer's disease: JAD 36*, 385–399. doi: 10.3233/JAD-122392.
37. Bamford, S.-M., and Walker, T. (2012). Women and dementia – Not forgotten. *Maturitas 73*, 121–126. doi: 10.1016/j.maturitas.2012.06.013.
38. Erol, R., Brooker, D., and Peel, E. (2016). The impact of dementia on women internationally: An integrative review. *Health Care for Women International 37*, 1320–1341. doi: 10.1080/07399332.2016.1219357.
39. Williams, L.A., Giddings, L.S., Bellamy, G., and Gott, M. (2017). 'Because it's the wife who has to look after the man': A descriptive qualitative study of older women and the intersection of gender and the provision of family caregiving at the end of life. *Palliative Medicine 31*, 223–230. doi: 10.1177/0269216316653275.
40. Fletcher, J.R. (2021). Structuring unequal relations: Role trajectories in informal dementia care. *Sociology of Health & Illness 43*, 65–81. doi: 10.1111/1467-9566.13194.
41. Bartlett, R., Gjernes, T., Lotherington, A.-T., and Obstefelder, A. (2018). Gender, citizenship and dementia care: A scoping review of studies to inform policy and future research. *Health & Social Care in the Community 26*, 14–26. doi: 10.1111/hsc.12340.
42. Williams, B. (2019). The big society: Ten years on. *Political Insight 10*, 22–25. doi: 10.1177/2041905819891369.
43. Dowling, E., and Harvie, D. (2014). Harnessing the social: state, crisis and (big) society. *Sociology 48*, 869–886. doi: 10.1177/0038038514539060.
44. DoH (2012). Prime Minister's challenge on dementia. GOV.UK. https://www .gov.uk/government/publications/prime-ministers-challenge-on-dementia.
45. GOV.UK (2013). Alzheimer's society launches dementia friends information sessions. *GOV.UK.* https://www.gov.uk/government/news/alzheimer-s-society -launches-dementia-friends-information-sessions.
46. Parkin, E., and Baker, C. (2021). *Dementia: Policy, Services and Statistics.* House of Commons Library.

47. Oliver, M. (1990). *The Politics of Disablement*. Macmillan Education.

48. Fletcher, J.R. (2021). Unethical governance: Capacity legislation and the exclusion of people diagnosed with dementias from research. *Research Ethics 17*, 298–308. doi: 10.1177/1747016120982023.

49. Kitwood, T.M. (1997). *Dementia Reconsidered: The Person Comes First*. Open University Press.

50. Sabat, S.R. (2001). *The Experience of Alzheimer's Disease: Life Through a Tangled Veil*. Wiley.

51. Gan, D.R.Y., Chaudhury, H., Mann, J., and Wister, A.V. (2021). Dementia-friendly neighborhood and the built environment: A scoping review. *The Gerontologist*, gnab019. doi: 10.1093/geront/gnab019.

52. Joy, M. (2021). Neoliberal rationality and the age friendly cities and communities program: Reflections on the Toronto case. *Cities 108*, 102982. doi: 10.1016/j.cities.2020.102982.

53. Conservative Party Manifesto 2019 (2019). https://www.conservatives.com/our-plan/conservative-party-manifesto-2019.

54. Pickett, J., Bird, C., Ballard, C., Banerjee, S., Brayne, C., Cowan, K., Clare, L., Comas-Herrera, A., Corner, L., Daley, S., et al. (2018). A roadmap to advance dementia research in prevention, diagnosis, intervention, and care by 2025. *International Journal of Geriatric Psychiatry 33*, 900–906. doi: 10.1002/gps.4868.

55. Dementia Discovery Fund (2022). https://svhealthinvestors.com/funds/the-dementia-discovery-fund.

56. WDC (2022). About us. World Dementia Council. https://worlddementiacouncil.org/about-us.

57. UK DRI (2021). About us. UK Dementia Research Institute. https://ukdri.ac.uk/about-us.

58. Lalli, G., Rossor, M., Rowe, J.B., and Strooper, B.D. (2021). The Dementia UK Ecosystem: A call to action. *The Lancet Neurology 20*, 699–700. doi: 10.1016/S1474-4422(21)00246-5.

59. UK DRI (2022). Dementia UK Ecosystem: Action through alliance. UK Dementia Research Institute. https://ukdri.ac.uk/news-and-events/dementia-ecosystem-uk-action-through-alliance.

60. APPG (2021). Fuelling the Moonshot: Unleashing the UK's potential through dementia research. Alzheimer's Society. https://www.alzheimers.org.uk/sites/default/files/2021-09/Fuelling_Moonshot_APPG.pdf.

61. GOV.UK (2022). Prime Minister launches "Dame Barbara Windsor Dementia Mission." GOV.UK. https://www.gov.uk/government/news/prime-minister-launches-dame-barbara-windsor-dementia-mission--2.

62. Brown, N., and Michael, M. (2003). A sociology of expectations: Retrospecting prospects and prospecting retrospects. *Technology Analysis & Strategic Management 15*, 3–18. doi: 10.1080/0953732032000046024.

63. Brown, N. (2003). Hope against hype - Accountability in biopasts, presents and futures. *Science & Technology Studies 16*, 3–21. doi: 10.23987/sts.55152.

64. Jaeger, J. (2022). The Cassava Sciences saga: Short sellers, 'gaming' the FDA, and the damaging ripple effects. *Compliance Week*. https://www.complianceweek.com/risk-management/the-cassava-sciences-saga-short-sellers-gaming-the-fda-and-the-damaging-ripple-effects/31416.article.

65. Taylor, K. (2016). *The Fragile Brain: The Strange, Hopeful Science of Dementia*. Oxford University Press.
66. ARUK (n.d.). #ShareTheOrange. Alzheimer's Research UK. https://www.alz heimersresearchuk.org/orange/.
67. Pitts-Taylor, V. (2010). The plastic brain: Neoliberalism and the neuronal self. *Health 14*, 635–652. doi: 10.1177/1363459309360796.
68. Spencer, B. (2022). Tories drop vow to double dementia funding. *The Sunday Times*. https://www.thetimes.co.uk/article/tories-drop-vow-to-double-dementia -funding-56mgvjs2w.
69. Pinches, F. (2022). UK Government pledges to deliver 'Dementia Moonshot' and fast-track the development of new treatments. Alzheimer's Research UK. https://www.alzheimersresearchuk.org/uk-government-pledges-to-deliver -dementia-moonshot/.
70. Fletcher, J.R., and Maddock, C. (2021). Dissonant dementia: Neuropsychiatry, awareness, and contradictions in cognitive decline. *Humanities and Social Sciences Communications 8*, 1–11. doi: 10.1057/s41599-021-01004-4.
71. Minkler, M. (1996). Critical perspectives on ageing: New challenges for gerontology. *Ageing & Society 16*, 467–487. doi: 10.1017/S0144686X00003639.
72. Estes, C.L. (2001). *Social Policy and Aging: A Critical Perspective*. SAGE.
73. CHPI (2019). Plugging the leaks in the UK care home industry – Strategies for resolving the financial crisis in the residential and nursing home sector. Centre for Health and the Public Interest.
74. Lovelace, B. (2020). Biogen's stock jumps 42% after FDA staff says it has enough data to support approving Alzheimer's drug. CNBC. https://www.cnbc .com/2020/11/04/biogens-stock-jumps-30percent-after-fda-says-it-has -enough-data-to-support-approving-alzheimers-drug-.html.
75. Philippidis, A. (2022). StockWatch: Biogen shares rebound as Alzheimer's drug aces phase III trial. *GEN Edge 4*, 728–732. doi: 10.1089/genedge.4.1.119.
76. Strauss, D. (2019). Biogen surges 42% after stunning reversal sees it revive plans for Alzheimer's treatment. Markets Insider. https://markets.businessinsider.com /news/stocks/biogen-stock-price-soars-on-plan-to-revive-alzheimers-treatment -2019-10-1028619410.
77. Fletcher, J.R. (2021). Chronological quarantine and ageism: COVID-19 and gerontology's relationship with age categorisation. *Ageing & Society 41*, 479–492. doi: 10.1017/S0144686X20001324.
78. Joy, M. (2021). Neoliberal rationality and the age friendly cities and communities program: Reflections on the Toronto case. *Cities 108*, 102982. doi: 10.1016/j. cities.2020.102982.
79. Joy, M. (2018). Problematizing the age friendly cities and communities program in Toronto. *Journal of Aging Studies 47*, 49–56. doi: 10.1016/j.jaging.2018.10.005.
80. Hansen, T.E.A., Praestegaard, J., Tjørnhøj-Thomsen, T., Andresen, M., and Nørgaard, B. (2022). Dementia-friendliness in Danish and international contexts: A critical discourse analysis. *The Gerontologist 62*, 130–141. doi: 10.1093/geront/gnab056.
81. Hebert, C.A., and Scales, K. (2019). Dementia friendly initiatives: A state of the science review. *Dementia 18*, 1858–1895. doi: 10.1177/1471301217731433.
82. Harris, P.B., and Caporella, C.A. (2019). Making a university community more dementia friendly through participation in an intergenerational choir. *Dementia 18*, 2556–2575. doi: 10.1177/1471301217752209.

83. Mathie, E., Antony, A., Killett, A., Darlington, N., Buckner, S., Lafortune, L., Mayrhofer, A., Dickinson, A., Woodward, M., and Goodman, C. (2022). Dementia-friendly communities: The involvement of people living with dementia. *Dementia*, 14713012211073200. doi: 10.1177/14713012211073200.

84. Darlington, N., Arthur, A., Woodward, M., Buckner, S., Killett, A., Lafortune, L., Mathie, E., Mayrhofer, A., Thurman, J., and Goodman, C. (2021). A survey of the experience of living with dementia in a dementia-friendly community. *Dementia 20*, 1711–1722. doi: 10.1177/1471301220965552.

85. Verbakel, E. (2018). How to understand informal caregiving patterns in Europe? The role of formal long-term care provisions and family care norms. *Scandinavian Journal of Public Health 46*, 436–447. doi: 10.1177/1403494817726197.

86. Lyman, K.A. (1989). Bringing the Social Back in: A Critique of the Biomedicalization of Dementia1. *The Gerontologist 29*, 597–605. doi: 10.1093/geront/29.5.597.

87. Wong, G., and Knapp, M. (2020). Should we move dementia research funding from a cure to its care? *Expert Review of Neurotherapeutics 20*, 303–305. doi: 10.1080/14737175.2020.1735364.

9 Conclusion

Promissory Sociopolitical Histories

In this concluding chapter, I bring together the various issues covered throughout the book to argue that a lack of robust critical engagement with the neuropsychiatric biopolitics of dementia lies at their centre. I begin by briefly summarising the story that I have told throughout the book as a whole. This begins with the remarkable rise of dementia research under the influence of the neuropsychiatric biopolitics of dementia and culminates in a contemporary political economy of dementia characterised by evaporating support and proliferating capital accumulation. My overall argument is that a more neurocritical dementia studies – by which I mean a dementia studies that is informed by the core premises of critical gerontology and critical psychiatry[1] as two fields that have resonant heritages of resisting similar biopolitics, is more robustly engaged with claims relating to ageing and cognition, and is more forthright in pinpointing biopolitical commitments – is uniquely positioned to resist problematic aspects of the neuropsychiatric biopolitics of dementia and reformulate a more salutogenic political economy of dementia.

This may all sound somewhat nebulous and idealistic, so I do two things to tighten it up a little. First, I show how historic responses to dementia, both deliberate and accidental, can offer us some inspiring blueprints for developing a new sociopolitics of dementia. In particular, new epidemiological evidence regarding historic public health developments and their potential long-term implications shows that we might be able to make inroads into the incidence rates of dementia. I also point to historic research movements that developed contextualised psychosocial understandings of dementia and used those understandings to achieve meaningful political transformations for older people experiencing cognitive decline. Second, I attend more closely and pragmatically to the range of things that we can all do right now in pursuit of precisely what I suggest above: resisting problematic aspects of the neuropsychiatric biopolitics of dementia and reformulating a more salutogenic political economy of dementia.

* * *

DOI: 10.4324/9781003398523-9

I began this book with an account of the meteoric rise of contemporary dementia research from the late 1970s onward, noting how reconfigurations of ageing and disease helped American stakeholders to unleash the vast potential of AD as a political entity. On the one hand, we can interpret this as a heartening tale of substantial resources being dedicated to solving a major source of human distress. On the other hand, the 1970s was a long time ago, and it seems as though almost none of the headline aims of the AD movement have been met or are even close to being met for that matter. Dementia studies, a heterogeneous amalgam of social scientific and humanities scholarship and activity, is sometimes represented as having arisen in the 1990s as a response to dehumanising (bio)medicalisation and the nefarious (bio)medical model of dementia. However, this is a limiting interpretation of the wider biopolitical nature of the phenomena in question and the embeddedness of dementia studies within that biopolitics.

In response, I have argued that those of us who identify with dementia studies could fruitfully focus on the neuropsychiatric biopolitics of dementia. An attentiveness to biopolitics requires that we unpack the ways in which particular imaginaries of dementia permeate public consciousness so that publics self-govern their conduct according to corresponding normative commitments. This extends beyond traditional (bio)medicalisation. It is effectively a means of bringing a particular order to life itself, manifest in the (self) governance of our relations with our brains, our minds, and ultimately our selves. This biopolitics relies on an imaginary of dementia as:

A syndrome of cognitive decline caused by discrete neuropathologies that are distinct from ageing, and ... not enough people are aware of this. Furthermore, because dementia is caused by disease, and biomedical sciences have cured some diseases, dementia is a technoscientific challenge that will be solved through technoscientific endeavours.[1]

In particular, I argue that the neuropsychiatric biopolitics of dementia is defined by three core claims: (1) that dementias are caused by discrete diseases of the brain, (2) that dementia is not a normal part of ageing and (3) that research will discover a cure. These messages are proliferated by a coalition of neuropsychiatric stakeholders. Far from being the terrain of neurologists and psychiatrists per se, the key progenitors of neuropsychiatric biopolitics are often governments and politicians, charities, celebrities, biotech enterprises and the media.

The neuropsychiatric biopolitics of dementia that is reproduced by this coalition of stakeholders has fundamentally reconfigured dementia. Through the conceptual mechanics of circularity, dementia has been remade in reference to hypothetical neuropathologies, often irrespective of scientific evidence, to the extent that contemporary iterations of dementia can be entirely stripped of the cognitive characteristics that have traditionally demarcated most people's experiences of dementia. Aducanumab stripped cognition away entirely, and lecanemab and donanemab are now artistically opera-tionalising and advertising clinically meaningless cognitive effects with the aid of media,[2] charities[3] and politicians.[4] These new dementias have been materially realised in strange new forms, such as paralysed worms and bio-marked prodromal patients, and have even been successfully treated by sev-eral interventions, the most notable being aducanumab and lecanemab. In these machinations, we find dementia manifest as a biopolitical entity that is almost entirely divorced from the experiences of cognitive impairment and consequent dysfunction that animated people affected by dementia and dementia researchers alike before the 1970s.

Perched astride the perimeter of neuropsychiatric biopolitics, a lot of the dementia studies tradition can feel rather awkwardly positioned in relation to dementia generally. There are several examples of areas where dementia studies can be too neuro-agnostic, participating in neuropsychiatric biopoli-tics in a relatively uncritical manner and hence becoming complicit in it. I have sat through countless presentations at associated conferences which open with appeals to the economic gravity of dementia as a syndrome result-ing from brain disease as opposed to ageing. These are tempting introductory clichés that serve a particular biopolitics every time they are used. In this book, I have focused on stigma, ethnicity and friendliness as topics where a broad collection of uncritical dementia studies scholarship strays beyond neuro-agnostic complicity and becomes an actively explicit extension of neu-ropsychiatric biopolitics. These are rapidly proliferating areas of dementia studies work, and I would argue that they need to be swiftly redressed. More broadly, these issues speak to the deeper need for nurturing an alertness to the neuropsychiatric biopolitics of dementia and critically reconsidering our own relatedness to that biopolitics in many different forms.

The need to do so is pressing because neuropsychiatric biopolitics has occasioned, and is in many cases hastening, the generation of a political economy of dementia that is increasingly disaggregated from, and even con-trary to, the interests of many people affected by dementia. In the wake of the 2008 financial crisis, this political economy has intensified post-1970s trends toward lower social support and heightened personal responsibility in the interests of capital accumulation. Formal support has been reduced to pro-viding information so that it falls to families to orchestrate material support, especially unpaid lone female carers. At the same time, demographic alarm-ism has been reinvigorated as a new demographic dividend, making dementia into an alluring speculative opportunity, with potential consumable interven-tions offering momentous returns on investment, often irrespective of what we might consider successful endpoints. Public, private and third-sector insti-tutions have coalesced around friendliness and promissory technoscience, and a lot of dementia studies work, especially regarding stigma, ethnicity and friendliness, purposefully resonates with a big friendly society ideology. There is a lot of good intention here, but it risks contributing to darkening prospects for people affected by dementia in the present and the future. With this in mind, I argue that a neurocritical dementia studies must resist the neuropsychiatric biopolitics of dementia if we are to successfully respond to dementia as a problem and successfully meet the aims that have headlined the development of dementia research generally.

9.1 Promissory Histories

It is easy to feel downhearted when considering the contents of this book in the round. The problems that we face are simultaneously hefty, pervasive and slippery. Indeed, I am relatively pessimistic about the prospects of the dementia economy and its repercussions for people affected by dementia, both today and far into the future. Nonetheless, I would argue that this is more of a motivation for trying harder than for giving up. As we approach the end of this book, I think it is important to highlight some reasons to be hopeful, alongside practical strategies through which dementia studies as a collective force and the individuals within it can push for improvements.

In this book, I have written at length about futures, and manipulations thereof, as being essential to shaping our presents. They make speculative futures more likely by catalysing capital and shutting down alternatives. However, our present dispositions toward the future are also responsive to deficit. If we simply cannot envisage a way out, then we are more likely to reconcile ourselves to our present conditions. The political scientist Barbara Prainsack has articulated this capacity for non-imagination to dictate the present:

> The absence of visions about what an alternative, better, future should look like creates facts on the ground. It makes us accept the status quo, or the supposedly "natural" course of things, as a given, and it makes us put up with its negative effects. In the worst case, it natural-ises specific distributions of power and agency, and suggests that these are beyond our control.[5]

With this in mind, it is vital that a neurocritical dementia studies does not simply pursue critique without construction in the sort of finger-wagging manner that critical scholars can inadvertently slide toward. We certainly want to avoid creating a vacuum of hope, exacerbating feelings of future-lessness that can so easily provoke anxiety and disaffection.[6] Hence, our critique must be matched with our own promissory sociopolitics, manifesting the same aesthetic of hopefulness that saturates the neuropsychiatric biopoli-tics of "research will discover a cure". Fortunately, I see two major reasons why our hopefulness can be firmly justified.

The first reason to be hopeful is that epidemiology is currently suggesting new strategies for responding to dementia in a genuinely substantial man-ner. It has become apparent over recent years that, while absolute numbers continue to rise amidst population ageing, age-specific dementia incidence has been in decline for over a decade (and perhaps two decades) in several high-income countries.[7–10] It is generally believed that this is due to a range of post-war transformations relating to public health in the mid-20th century. Improvements in areas such as education, housing, living standards, health-care access and nutrition may have collectively contributed to political econo-mies that were more conducive to cognitive health.[11] The people who lived through these post-war improvements are now arriving at the high-risk ages for dementia, so declining incidence today partially reflects political determi-nants in the mid-20th century. While our contemporary drug pipeline falters, it turns out that we might have a wider range of partial anti-dementia inter-ventions at our disposal and that our ancestors were already implementing some of those strategies 70 years ago. Well done them. Not so well done us.

Today, despite a greatly expanded focus on addressing dementia, we find ourselves beset by the erosion of salutogenic political determinants. The political economy of dementia that I characterised in the previous chapter is ultimately a small-scale manifestation of the larger phenomena that have come to shape our contemporary political economy more generally. Lower collective social support, greater reliance on personal luck and an emphasis on private capital accumulation are not unique to the world of dementia. There are many particular ways in which this political economy has impacted and is still impacting factors that we know are pivotal to future dementia rates. For example, children have missed years of school due to political responses to COVID, particularly in the poorest families who lack access to digital technologies. A report in 2022 by UNICEF, UNESCO and the World Bank found that COVID policies resulted in a global increase in illiteracy among 10-year-olds from 53% to 70%.[12] In the UK, food bank use has increased from under 26,000 people in 2008–2009 to over 2.5 million in 2020–2021, as millions struggle to access nutrition.[13] There is also growing healthcare inaccessibility as waiting lists increase and a greater range of services are privatised. As an example, in recent years, it has become increasingly difficult to have ear wax removed on the NHS, with most people now having to pay a private clinic for the service, contradicting NICE guidance.[14] Similarly, NHS dentistry is now hard to come by. A 2022 survey revealed that 90% of dentists were not accepting NHS patients, with whole regions becoming "dentistry deserts" and members of the public performing DIY dentistry, including removing their own teeth.[15] Both hearing impairment[16–18] and bad oral hygiene[19, 20] are risk factors for dementia, so by ignoring them today, we may be contributing to future dementias.

I have written a lot in this book about the ways in which promissory futures of dementia have immediate material consequences and are there-fore influencing our present. It is important to recognise that, through the political decisions highlighted above, our present is simultaneously dictating the future of dementia. Of course, some long-term effects are almost impos-sible to predict with confidence. But some are relatively straightforward. Decreased access to education and healthcare almost certainly means that some people alive today will go on to develop more pronounced cognitive impairments than they would otherwise have experienced. Mid-20th-century political and economic transformations likely set the scene for declining dementia incidence in the early 21st century. Early 21st-century transformations are similarly constraining the incidence rates of the late 21st century. If the contemporary epidemiological evidence is reliable (and while it certainly looks convincing, this remains a big "if"), then our present political economy is likely already driving some increases in dementia incidence and severity in our future.

This observation is a poignant reminder of the manner in which our contemporary political economy of dementia can disaggregate the efficacy and successfulness of anti-dementia interventions, particularly when those interventions are (un)conducive to other political and economic interests. As I outlined in Chapter 5, aducanumab has shown us that an intervention does not need to be clinically effective to be successful. Contemporary backward steps regarding public cognitive health show us that effective interventions will not necessarily be successfully pursued and implemented. Hence, our political economy of dementia not only answers to interests beyond simply addressing dementia, but it can also place greater emphasis on those additional interests, pursuing them even when they are at odds with addressing dementia. This is a core contention of a neurocritical dementia studies – the neuropsychiatric biopolitics of dementia is not inherently concordant with medicine or science and can often be at odds with them, particularly when beholden to opposing financial and moral interests.

There are, however, serious attempts to learn from the observation that historic public health circumstances have some potential to shape contemporary dementia incidence. These efforts are primarily concentrated in a prevention agenda of epidemiological scholarship that has developed rapidly over the past decade. This effort has been spearheaded by the publication of two special Lancet Commission Reports in 2017[21] and 2020[22] led by professor of psychiatry Gill Livingston. These reports stratified dementia risk percentages according to specific risk factors. The more recent report attributed 40% of contemporary dementia prevalence to the following modifiable risk factors: poor education (7%), hearing loss (8%), traumatic brain injury (3%), hypertension (2%), alcohol (1%), obesity (1%), smoking (5%), depression (4%), isolation (4%), inactivity (2%), pollution (2%) and diabetes (1%). Predictably, the headline claim that 40% of dementia was potentially preventable translated into a plethora of media headlines regarding the need for people to change their lifestyles today to reduce their dementia risk.[23–25] There is evidently some attempt to conjure a more public health-focused approach here, but from a critical perspective, this type of depoliticised DIY public health messaging is unlikely to be a positive strategy for dementia intervention.

The flourishing prevention agenda is, on the one hand, well-intentioned and grounded in a reasonable epidemiological evidence base (at least by the standards of neuropsychiatric biopolitics). On the other hand, there is at best a political naivety to a lot of these endeavours, if not outright complicity in the very processes that are contributing to pathogenic determinants of dementia. Indeed, some of the concurrent scholarship manifests attributes of an uncritical dementia studies that I argue against. The misrepresentation of public health as a matter of personal lifestyle choice can easily distract us from paying attention to the social determinants of health as structural problems with structural solutions. This is a matter of interpretation as much as it is a matter of embracing the existing evidence base regarding things that appear to have worked in recent history. 20th-century gains regarding 21st-century dementia did not come about because proactive individuals made post-war resolutions to be less depressed and hit their heads less often. Those gains emerged, organically and unwittingly, as a happy accident of political economic phenomena far beyond the personal willpower of the individuals who have subsequently benefitted. Rather than trying to force the lessons of epidemiology to fit an ill-suited self-help fetish, we could send children to decent schools away from busy roads and provide them with nutritious meals (perhaps via some form of "moonshot").

As well as guarding against simplistically autonomous misunderstandings of public health – e.g. in terms of an individual quitting smoking and eating kale – it is also important that the prospects for well-designed and well-implemented public health approaches to dementia are not sensationalised. Of course, 40% fewer cases of dementia by the late 21st century would be a fantastic result, but that does mean that 100% of cases will remain in the present and 60% of cases will remain in the distant future, even assuming that interventions are fully effective. It is also important to take the 40% claim with a large pinch of salt. This epidemiological work is relatively recent and will undoubtedly be subject to considerable revision over the next decade. Establishing causality is essentially impossible, and headline stats are, to some extent, arbitrary. Long-term percentage reduction via political economy, however fruitful that could be, is ultimately a far cry from the immediate eradication of dementia that is espoused by promissory technoscience. Advocates of preventative approaches are rightly critiqued for overplaying their prospects. If we stopped all pollution, depression, hearing loss, etc., tomorrow, we would still not abolish dementia per se, far from it. Indeed, one result of this would be that more people would live longer, which could even push prevalence in the opposite direction, given the age-associated nature of dementia.

An openness to the limits of such approaches is itself important. The message here is not some irresponsible "we will beat dementia" hype, but rather a pragmatic one of less dementia, less severe dementia, and less impairing dementia, which is better dealt with when it does occur. Ultimately, post-war political economies may have reduced incidence, but they could also offer a better way of responding, via robust social support systems, to the cognitive decline that will inevitably still characterise many people's later lives. We could have our cake and eat it, with political economies that simultaneously lower incidence and improve experiences of the dementias that are left over. Political transformations could target societies that not only lessen dementia but are also better equipped for those dementias that will inevitably still occur. Win–win, albeit by degrees. This is the realistic promise of a future political economy of dementia, if we so choose – a world with lower age-specific dementia incidence and where the dementia that does occur is responded to with rigorous and reliable support. It is no utopia, but it is preferable to our contemporary circumstances. More importantly, it is feasible and likely to be somewhat effective based on available evidence.

The core idea here is not only of dementia being in context but dementia being of context. This is not a new approach by any means. In the mid-20th century, before the NIA made Katzman's de-aged AD a household name and far before Kitwood centred in on relationships, overlapping American traditions of social psychiatry and social gerontology developed psychosocial understandings of dementia as mental deterioration bound up with societal contexts of ageing. Scholars were alert to the growing numbers of older people labelled as senile and/or insane, alongside the already well-known discrepancies between neurophysiology and cognitive impairment. Based on these observations, they concluded that dementia would become a substantial social problem if governments did not implement policy programmes dedicated to later-life well-being. These programmes would need to bolster healthcare access, financial stability and intergenerational cohesion in rapidly modernising environments.[26, 27]

Though operating under the monikers of social psychiatry and social gerontology, we might readily interpret these arguments as fundamentally critical in nature. Breaking away from the early 20th-century European psychiatry of Alzheimer and Kraepelin, these scholars were alert to the ways in which dementia was socio-politically constituted and the concerning direction of travel.[28] With this in mind, they deconstructed the normative commitments at stake in contemporary approaches to dementia and responded by advocating for political transformation as a means of addressing the problem.[29] They were somewhat successful in doing so. In the 1960s, their work informed the development of programmes such as Medicare and the Older Americans Act, expanding healthcare coverage and a range of social services to at-risk older people.[30] The advent of the neuropsychiatric biopolitics of dementia in the late 1970s, coinciding with the decline of activist government, undermined these fledgling forms of critical thinking on dementia as it rapidly became the predominant institutional and public approach to understanding cognitive decline in later life. Nonetheless, we did it once, and we can do it again.

We might ask what these two things have in common: (1) contemporary epidemiological evidence regarding post-war political economies that have proved protective against dementia and (2) mid-20th-century social psychiatric and social gerontological work on dementia as a psycho-socio-political problem requiring public reform. The answer is that both of these phenomena offer a type of promissory history. By this, I mean that we can echo the promissory strategies that typify contemporary technoscience – i.e. making futures more certain by appealing to the inevitability of scientific advance – by similarly appealing to real historic developments as firm evidence for our own futures. What this promissory history lacks when compared with the emotive appeal of promissory technoscience, it makes up for in its basis in reality. These things happened relatively recently and are entirely within our technical capabilities. If nothing else, a neurocritical dementia studies can take heart from these histories. Despite the pessimism I attested to at the beginning of this section, from a certain perspective, dementia is something that we are already sufficiently equipped to meaningfully respond to in a range of ways that can effectively improve the lives of those affected.

9.2 Neurocritical Dementia Studies

This text is not meant to be a grand treaty advocating momentous societal change. My intention is to coax those who identify with dementia studies into adopting a more neurocritical stance. Yet that aim remains a little vague and expansive, so as I draw to a close and attempt to summarise, I want to attend more practically to the things that we can do to move the dial, even if only by a little. You might ask, why focus on dementia studies at all? It may seem a little unfair to lay problems at the door of a loose collection of heterogeneous ideas and practices that has so often strove to resist these types of problems. I focus on dementia studies specifically because I believe that it, or more specifically, *we*, have a particular power (and perhaps a particular responsibility) as an unusual group of biopolitics-adjacent stakeholders. That is, in the real world, it is nigh on impossible to professionally engage with dementia and not be somehow affected by its biopolitical gravity. We have one foot in the tent, in terms of the indebtedness of our very existence, as people who speak to something called "dementia", to that biopolitics. We have one foot outside the tent, in terms of our rich heritage of examining and resisting the political constitution of problematic experiences of dementia in many different forms. Rather than decrying systems and advocating vague political change, I want to zero in on what I would like to cultivate as strands of thought and action that can intersect a wide array of dementia studies. I would personally frame this as a form of solidarity with people affected by dementia, which is ultimately what I believe dementia studies is and should be.

What to do? First, our personal politics can be decidedly anti-dementia. In light of contemporary epidemiological evidence regarding the political economic determinants of dementia, it is reasonably straightforward to vote for parties with anti-dementia policies and to participate in action that seeks to further those policies. First and foremost are policies to widen access to education and healthcare. If public policy gets those two things right, it will be making dents in future dementia incidence. Then there are concurrent policies relating to social support for carers and disabled and older people. Widening access (and access is not the same as availability) to real-world practical support services (by which I mean human and physical infrastructural support, not to be conflated with research funding or awareness raising) is not an absolute guarantee of success, but it is our best bet. Reasonably attainable; reasonably likely to be effective. Of course, we all quite rightly have many more political concerns than just dementia, but a "dementia-friendly" citizen has the above issues in mind when pursuing their own politics.

To support this approach to a more personal politics of dementia, it could be helpful to develop a dedicated dementia assessment of party manifestos going into each election and perhaps even related analyses of major policy changes as they are being developed. This could be produced and promoted by a broad coalition of critical dementia studies scholars and, crucially, people affected by dementia. Some organisations, e.g. Age Scotland,[31] have already begun to develop such manifestos, but it would be a mistake to leave such work to specific organisations given the influence of lobbying by different interest groups in the political economy of dementia. The simple existence of an up-to-date and accessible dementia manifesto could help to nurture a general appreciation of the status of dementia as a fundamentally political entity. Importantly, such an assessment must not naively conflate commitments to research funding with a commitment to improving the lives of people affected by dementia. This is one reason why the involvement of people affected by dementia in dementia studies is so important, because their interests will not always be neatly aligned with the interests of other dementia studies stakeholders.

At a more intimate level, we can do a better job of curating our content, be that presentations, publications or social media. We must be highly alert to the manner in which things like stigma, minoritised ethnic awareness, friendly communities, celebrity research appeals and various other enterprises that rely on and reproduce the neuropsychiatric biopolitics of dementia distract us from the things that we have solid scientific evidence about. Instrumentally, awareness raising can be a rewarding gravy train to ride, but the neurocritical dementia studies scholar must be aware of the biopolitics that it serves. Before spreading awareness that we think we have and others need, we should reflect on where our own awareness comes from and what makes it better than the awarenesses of others. This is especially true for those scholars demarcating minoritised ethnic groups as being uniquely in need of our attention. Regarding ethnicity, we could engage with people affected by dementia based on a foundational assumption that they have meaningful experiences that we can learn from rather than defining them as somehow problematic and seeking to change them. Frankly, to do otherwise, via rubrics of race and ethnicity, is racist.

In essence, this entire book is replete with cautionary tales and examples of things we can avoid doing as a means of nurturing forms of neurocriticality. Do not absentmindedly refer to "stigma" as a sort of vague catchall term for badness and/or ignorance. Do not assume that telling the public about brain diseases will mitigate that stigma. Do not reiterate the throwaway biopolitical claims that litter too many introductions and conclusions. Call out biopolitical claims. Refute them in reference to the scientific evidence base. Ask what "normal ageing" is. Ask why hallmark neuropathologies and cognitive impairment are not neatly correlated. Ask how many of the billions allocated to dementia research have directly benefitted people affected by dementia. Ask how their well-being has been materially enhanced by friendliness and oranges and moonshots. Ask what qualifies a study of worm proteins to be described as "dementia research". Ultimately, all of this micro-criticality can help to disaggregate the neuropsychiatric biopolitics of dementia as a normative project.

In arguing that the neuropsychiatric biopolitics of dementia is antithetical to *good* science, I am not naively championing science as an idyllic alternative to biopolitics, producing objective measurements of an immutable world. I am well aware of the many ways in which even "legitimate" science can be read as a form of politics in and of itself. The entire social studies of science discipline has developed around investigating the ways in which, just like any other aspect of human life, the production of scientific knowledge is an amalgam of messy practices, value judgements and political struggle. These observations refute simplistic imaginings of what science is, but they do not undermine science as an entity per se nor refute its value. Science, broadly conceived, has long enabled us to make sense of the world in deeply meaningful and useful ways. Science as a general concept can encapsulate a wonderous means of being in the world, combining the curiosity to understand and the conviction to enact change.

With this in mind, biopolitics is not inherently problematic because it is somehow a corruption of something called science that is otherwise pure. Science is biopolitics, and biopolitics is science. We define and study phenomena that matter to us in ways that we think will produce results that will matter and deftly leverage capital of various forms to suit those ends. There is a reason that dementia research is a far bigger field than pocket-fluff research. Dementia matters a lot to a lot of us. Rather than being bad because it is not science, the neuropsychiatric biopolitics of dementia can be viewed as being partially bad because it has some troubling features and repercussions, and a neurocritical dementia studies should attend to these. Science and medicine are not apolitical or value-neutral (though, of course, some like to pretend that they are), nor should they be. The neuropsychiatric biopolitics of dementia is not inherently problematic because it contradicts basic scientific evidence, clinical realities and the experiences of people affected by dementia (though it can be and is problematic for these reasons in various instances). It is more decidedly troublesome because it does these things in the interests of capital accumulation, too often at the expense of people affected by dementia. This is more a question of degrees than a neat good-science versus bad-biopolitics binary, but they are degrees that matter.

To be neurocritical is to recognise that various facets of dementia studies could benefit from more robust engagements with neuroscience, cognitive science, geriatric psychiatry and epidemiology. This would firstly enable us to better contest the neuropsychiatric biopolitics that manipulates science and medicine to achieve political ends. When a charity or politician pontificates about normal ageing, discrete neuropathologies and future cures, a neurocritical dementia studies could offer balancing arguments, not based on archaic and limited (bio)medicalisation critiques, but instead based on a weight of neurological, cognitive and epidemiological evidence that has too often been corrupted, if not flatly ignored by neuropsychiatric biopolitical stakeholders. That evidence may have various flaws, but it is the best we have. Crucially, that evidence can be made conducive to arguments for a neurocritical sociopolitics of dementia, centring on systemic support for both contemporary and future people affected by dementia. This is surely preferable to a neuropsychiatric biopolitics that results in a few stakeholders accruing capital at the expense of people affected by dementia. Hence, a neurocritical dementia studies should strive to expose the contradictions between the neuropsychiatric biopolitics of dementia and the wider social and natural sciences of ageing and cognition.

Just as I do not want to naively venerate science as a value-neutral apolitical pursuit, I do not want to suggest that dementia should be depoliticised, or at least that we should somehow pretend that dementia could ever be apolitical. In fact, quite the opposite. One of our most potent responses to the neuropsychiatric biopolitics of dementia should be to provide an alternative. To my mind, we are the best-placed group of stakeholders for charting a way out of the contemporary dementia quagmire. Critical dementia studies could develop a distinct sociopolitics of dementia. Indeed, it has already done so to a large extent, albeit in a piecemeal fashion and too often limited by historical concerns of (bio)medicalisation and dehumanisation, coupled with an agnosticism toward neuropsychiatric biopolitics. These issues matter greatly but also risk distracting from the bigger picture. Our challenge is principally to refine our heterogeneous work as a more coherent and explicitly resistive alternative to the neuropsychiatric biopolitics of dementia and the political economy of dementia that it supports. As discussed above, we can find significant inspiration in a type of promissory history revolving around post-war public health and mid-20th-century social psychiatry and social gerontology. It is attainable.

So far, I have outlined a range of strategies that, in my opinion, at least, are fairly easy to achieve. There is the simple act of reinforcing and spreading our alertness to the sociopolitical determination of dementia and articulating this more explicitly and coherently right across our diverse projects. We can advocate for anti-dementia political economies that are conducive to support in the present and hopefully to lower incidence in the future. We can avoid uncritically reiterating biopolitical claims regarding the nature of dementia and dementia research. We can reflect more critically on our uses of concepts such as stigma and awareness and the manner in which we position different groups of people in relation to those concepts and to dementia itself. We can overcome neuro-agnosticism by engaging more robustly with the relevant sciences, drawing on those engagements to challenge suspect biopolitics and strengthen realistic and positive promissory sociopolitics of dementia. We can learn from history to promote alternative promissory futures of dementia, echoing the hopefulness of promissory technoscience and bolstering it with a firmer evidence base.

Those things are relatively easy to commit to. More challenging is a critical reworking of the relationship between institutionalised dementia studies and the broader dementia economy. As I have repeatedly noted throughout this book, the development of dementia studies as an institutional entity is inseparable from the wider development of the political economy of dementia over recent decades, all flourishing under the influence of neuropsychiatric biopolitics. We need to recognise our embeddedness within a dementia economy that is too often set up to benefit certain stakeholders, including research institutions and, to varying extents, researchers themselves, more than people affected by dementia. A portion of our success is either directly or indirectly attributable to the neuropsychiatric biopolitics of dementia and the political economy of dementia that it supports. Much of what I have suggested above is a means of addressing the indirect relatedness of dementia studies and neuropsychiatric biopolitics, but our direct, especially financial, links to that biopolitics must also be subject to critical, and perhaps uncomfortable, scrutiny.

This critical effort must begin with the major dementia-related organisations that operate as middlemen between public funding and research programmes. It is tempting to cast the Alzheimer's Association as a leading villain in light of its questionable political and financial entanglements with Biogen and aducanumab,[32] not to mention other serious questions. However, the Alzheimer's Association is not unique in this respect. Let us not forget that former British prime minister David Cameron is the president of ARUK. He is the same man who oversaw deep retrenchments of social care provision,[33] worsening healthcare access,[34] increased child poverty[35] and huge food bank expansion.[36] In my view, as far as any one individual has likely contributed to increasing the future incidence of dementia, he is relatively uniquely positioned. Having done so, he quickly progressed to lobbying for funding for biopolitical advertising campaigns such as #ShareTheOrange and promissory technoscience enterprises more broadly. Hence, ARUK and its stakeholders should not get off the hook amidst more prominent criticism of the Alzheimer's Association.

In 2020, the Alzheimer's Society chief executive Jeremy Hughes stepped down from his role amidst controversies regarding staff bullying and related six-figure staff payoffs. This catalysed wider criticisms regarding the charity's broader trajectory through the 2010s, away from supporting people affected by dementia and toward friendliness and awareness as a more politically and

financially productive strategy. The Alzheimer's Society has recently partnered with the Football Association, which in recent years has found itself
under mounting public pressure regarding the links between football-related
brain injury and dementia. The partnership focuses on spreading awareness
and making football clubs dementia-friendly. A cynic might wonder whether
the FA has purchased friendliness from the Alzheimer's Society as a distrac-
tion from the substantial role that the organisation appears to play in causing dementia. These organisations undoubtedly do a great deal of good in
many different ways, but they are also key stakeholders in a murky political
economy of dementia that has some regrettable attributes.

A great deal of laudable dementia studies work is funded because of
campaigns such as #ShareTheOrange and Dementia Friends, or because of
partnerships with organisations like Biogen or the FA. We are by no means
distinct from or morally above the contemporary political economy of dementia. There are hence difficult questions to be asked about the nature of capital accrual in dementia studies specifically. Personally, I have so far avoided
dementia-related funding, being supported instead by broader social science
research grants. However, it is probably not feasible, nor expedient, to reac-
tively turn our backs on every problematic stakeholder. Moreover, I am not
a martyr. I have to earn a living the same as everyone else, and if it were a
choice between a dementia grant or unemployment, I would take the money.
To be clear, what I mean by this is that, in a precarious and largely well-
intentioned sector, researchers should not be personally blamed for receiving
funding that relies on the neuropsychiatric biopolitics of dementia. Hence,
while I think that we should reflect on our funding practices, I do not think
that dementia studies should automatically shun potentially ill-gotten investments. Instead, scholars might collectively work to reconfigure the relations
between dementia studies and funders who are firmly embedded within the
neuropsychiatric biopolitics of dementia. We should hold funders to account,
and funders should be receptive. That work begins with the forthright articulation of relevant concerns, which I have hopefully managed to achieve, at
least to some extent, herein.

* * *

As I have admitted above, I am pessimistic about the overall trajectory of
dementia as a biopolitical entity and the political economy that it nurtures.
I see a bad situation worsening. However, I think that it is important to
end on a positive note, for myself as much as anything else. The positive is
dementia studies. The field is far from perfect, but the fact that it exists at
all is a reason for hope. One of my greatest privileges has been teaching service providers about sociopolitical facets of dementia and seeing them grap-
ple with their preconceptions, especially when they return to tell me about
the positive ways in which they have adapted their practice, sometimes to
great effect. Moreover, every time I attend one of the many dementia studies

initiatives that are meaningfully including people affected by dementia, if not being run by them independently, I am reinvigorated by the sense in which we are collectively imposing a countercultural dementia on, and often in spite of, the world. This is good by itself, but how much more impressive is it that we have achieved so much while working within the wider context outlined in this book. We might be fighting the tide, but we are at least making waves.

Note

1 I limit myself to these two fields because they speak so directly to neuropsychiatric biopolitics and are relatively untapped, but critical dementia studies as a whole requires engagement with a far wider array of scholarships.

References

1. Fletcher, J.R., and Maddock, C. (2021). Dissonant dementia: Neuropsychiatry, awareness, and contradictions in cognitive decline. *Humanities and Social Sciences Communications 8*, 1–11. doi: 10.1057/s41599-021-01004-4.
2. Gregory, A. (2023). New Alzheimer's drug slows cognitive decline by 35%, trial results show. *The Guardian*. https://www.theguardian.com/society/2023/may/03/new-alzheimers-drug-slows-cognitive-decline-by-35-trial-results-show.
3. Alzheimer's Society (2023). Positive news today that breakthrough #alzheimers drug #donanemab slows the disease. @RichJamesOakley says this could be "the beginning of the end of Alzheimer's disease." Twitter. https://twitter.com/alzheimerssoc/status/1653723227988869121.
4. Cameron, D. (2023). Victory against dementia is within our grasp. *The Telegraph*. https://www.telegraph.co.uk/news/2023/05/04/victory-against-dementia-is-within-our-grasp/.
5. Prainsack, B. (2023). The Roots of Neglect: Towards a Sociology of Non-Imagination. *Tecnoscienza: Italian Journal of Science & Technology Studies 13*, 13–34.
6. Tutton, R. (2022). The Sociology of Futurelessness. *Sociology*, 00380385221122420. doi: 10.1177/00380385221122420.
7. Ahmadi-Abhari, S., Guzman-Castillo, M., Bandosz, P., Shipley, M.J., Muniz-Terrera, G., Singh-Manoux, A., Kivimäki, M., Steptoe, A., Capewell, S., O'Flaherty, M., et al. (2017). Temporal trend in dementia incidence since 2002 and projections for prevalence in England and Wales to 2040: Modelling study. *BMJ 358*, j2856. doi: 10.1136/bmj.j2856.
8. Grasset, L., Brayne, C., Joly, P., Jacqmin-Gadda, H., Peres, K., Foubert-Samier, A., Dartigues, J.-F., and Helmer, C. (2016). Trends in dementia incidence: Evolution over a 10-year period in France. *Alzheimer's & Dementia 12*, 272–280. doi: 10.1016/j.jalz.2015.11.001.
9. Sposato, L.A., Kapral, M.K., Fang, J., Gill, S.S., Hackam, D.G., Cipriano, L.E., and Hachinski, V. (2015). Declining incidence of stroke and dementia: Coincidence or prevention opportunity? *JAMA Neurology 72*, 1529–1531. doi: 10.1001/jamaneurol.2015.2816.
10. Taudorf, L., Nørgaard, A., Islamoska, S., Jørgensen, K., Laursen, T.M., and Waldemar, G. (2019). Declining incidence of dementia: A national registry-based

study over 20 years. *Alzheimer's & Dementia 15*, 1383–1391. doi: 10.1016/j. jalz.2019.07.006.

11. George, D.R., and Whitehouse, P.J. (2021). *American Dementia: Brain Health in an Unhealthy Society*. Johns Hopkins University Press.

12. The World Bank, UNESCO, and UNICEF (2021). The state of the global education crisis: A path to recovery. *The World Bank*. https://www.worldbank .org/en/topic/education/publication/the-state-of-the-global-education-crisis-a -path-to-recovery.

13. Clark, D. (2021). UK foodbank users 2021. *Statista*. https://www.statista.com/ statistics/382695/uk-foodbank-users/.

14. RNID (2022). Our ear wax removal campaign. Royal National Institute for Deaf People. https://rnid.org.uk/get-involved/campaign-with-us/ear-wax -removal-campaign/.

15. UK Parliament (2022). MPs to examine struggle to access NHS dentistry services. UK Parliament. https://committees.parliament.uk/committee/81/health -and-social-care-committee/news/175008/mps-to-examine-struggle-to-access -nhs-dentistry-services/.

16. Ford, A.H., Hankey, G.J., Yeap, B.B., Golledge, J., Flicker, L., and Almeida, O.P. (2018). Hearing loss and the risk of dementia in later life. *Maturitas 112*, 1–11. doi: 10.1016/j.maturitas.2018.03.004.

17. Thomson, R.S., Auduong, P., Miller, A.T., and Gurgel, R.K. (2017). Hearing loss as a risk factor for dementia: A systematic review. *Laryngoscope Investigative Otolaryngology 2*, 69–79. doi: 10.1002/lio2.65.

18. Yeo, B.S.Y., Song, H.J.J.M.D., Toh, E.M.S., Ng, L.S., Ho, C.S.H., Ho, R., Merchant, R.A., Tan, B.K.J., and Loh, W.S. (2023). Association of hearing aids and cochlear implants with cognitive decline and dementia: A systematic review and meta- analysis. *JAMA Neurology 80*, 134–141. doi: 10.1001/jamaneurol.2022.4427.

19. Noble, J.M., Scarmeas, N., and Papapanou, P.N. (2013). Poor oral health as a chronic, potentially modifiable dementia risk factor: Review of the literature. *Current Neurology and Neuroscience Reports 13*, 384. doi: 10.1007/ s11910-013-0384-x.

20. Daly, B., Thompsell, A., Sharpling, J., Rooney, Y.M., Hillman, L., Wanyonyi, K.L., White, S., and Gallagher, J.E. (2017). Evidence summary: The relationship between oral health and dementia. *British Dental Journal 223*, 846–853. doi: 10.1038/sj.bdj.2017.992.

21. Livingston, G., Sommerlad, A., Orgeta, V., Costafreda, S.G., Huntley, J., Ames, D., Ballard, C., Banerjee, S., Burns, A., Cohen-Mansfield, J., et al. (2017). Dementia prevention, intervention, and care. *The Lancet 390*, 2673–2734. doi: 10.1016/S0140-6736(17)31363-6.

22. Livingston, G., Huntley, J., Sommerlad, A., Ames, D., Ballard, C., Banerjee, S., Brayne, C., Burns, A., Cohen-Mansfield, J., Cooper, C., et al. (2020). Dementia prevention, intervention, and care: 2020 report of the Lancet Commission. *The Lancet 396*, 413–446. doi: 10.1016/S0140-6736(20)30367-6.

23. Davis, N. (2020). Lifestyle changes could delay or prevent 40% of dementia cases – Study. *The Guardian*. https://www.theguardian.com/society/2020/jul/30 /lifestyle-changes-could-delay-or-prevent-40-of-dementia-cases-study.

24. Klein, A. (2020). These are the 12 ways you can drastically cut your dementia risk. *New Scientist*. https://www.newscientist.com/article/2250401-these-are -the-12-ways-you-can-drastically-cut-your-dementia-risk/.

25. University of Southern California - Health Sciences Forty percent of dementia cases could be prevented or delayed by targeting 12 risk factors throughout life. *ScienceDaily.* https://www.sciencedaily.com/releases/2020/07/200730123651.htm.

26. Ballenger, J.F. (2017). Framing confusion: Dementia, society, and history. *AMA Journal of Ethics 19*, 713–719. doi: 10.1001/journalofethics.2017.19.7.mhst1-1707.

27. Burch, S., and Longmore, P.K. (2009). *Encyclopedia of American Disability History.* Facts on File.

28. Ballenger, J. (2000). Beyond the characteristic plaques and tangles: Mid-twentieth century US psychiatry and the fight against senility. In *Concepts of Alzheimer Disease: Biological, Clinical, and Cultural Perspectives*, P. J. Whitehouse, K. Maurer, and J. F. Ballenger, eds. Johns Hopkins University Press.

29. Ballenger, J. (2006). Progress in the history of Alzheimer's disease: The importance of context. In *Alzheimer's Disease: A Century of Scientific and Clinical Research*, G. Perry, J. Avila, J. Kinoshita, and M. A. Smith, eds. IOS Press.

30. Kaplan, D.B., and Andersen, T.C. (2013). The transformative potential of social work's evolving practice in dementia care. *Journal of Gerontological Social Work 56*, 164–176. doi: 10.1080/01634372.2012.753652.

31. Age Scotland (2021). *A Manifesto: For Human Rights for People Living with Dementia and Unpaid Carers.* Age Scotland.

32. Alzheimer's Association (2022). Our commitment to transparency. Alzheimer's Association. https://alz.org/about/transparency.

33. The King's Fund (2023). Social care 360: Expenditure. https://www.kingsfund.org.uk/publications/social-care-360/expenditure.

34. Hiam, L., Dorling, D., and McKee, M. (2020). Things fall apart: The British health crisis 2010–2020. *British Medical Bulletin 133*(1), 4–15.

35. Joseph Rowntree Foundation (2023). Overall UK Poverty rates. https://www.jrf.org.uk/data/overall-uk-poverty-rates#:~:text=In%202020%2F21%2C%20around%20one,living%20in%20poverty%20(27%25).

36. The Trussel Trust (2015). Foodbank use tops one million for first time. https://www.trusselltrust.org/wp-content/uploads/sites/2/2015/06/Trussell-Trust-foodbank-use-tops-one-million.pdf.

Index

For Product Safety Concerns and Information please contact our EU
representative GPSR@taylorandfrancis.com
Taylor & Francis Verlag GmbH, Kaufingerstraße 24, 80331 München, Germany

www.ingramcontent.com/pod-product-compliance
Lightning Source LLC
Chambersburg PA
CBHW060241220326
41598CB00027B/4006